THIRD EDITION

CLINICAL APPLICATIONS OF PATHOPHYSIOLOGY

An Evidence–Based Approach

Valentina L. Brashers, MD

Professor of Nursing
Attending Physician in Internal Medicine
University of Virginia
Charlottesville, Virginia

MOSBY

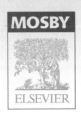

ELSEVIER

MOSBY
ELSEVIER

11830 Westline Industrial Drive
St. Louis, Missouri 63146

CLINICAL APPLICATIONS OF
PATHOPHYSIOLOGY: An Evidence-Based Approach
Copyright © 2006 by Mosby, Inc., an affiliate of Elsevier Inc.

ISBN-13: 978-0-323-04530-8
ISBN-10: 0-323-04530-8

Previous editions copyrighted 1998, 2002

ISBN-13: 978-0-323-04530-8
ISBN-10: 0-323-04530-8

Managing Editor: Brian Dennison
Developmental Editor: Betsy Stream
Publishing Services Manager: Jeff Patterson
Senior Project Manager: Mary G. Stueck
Design Direction: Andrea Lutes

Printed in the United States of America

Last digit is the print number: 9 8 7 6

Contributors

Leslie Buchanan, RN, MSN, ENP
University of Virginia Health System
Charlottesville, Virginia

Suzanne M. Burns, RN, MSN, ACNP, CCRN
Professor of Nursing and APN 2
University of Virginia School of Nursing
University of Virginia Health System
Charlottesville, Virginia

Eugene C. Corbett, Jr., MD, FACP
Brodie Professor of Medicine
Associate Professor of Nursing
University of Virginia
Charlottesville, Virginia

Mikel Gray, PhD, CUNP, CCCN, FAAN
Professor of Nursing
University of Virginia School of Nursing;
Nurse Practitioner
Department of Urology
University of Virginia Health System
Charlottesville, Virginia

Kathleen R. Haden, RN, MSN, CS, ANP-C
Nurse Practitioner
Hematology Oncology Patient Enterprises, P.C.;
Clinical Adjunct Faculty
University of Virginia
Charlottesville, Virginia;
Clinical Adjunct Faculty
Purdue University
Lafayette, Indiana

Amy M. Hiles, RN, MSN, APN-BC, CNE
Clinical Faculty
University of Virginia School of Nursing
Charlottesville, Virginia

Richard P. Keeling, MD
CEO, Keeling & Associates, Inc.;
Senior Fellow
National Center for Science and Civic
  Engagement
New York, New York

Gail L. Kongable, MSN, FNP, MPH
Associate Professor of Research
University of Virginia Health Sciences
Charlottesville, Virginia

Patrice Y. Neese, RN, MSN, CS, ANP
Nurse Practitioner
University of Virginia Health System
Department of Surgery
Charlottesville, Virginia

Lucy R. Paskus, RN, MSN, CPNP
St. Vincent Children's Hospital
Indianapolis, Indiana

Kathryn B. Reid, PhD, RN, CCRN, APRN-BC
Assistant Professor
University of Virginia School of Nursing
Charlottesville, Virginia

Juanita Reigle, MSN, ACNP
Acute Care Nurse Practitioner and Associate
  Professor of Nursing
University of Virginia Health System
Charlottesville, Virginia

Preface

Welcome to the third edition of *Clinical Applications of Pathophysiology: An Evidence-Based Approach.* As with the previous editions, the purpose of this book is to provide a summary of the pathophysiology of selected common diseases or illnesses and the application of that information to clinical assessment, diagnosis, and management. Case studies are provided to reinforce the skills learned in each chapter, and an up-to-date list of suggested readings is included. Instructors who adopt the book for course use may obtain the Solutions from their Elsevier sales representative or by calling Faculty Support at 1-800-222-9570.

This text is designed to be used by the health care clinician, student, and educator. By understanding the underlying pathophysiologic processes, the reader can better predict clinical manifestations, choose evaluative studies, initiate appropriate therapies, and anticipate potential complications. In addition, insights into the underlying disease process can prepare the practitioner for the use of new and innovative interventions and drugs.

This book is organized by body system, with 27 selected diagnoses that are not only common to clinical practice but represent concepts of pathophysiology, evaluation, and management that can be applied to many other illnesses.

The first section contains a concise summary of the disease, including Definition, Epidemiology, Pathophysiology, Patient Presentation, Differential Diagnosis, Keys to Evaluation, and Keys to Management. Figures and tables illustrate important points. This information is followed by a unique "Pathophysiology → Clinical Link" diagram that emphasizes how an understanding of the pathophysiologic principles can guide patient care. A list of selected recent articles is included for each chapter.

The second section of each chapter contains a representative case study in a fill-in-the-blank format that can be used by clinicians and students to practice their skills and by educators to evaluate their students.

Valentina L. Brashers

Acknowledgments

This book would not exist without the generous and kind support of Kathy McCance and Sue Huether of the University of Utah. They not only encouraged me to write the first edition of this book but also supported me in developing this much-improved third edition. I have used their nationally-renowned text *Pathophysiology: The Biologic Basis of Disease in Adults and Children* in my classes for years, and am honored to be a contributing author to their outstanding scholarly works. They set the standard for the teaching of pathophysiology, and I am grateful for the opportunity to learn from them both. They are the very best of mentors, role models, and friends.

This third edition would not have been possible without the hard work and support of Managing Editor Brian Dennison at Elsevier who has joined me in my commitment to turning out the very best and most accurate book possible. Mary Stueck and Betsy Stream did an outstanding job of finalizing the chapters and getting them ready for this exciting new third edition.

I am endlessly grateful to the expert clinical nurses who contributed many of the case studies for this book. Their expertise has guided my teaching, my writing, and my practice for many years. I would also like to thank my students for their enthusiasm for pathophysiology; they are my inspiration and my reason for coming to work each day. I would like to especially thank Mikel Gray for his hard work and scholarly contribution to the chapter on urinary tract infection. Eugene Corbett, Jr. and Richard Keeling, provided their valuable expertise to this book. They have my respect and gratitude for all their contributions to my teaching and writing.

My colleagues at the University of Virginia School of Nursing have been supportive in both word and deed of my unique role in the School. It is my privilege to work with such a knowledgeable, dedicated, and caring group of professionals. I would like to thank my Dean, Jeanette Lancaster, who has always given me the opportunity to express my energies and ideas in creative ways.

Finally, I would like to thank my family and friends, especially Patty, for putting up with my long hours and distracted ways for yet another edition of this book.

Contents

Hypertension

DEFINITION

- Hypertension (HTN) is defined as sustained abnormal elevation of the arterial blood pressure.
- The Seventh Report of the Joint National Committee on Detection, Evaluation, and Treatment of High Blood Pressure (JNC VII) defines high blood pressure in adults as follows:

Category	Systolic (mm Hg)		Diastolic (mm Hg)
Normal	<120	*and*	<80
Prehypertension	120-139	*or*	80-89
Stage 1 hypertension	140-159	*or*	90-99
Stage 2 hypertension	≥160	*or*	≥100

- The category "Prehypertension" indicates the group at risk for developing HTN for which there is an opportunity to prevent progression with life-style modification.
- Approximately 95% of hypertension is called primary (essential) HTN; 5% is termed secondary HTN.
- There are many processes contributing to primary HTN (see following).
- Secondary HTN can be caused by renal parenchymal disease, renal vascular disease, adrenocortical disease (Cushing disease or hyperaldosteronism), pheochromocytoma, hyperthyroidism, hyperparathyroidism, and some drugs such as oral contraceptives.

EPIDEMIOLOGY

- Hypertension is the most common primary diagnosis in the United States; approximately 65% of Americans older than the age of 60 have hypertension.
- HTN is a risk factor for coronary artery disease, congestive heart failure, stroke, and renal failure.
- Each 20-mm Hg increase in systolic pressure or 10-mm Hg increase in diastolic pressure above normal increases cardiovascular risk twofold.
- Blacks tend to develop more severe HTN at an earlier age and have nearly twice the risk of stroke and myocardial infarction (MI) as whites.
- In people older than age 55, systolic hypertension is a more important cardiovascular risk factor than is diastolic hypertension.
- Patient awareness and adequacy of management remain surprisingly low.
- The National Health and Nutrition Examination Survey (NHANES) IV found a significant reduction in morbidity and mortality attributable to hypertension due to improved awareness and management, but this decline is leveling off, especially in minority populations.
- Risk factors in all populations include age, obesity, sedentary life-style, family history, smoking, alcohol, high sodium intake (especially in blacks, older adults, and those with diabetes), and low potassium or magnesium intake (especially in blacks). The use of nonsteroidal anti-inflammatory agents (NSAIDs) has also been associated with a significant increased risk for HTN.

PATHOPHYSIOLOGY

- Primary hypertension results from a complicated interaction between genetics and the environment mediated by a host of neurohormonal mediators.
- A sustained increase in blood pressure is the result of increased peripheral resistance, increased blood volume, or both.
- *Genetics:* Heritability accounts for an estimated 30% to 40% of primary hypertension cases.
  - Genes that have been implicated include angiotensin II receptor, angiotensinogen and renin genes; endothelial nitric oxide synthetase genes; G protein receptor kinase gene; adrenergic receptor genes; calcium transport and sodium-hydrogen antiporter genes (affect salt sensitivity); and genes that are associated with insulin resistance, obesity, hyperlipidemia, and hypertension as a cluster of traits.
  - Adducin is a membrane-skeleton protein that plays an important role in the determination of cellular morphology and motility and in the regulation of membrane ion transport. It interacts with Na^+, K^+ ATPase and thus regulates the sodium-potassium pump. Mutations (e.g., ADD1 Gly460Trp) of the gene that codes for adducin cause an increase in tubular renal reabsorption of sodium and are associated with an approximately 50% to 70% increase in risk for hypertension in whites. The presence of an adducin gene mutation indicates that the affected individual is more likely to be salt sensitive and to respond more effectively to diuretic treatment of his or her hypertension.
- Contributing factors to the pathophysiology of primary hypertension include:
  - Increased activity of the sympathetic nervous system (SNS).
    1. Results from genetic changes in receptors plus sustained serum catecholamine levels.
    2. Increases cardiac contractility and heart rate and induces arteriolar vasoconstriction.
    3. Also contributes to structural changes in blood vessels (vascular remodeling), renal sodium retention, insulin resistance, increased renin and angiotensin levels, and procoagulant effects.
  - Increased activity of the renin-angiotensin-aldosterone system (RAA).
    1. Directly vasoconstricts but also increases SNS activity and decreases vasodilatory prostaglandins and nitric oxide levels.
    2. Causes renal sodium retention (shifts pressure-natriuresis relationship) (Figure 1-1).
    3. Mediates arteriolar remodeling (structural changes in vessel walls).
    4. Mediates end-organ damage to heart (hypertrophy), blood vessels, and kidneys.
  - Defects in natriuretic hormone function (atrial natriuretic peptide [ANP]), brain natriuretic peptide (BNP), C-type natriuretic peptide (CNP), and urodilantin.
    1. Modulate renal sodium (Na^+) excretion and decrease vasomotor tone.
    2. Function of these hormones is affected by excessive sodium intake; inadequate dietary intake of potassium, magnesium, and calcium; and obesity.
    3. Dysfunction results in increased vascular tone and a shift in the pressure-natriuresis relationship leading to salt and water retention and increased blood volume.
  - Inflammation.
    1. Changes in neurohumoral function lead to endothelial dysfunction and tissue ischemia, which stimulate the release of inflammatory mediators such as prostaglandins and thromboxanes.
    2. Chronic inflammation leads to vascular remodeling and preglomerular arteriopathy, which can contribute to salt and water retention and renal dysfunction.
  - Obesity.
    1. Causes changes in systemic hemodynamics that may contribute to hypertension.
    2. Associated with increased activity of the sympathetic nervous system (perhaps due to high levels of leptin), and the RAA system.
    3. Obesity is also linked to endothelial dysfunction (increased endogenous vasoconstrictors and insulin resistance).

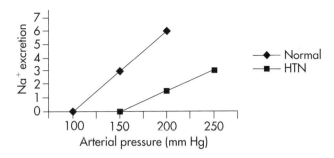

FIGURE **1-1 Pressure-Natriuresis Relationship.** (From Crowley, A. W., & Roman, R. J. (1996). The role of the kidney in hypertension. *Journal of the American Medical Association, 275,* 1581.)

- Endothelial dysfunction.
    1. Decreased production of vasodilators such as nitric oxide and increased production of vasoconstrictors such as endothelin.
    2. Dysfunction of the endothelium also contributes to vascular remodeling.
- Insulin resistance.
    1. Hypertension is common in diabetes, and insulin resistance is found in many hypertensive patients without clinical diabetes.
    2. Insulin resistance is associated with decreased endothelial release of nitric oxide and other vasodilators and has direct effects on renal function.
    3. Insulin resistance and high insulin levels increase SNS and RAA activity.
- These mechanisms explain elevations in peripheral resistance due to an increase in vasoconstrictors or a decrease in vasodilators and are felt to mediate changes in what is called the "pressure-natriuresis relationship" which states that hypertensive individuals have less renal sodium excretion for a given increase in blood pressure (Figure 1-1).
- Chronic hypertension both results from, and contributes to, vascular remodeling. Within the walls of arteries and arterioles, smooth muscle cells undergo hypertrophy and hyperplasia with associated fibrosis of the tunica intima and media. Once significant fibrosis has occurred, reduced blood flow and dysfunction of the organs perfused by these affected vessels is the inevitable result. Target organs for hypertensive vascular disease include the kidney, brain, heart, extremities, and eyes.
- The pathophysiology of essential hypertension is summarized in Figure 1-2.
- An understanding of this pathophysiology supports the current interventions employed in the management of HTN such as salt restriction, weight loss and diabetic control, SNS blockers, RAA blockers, nonspecific vasodilators, diuretics, and new drugs that modulate ANP and endothelin.

PATIENT PRESENTATION

History

Family history; childhood history of increased blood pressure (BP); other cardiac risk factors such as diabetes or dyslipidemia; history of stroke; smoking; alcohol abuse; high salt intake; recent changes in weight or obesity; medications, herbal remedies, or illicit drugs.

Symptoms

Usually asymptomatic in early stages; if BP rises acutely, patient may develop epistaxis, headache, blurred vision, tinnitus, dizziness, transient neurologic deficits, or angina; if more slowly progressive, the patient may present with symptoms related to end-organ damage such as congestive heart failure, stroke, renal failure, or retinopathy.

Examination

Systolic or diastolic HTN; skin for striae; retinopathy with vasoconstriction, arterial nicking, hemorrhages, or exudates; focal neurologic deficits; cardiomegaly (displaced point of maximal

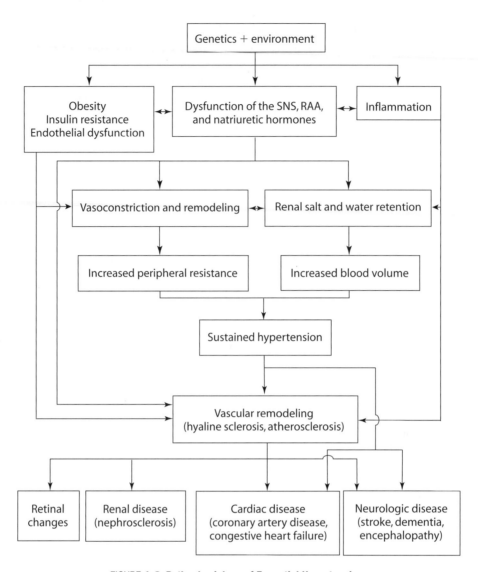

FIGURE **1-2** **Pathophysiology of Essential Hypertension.**

impulse [PMI]), heave, gallops (S_3 or S_4); decreased peripheral pulses or bruits; abdominal bruits or masses; peripheral or pulmonary edema; if severe or sudden HTN, look for encephalopathic changes with cerebral edema and papilledema.

DIFFERENTIAL DIAGNOSIS

- First differentiate an isolated increase in blood pressure from true HTN (see Keys to Assessment).
- Then rule out secondary HTN.
    - Renal vascular or parenchymal disease.
    - Cushing disease or primary hyperaldosteronism.
    - Pheochromocytoma.
    - Hyperthyroidism.
    - Hyperparathyroidism.

KEYS TO ASSESSMENT

- Goals of evaluation are to establish the true diagnosis of HTN, rule out secondary HTN, assess for end-organ damage, and evaluate for overall cardiovascular and neurovascular risk profile.

- Diagnosis requires the measurement of blood pressure on at least two separate occasions averaging two readings at least 2 minutes apart, with the patient seated, the arm supported at heart level, after 5 minutes rest, with no smoking or caffeine intake in the past 30 minutes.
- The American Heart Association updated its recommendations for the diagnosis of hypertension in 2004 to include 24-hour ambulatory blood pressure monitoring in selected patients due to its better correlation with end-organ damage and its ability to screen out "white coat HTN" (occurs only in the clinic). It also detects those patients who fail to have a nocturnal decrease in blood pressure and who may be at higher cardiovascular risk. It is especially recommended for patients with drug resistance, hypotensive symptoms with medications, episodic HTN, and autonomic dysfunction. Home blood pressure monitoring with approved devices can also aid in the management of hypertension.
- Isolated systolic hypertension is the most important risk factor for stroke and cardiovascular disease and must be recognized and managed; in the older adult the pulse pressure is also an indicator of cardiovascular risk.
- Review history carefully for symptoms of underlying causes of secondary hypertension and for the use of medications such as oral contraceptives and NSAIDs.
- Examine for abdominal masses, bruits, manifestations of Cushing disease (truncal obesity, striae), manifestations of pheochromocytoma (tachycardia, sweating, tremor).
- Funduscopic, vascular, cardiac, pulmonary, extremity, and neurologic examination.
- Laboratory: Urinalysis, chemistries including sodium, potassium, fasting glucose, blood urea nitrogen (BUN) and creatinine (Cr), serum calcium and magnesium, lipid profile, electrocardiogram (ECG).
- Microalbuminuria is an important indicator of early hypertensive renal disease.
- Consider more specific tests such as renin, cortisol, urine catecholamines, renal ultrasound, echocardiogram, and vascular studies if history, physical, and severity of HTN indicate possible secondary cause or significant end-organ involvement.
- A comprehensive review of life-style issues is key to designing a management program that is effective and suited to the individual needs of the patient (thus improving adherence).

KEYS TO MANAGEMENT

- The primary goal of prevention and treatment of hypertension is to reduce cardiovascular and renal morbidity and mortality.
- *Prevention:* Target persons with prehypertension, a family history of HTN, and one or more life-style contributors to age-related increases in BP such as obesity, high sodium intake, physical inactivity, and excessive alcohol intake.
- Decisions on therapy for hypertensive patients are based on the following:
  - The degree of blood pressure elevation.
  - The presence of "compelling indications" such as heart failure, ischemic heart disease, coronary artery disease, stroke, diabetes, or renal disease.
- Patient education.
  - Successful adherence to antihypertensive recommendations requires a patient-centered interdisciplinary approach to care.
  - A clear explanation of the rationale behind treatment and the potential side effects of the medication is essential. In addition, help with the cost of the medications may be indicated.
- Life-style modification.
  - Weight reduction (single most effective method of prevention; individualize the program).
  - Exercise (regular aerobic exercise to achieve moderate physical fitness).
  - Low-salt diet (goal of 2.4 g salt/day); increase potassium, calcium, and magnesium intake (Dietary Approaches to Stop Hypertension [DASH] eating plan is recommended).
  - Decrease alcohol intake (no more than two 12-oz servings of beer, 10 oz of wine, or 1 oz of whiskey per day for men; half that amount for women).
  - Cessation of smoking.

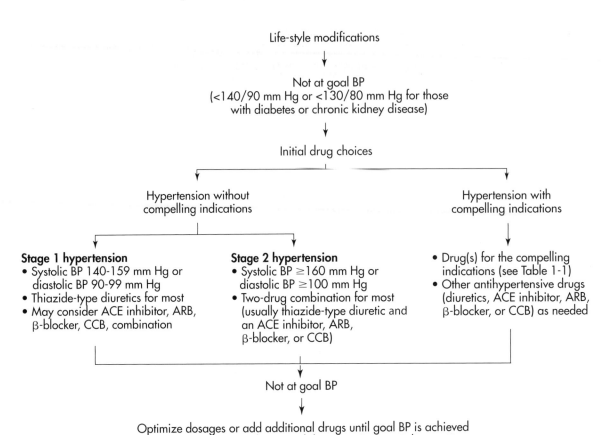

FIGURE **1-3 Overview of Hypertension Management.** (From Chobanian, A.V., Bakris, G. L., Black, H. R., Cushman, W. C., Green, L. A., Izzo, J. L. Jr, Jones, D. W., Materson, B. J., Oparil, S., Wright, J. T. Jr., & Roccella, E. J. (2003). The Seventh Report of the Joint National Committee on Prevention, Detection, Evaluation, and Treatment of High Blood Pressure: The JNC 7 Report. *Journal of the American Medical Association,* 289, 2560-2571.)

- Pharmacologic intervention (overview as recommended by JNC VII; Figure 1-3).
  - JNC VII recommends that a thiazide-type diuretic should be used in the treatment of most individuals with uncomplicated hypertension, either alone or in combination with drugs from another class of antihypertensive.
  - Compelling indications such as heart failure, ischemic heart disease, known coronary artery disease, stroke, diabetes, left ventricular hypertrophy, or renal disease require the addition or substitution of other antihypertensive drug classes such as angiotensin-converting enzyme (ACE) inhibitors, angiotensin receptor blockers (ARB), β-blockers (BB), or calcium channel blockers (CCB) (Table 1-1).
  - Most patients will require two or more antihypertensive medications in combination. If the initial blood pressure is greater than 20 mm Hg systolic or 10 mm Hg diastolic above the target pressures, initiation of therapy with two agents, one of which is a thiazide-type diuretic, is suggested. Fixed-dose combinations of two agents from different classes often contain very low doses of each agent, thus minimizing adverse effects while providing good antihypertensive efficacy (e.g., low-dose diuretic + ACE inhibitor).
- *Follow-up:* Once antihypertensive drug therapy is initiated, individuals should return for follow-up at approximately monthly intervals. After BP is at goal and stable, follow-up visits can usually be at 3- to 6-month intervals. Serum potassium and creatinine should be monitored at least one to two times a year. More frequent visits will be necessary for patients with complicating comorbid conditions.

TABLE **1-1** Compelling Indications* for Individual Drug Classes

Compelling Indication	Recommended Drugs					
	Diuretic	BB[†]	ACEI[†]	ARB[†]	CCB[†]	Aldo ANT[†]
Heart failure	X	X	X	X		X
Post myocardial infarction		X	X			X
High coronary risk	X	X	X		X	
Diabetes	X	X	X	X	X	
Chronic kidney disease			X	X		
Recurrent stroke prevention	X		X			

From Chobanian A. V., Bakris, G. L., Black, H. R., Cushman, W. C., Green, L. A., Izzo, J. L. Jr., Jones, D. W., Materson, B. J., Oparil, S., Wright, J. T. Jr., & Roccella, E. J. (2003). The Seventh Report of the Joint National Committee on Prevention, Detection, Evaluation, and Treatment of High Blood Pressure: The JNC 7 report. *Journal of the American Medical Association*, 289, 2560-2571.
*Compelling indications for antihypertensive drugs are based on benefits from outcome studies or existing clinical guidelines; the compelling indication is managed in parallel with the BP.
[†]Drug abbreviations: *ACEI*, angiotensin converting enzyme inhibitor; *ARB*, angiotensin receptor blocker; *Aldo ANT*, aldosterone antagonist; *BB*, β-blocker; *CCB*, calcium channel blocker.

- After 1 year of successful blood pressure control, especially if there has been significant life-style modification, patients with uncomplicated HTN can be considered for step-down therapy.
- The future:
  - New more effective and safer antihypertensives are being developed each year.
  - Pharmacogenetics will provide an accurate method for determining which individuals are more likely to respond best to certain drug choices.

PATHOPHYSIOLOGY →	CLINICAL LINK
What is going on in the disease process that influences how the patient presents and how he or she should be managed?	*What should you do now that you understand the underlying pathophysiology?*
Patients with prehypertension are at increased risk for developing HTN and its many sequelae.	It is critical to identify at-risk patients (family history, race, older age, smoker, high-salt diet, diabetes, dyslipidemia) and intervene with life-style modification.
The pathophysiology of the hemodynamic manifestations of HTN includes increased peripheral resistance and increased circulating blood volume.	HTN results in increased work for the heart, making cardiac complications such as hypertrophy and ischemia more likely, and hypertension will usually respond to a combination of vasodilators and diuretics.
Renal parenchyma disease, renal artery stenosis, and adrenal diseases result in hormonally induced increases in peripheral resistance and circulating volume and therefore HTN.	The initial assessment of a patient with HTN should include evaluation for possible secondary causes, including a careful physical examination (rule out abdominal bruits or masses, striae) and laboratory tests (chemistries, urinalysis, BUN, and Cr).
One of the most important mediators of primary HTN is the overactivity of the RAA system; angiotensin II has been implicated in the pathogenesis of other HTN-related diseases such as congestive heart failure, MI, and diabetic renal disease.	ACE inhibitors and angiotensin II receptor blockers are effective in many patients with HTN and are specifically indicated in patients with congestive heart failure, MI with systolic dysfunction, and diabetes.
The proposed mechanisms of primary HTN include effects on the pressure-natriuresis relationship. This relationship is also influenced by calcium, potassium, and magnesium intake.	Recent studies have reconfirmed the importance of salt restriction for most patients (especially blacks, older adults, and those with diabetes) in uncomplicated HTN. Adequate potassium, calcium, and magnesium intake is recommended.
Insulin resistance and associated endothelial dysfunction have been implicated as a cause of primary hypertension even in the absence of diabetes, and is influenced by activity of the RAA and SNS.	Treatment of insulin resistance with hypoglycemic agents can reduce blood pressure in many patients with diabetes, and treatment of hypertension with ACE inhibitors can improve insulin sensitivity and protect against renal damage in diabetes.
HTN is usually asymptomatic and target organ damage develops slowly.	Patient education about HTN and its potential complications improves adherence to therapy.

SUGGESTED READINGS

Aronow, W. S. & Frishman, W. H. (2004). Treatment of hypertension and prevention of ischemic stroke. *Current Cardiology Reports*, 6, 124-129.

Aviv, A., Hollenberg, N. K., & Weder, A. (2004). Urinary potassium excretion and sodium sensitivity in blacks. *Hypertension*, 43, 707-713.

Bakris, G. L. (2004). The importance of blood pressure control in the patient with diabetes. *American Journal of Medicine*, 116(suppl 5A), 30S-38S.

Ball, S. G. & White, W. B. (2003). Debate: angiotensin-converting enzyme inhibitors versus angiotensin II receptor blockers—a gap in evidence-based medicine. *American Journal of Cardiology*, 91, 15G-21G.

Bianchi, G. & Tripodi, G. (2003). Genetics of hypertension: the adducin paradigm. *Annals of the New York Academy of Sciences*, 986, 660-668.

Black, H. R. (2004). Evolving role of aldosterone blockers alone and in combination with angiotensin-converting enzyme inhibitors or angiotensin II receptor blockers in hypertension: a review of mechanistic and clinical data. *American Heart Journal*, 147, 564-572.

Centers for Disease Control and Prevention. (2005). Racial/ethnic disparities in prevalence, treatment, and control of hypertension—United States, 1999-2002. *Morbidity & Mortality Weekly Report*, 54, 7-9.

Chobanian, A. V., Bakris, G. L., Black, H. R., Cushman, W. C., Green, L. A., Izzo, J. L. Jr., Jones, D. W., Materson, B. J., Oparil, S., Wright, J. T. Jr., & Roccella, E. J. (2003). The Seventh Report of the Joint National Committee on Prevention, Detection, Evaluation, and Treatment of High Blood Pressure: The JNC 7 Report. *Journal of the American Medical Association*, 289, 2560-2571.

Chua, D. Y. & Bakris, G. L. (2004). Clinical implications of blockade of the renin-angiotensin system in management of hypertension. *Contributions to Nephrology*, 143, 105-116.

Correia, M. L. & Haynes, W. G. (2004). Leptin, obesity and cardiovascular disease. *Current Opinion in Nephrology & Hypertension*, 13(2), 215-223.

Davis, B. R., Furberg, C. D., Wright, J. T., Jr., Cutler, J. A., Whelton, P., & ALLHAT Collaborative Research Group. (2004). ALLHAT: setting the record straight. *Annals of Internal Medicine*, 141, 39-46.

Davy, K. P. & Hall, J. E. (2004). Obesity and hypertension: two epidemics or one? *American Journal of Physiology—Regulatory Integrative & Comparative Physiology*, 286, R803-R813.

Epstein, B. J. & Gums, J. G. (2005). Angiotensin receptor blockers versus ACE inhibitors: prevention of death and myocardial infarction in high-risk populations. *Annals of Pharmacotherapy*, 39, 470-480.

Epstein, M. & Campese, V. M. (2004). Evolving role of calcium antagonists in the management of hypertension. *Medical Clinics of North America*, 88, 149-165.

Francos, G. C. & Schairer, H. L. Jr. (2003). Hypertension. Contemporary challenges in geriatric care. *Geriatrics*, 58, 44-49.

Frohlich, E. D. (2004). Target organ involvement in hypertension: a promise of prevention and reversal. *Medical Clinics of North America*, 88, 209-221.

Grisk, O. & Rettig, R. (2004). Interactions between the sympathetic nervous system and the kidneys in arterial hypertension. *Cardiovascular Research*, 61, 238-246.

Hall, J. E. (2003). The kidney, hypertension, and obesity. *Hypertension*, 41, 625-633.

Hollenberg, N. K. (2004). Renal function in the patient with hypertension. *Medical Clinics of North America*, 88, 131-140.

Hooper, L., Bartlett, C., Davey, S. G., & Ebrahim, S. (2004). Advice to reduce dietary salt for prevention of cardiovascular disease. [Update of *Cochrane Database Systematic Reviews* 2003;(3):CD003656; PMID: 12917977.] *Cochrane Database of Systematic Reviews* CD003656.

Hooper, L., Bartlett, C., Davey, S. M., & Ebrahim, S. (2003). Reduced dietary salt for prevention of cardiovascular disease [Update of *Cochrane Database Systematic Reviews* 2003;(1):CD003656; PMID: 12535482.] *Cochrane Database of Systematic Reviews* CD003656.

Jamerson, K. A. (2004). The disproportionate impact of hypertensive cardiovascular disease in African Americans: getting to the heart of the issue. *Journal of Clinical Hypertension*, 6, 4-10.

Jurgens, G. & Graudal, N. A. (2004). Effects of low sodium diet versus high sodium diet on blood pressure, renin, aldosterone, catecholamines, cholesterols, and triglyceride. [Update of *Cochrane Database Systematic Reviews* 2003;(1): CD004022; PMID: 12535503]. *Cochrane Database of Systematic Reviews* CD004022.

Kaplan, N. M., Gidding, S. S., Pickering, T. G., & Wright, J. T. Jr. (2005). Task force 5: systemic hypertension. *Journal of the American College of Cardiology*, 45, 1346-1348.

Kearney, P. M., Whelton, M., Reynolds, K., Muntner, P., Whelton, P. K., & He, J. (2005). Global burden of hypertension: analysis of worldwide data. *Lancet*, 365, 217-223.

Kelham, C. L. (2005). Self monitoring of blood pressure at home: informed self regulation of drug treatment could be next step. *British Medical Journal*, 330, 148.

Kenchaiah, S. & Pfeffer, M. A. (2004). Cardiac remodeling in systemic hypertension. *Medical Clinics of North America*, 88, 115-130.

Kjeldsen, S. E., Os, I., Hoieggen, A., Beckey, K., Gleim, G. W., & Oparil, S. (2005). Fixed-dose combinations in the management of hypertension: defining the place of angiotensin receptor antagonists and hydrochlorothiazide. *American Journal of Cardiovascular Drugs*, 5, 17-22.

Krousel-Wood, M. A., Muntner, P., He, J., & Whelton, P. K. (2004). Primary prevention of essential hypertension. *Medical Clinics of North America*, 88, 223-238.

Kumagai, H., Onami, T., Iigaya, K., Takimoto, C., Imai, M., Matsuura, T., Sakata, K., Oshima, N., Hayashi, K., & Saruta, T. (2004). Involvement of renal sympathetic nerve in pathogenesis of hypertension. *Contributions to Nephrology*, 143, 32-45.

Kunhiraman, B. P., Jawa, A., & Fonseca, V. A. (2005). Potential cardiovascular benefits of insulin sensitizers. *Endocrinology & Metabolism Clinics of North America*, 34, 117-135.

Liebson, P. R. (2003). ALLHAT and AFFIRM. *Preventive Cardiology*, 6, 54-60.

Livingston, E. H. & Ko, C. Y. (2005). Effect of diabetes and hypertension on obesity-related mortality. *Surgery*, 137, 16-25.

Manunta, P. & Bianchi, G. (2004). Low-salt diet and diuretic effect on blood pressure and organ damage. *Journal of the American Society of Nephrology*, 15(suppl 1), S43-S46.

McDonough, A. A., Leong, P. K., & Yang, L. E. (2003). Mechanisms of pressure natriuresis: how blood pressure regulates renal sodium transport. *Annals of the New York Academy of Sciences*, 986, 669-677.

Moser, M. & Setaro, J. (2004). Continued importance of diuretics and beta-adrenergic blockers in the management of hypertension. *Medical Clinics of North America*, 88, 167-187.

Nabel, E. G. (2003). Cardiovascular disease. *New England Journal of Medicine*, 349, 60-72.

Natali, A. & Ferrannini, E. (2004). Hypertension, insulin resistance, and the metabolic syndrome. *Endocrinology & Metabolism Clinics of North America*, 33, 417-429.

O'Brien, E. (2003). Ambulatory blood pressure monitoring in the management of hypertension. *Heart (British Cardiac Society)*, 89, 571-576.

Ogihara, T., Asano, T., & Fujita, T. (2003). Contribution of salt intake to insulin resistance associated with hypertension. *Life Sciences*, 73, 509-523.

Onusko, E. (2003). Diagnosing secondary hypertension. *American Family Physician*, 67, 67-74.

O'Shaughnessy, K. M. & Karet, F. E. (2004). Salt handling and hypertension. *Journal of Clinical Investigation*, 113, 1075-1081.

Papademetriou, V. (1924). Hypertension and cognitive function. Blood pressure regulation and cognitive function: a review of literature. *Geriatrics*, 60, 20-22.

Perez del Villar, C., Garcia Alonso, C. J., Feldstein, C. A., Juncos, L. A., & Romero, J. C. (2005). Role of endothelin in the pathogenesis of hypertension. *Mayo Clinic Proceedings*, 80, 84-96.

Phillips, M. I. & Kimura, B. (2005). Antisense therapeutics for hypertension: targeting the renin-angiotensin system. *Methods in Molecular Medicine*, 106, 51-68.

Pickering, T. G., Hall, J. E., Appel, L. J., Falkner, B. E., Graves, J. W., Hill, M. N., Jones, D. H., Kurtz, T., Sheps, S. G., Roccella, E. J., Council on High Blood Pressure Research Professional and Public Education Subcommittee, American Heart Association. (2005). Recommendations for blood pressure measurement in humans: an AHA scientific statement from the Council on High Blood Pressure Research Professional and Public Education Subcommittee. *Journal of Clinical Hypertension*, 7(2), 102-109.

Pontremoli, R., Leoncini, G., & Parodi, A. (2005). Use of nifedipine in the treatment of hypertension. *Expert Review of Cardiovascular Therapy*, 3, 43-50.

Ram, C. V. (2003). Management of refractory hypertension. *American Journal of Therapeutics*, 10, 122-126.

Reaven, G. M. (2003). Insulin resistance/compensatory hyperinsulinemia, essential hypertension, and cardiovascular disease. *Journal of Clinical Endocrinology & Metabolism*, 88, 2399-2403.

Safar, M. E. & Benetos, A. (2003). Factors influencing arterial stiffness in systolic hypertension in the elderly: role of sodium and the renin-angiotensin system. *American Journal of Hypertension*, 16, 249-258.

Safar, M. E. & Smulyan, H. (2004). Hypertension in women. *American Journal of Hypertension*, 17, 82-87.

Savoia, C. & Schiffrin, E. L. (2004). Significance of recently identified peptides in hypertension: endothelin, natriuretic peptides, adrenomedullin, leptin. *Medical Clinics of North America*, 88, 39-62.

Scaglione, R., Argano, C., Di Chiara, T., & Licata, G. (2004). Obesity and cardiovascular risk: the new public health problem of worldwide proportions. *Expert Review Cardiovascular Therapy*, 2, 203-212.

Sowers, J. R. & Frohlich, E. D. (2004). Insulin and insulin resistance: impact on blood pressure and cardiovascular disease. *Medical Clinics of North America*, 88, 63-82.

Staessen, J. A., Wang, J., Bianchi, G., & Birkenhager, W. (2003) Essential hypertension. *Lancet*, 361, 1629-1641.

Stokes, G. S. (2004). Systolic hypertension in the elderly: pushing the frontiers of therapy—a suggested new approach. *Journal of Clinical Hypertension*, 6, 192-197.

Strazzullo, P., Galletti, F., & Barba, G. (2003). Altered renal handling of sodium in human hypertension: short review of the evidence. *Hypertension*, 41, 1000-1005.

Tanira, M. O. & Al Balushi, K. A. (2005). Genetic variations related to hypertension: a review. *Journal of Human Hypertension*, 19, 7-19.

Thurman, J. M. & Schrier, R. W. (2003). Comparative effects of angiotensin-converting enzyme inhibitors and angiotensin receptor blockers on blood pressure and the kidney. *American Journal of Medicine*, 114, 588-598.

Verdecchia, P., Angeli, F., & Gattobigio, R. (2004). Clinical usefulness of ambulatory blood pressure monitoring. *Journal of the American Society of Nephrology*, 15(suppl 1), S30-S33.

Watkins, P. J. (2003). Cardiovascular disease, hypertension, and lipids. *British Medical Journal*, 326, 874-876.

Whaley-Connell, A. & Sowers, J. R. (2005). Hypertension management in type 2 diabetes mellitus: recommendations of the Joint National Committee VII. *Endocrinology & Metabolism Clinics of North America*, 34, 63-75.

Hypertension

INITIAL HISTORY

- 47-year-old black male, banking executive.
- Coming in for physical examination after having his blood pressure checked at a health fair and being told it was high.
- No specific complaints.

Question 1. *What questions would you like to ask this patient?*

ADDITIONAL HISTORY AND FAMILY HISTORY

- No other health problems, on no medications.
- Father and older brother both have hypertension.
- Paternal grandparents each have history of MI and stroke at young age.
- Denies cardiac or neurologic symptoms.

Question 2. *Are there other questions you would like to ask this patient?*

MORE HISTORY

- Eats significant amounts of prepackaged foods and snack foods.
- Nonsmoker, drinks an average of three or four beers most evenings.
- Has gained 12 pounds over the past year due to physical inactivity.
- Last cholesterol checked 3 years ago; can only remember that his total cholesterol was 252 mg/dL; has "tried" to watch his diet.

Question 3. *What are his risk factors for HTN?*

PHYSICAL EXAMINATION

- Mildly obese male in no distress.
- T = 37 orally; P = 95 and regular; RR = 14; BP = 156/98 in both arms (sitting).

HEENT, Neck
- PERRLA, fundi with vasoconstriction but with no nicking, hemorrhages, or exudates.
- Pharynx clear.
- Neck supple without bruits or thyromegaly.

Lungs
- Good lung expansion bilaterally.
- Percussion without dullness throughout.
- Breath sounds clear.

Cardiac
- RRR, PMI fifth ICS at midclavicular line.
- No murmurs.
- Soft S_4 gallop heard at apex.

Abdomen
- Mildly obese.
- No abdominal bruits heard.
- Soft without tenderness or organomegaly, liver 8 cm at midclavicular line.
- No masses felt.

Extremities
- No edema; no clubbing; no bruits.
- Pulses full in all extremities.

Neurologic
- Alert and oriented.
- Strength 5/5 throughout.
- DTR 2+ and symmetric.
- Sensory intact to pinprick and light touch throughout.
- Proprioception normal.
- Gait steady.

Question 4.   *What are the pertinent positives and negatives on the physical examination and what might they mean?*

Question 5.   *What should be done now?*

Question 6. *How should he prepare for his next visit, and how should his blood pressure be measured when he returns?*

PATIENT'S RETURN VISIT

- Patient continues to feel well, no complaints.
- BP = 156/94 both arms, sitting with arm elevated to heart level.
- Rest of examination unchanged.

Question 7. *What now?*

PATIENT'S THIRD RETURN VISIT

- Still no complaints.
- BP = 158/97.
- Rest of examination unchanged.

Question 8. *What now? Would you order laboratory tests? If so, what?*

LABORATORY RESULTS

- All blood chemistries, including sodium, potassium, BUN, Cr, and calcium are normal.
- Complete blood count normal.
- Urinalysis negative for protein or glucose, microscopy without cells or cellular casts.
- Total cholesterol and LDL elevated; HDL slightly low.
- ECG shows increased QRS voltage in the chest leads.

Question 9. *What do the laboratory results mean?*

Question 10. *How should this patient be managed?*

Dyslipidemia and Atherosclerosis

DEFINITION

- Dyslipidemia, as defined by the National Cholesterol Education Program III (NCEP III) includes those changes in the lipid profile that are associated with an increased risk for atherosclerosis.

	Optimal	Near Optimal	Desirable	Borderline	High	Very High
Total cholesterol			<200	200-239	≥240	
LDL cholesterol	<100	100-129		130-159	160-189	≥190
TG			<150	150-199	200-499	≥500

	High	Low
HDL cholesterol	≥60	<40

HDL, High-density lipoprotein; *LDL*, low-density lipoprotein; *TG*, triglycerides.

- Follow-up reports to NCEP III published in 2004 suggest that treatment goals for those at high risk for atherosclerotic disease should be even more stringent, including an optimal LDL of less than 70 mg/dL.
- Atherosclerosis is a chronic inflammatory disease characterized by thickening and hardening of the arterial wall. Lesions contain lipid deposits and become calcified, leading to vessel obstruction, platelet aggregation, and abnormal vasoconstriction.

EPIDEMIOLOGY

- Hyperlipidemia.
  - The American Heart Association states that for people older than the age of 20, approximately 50% of whites, and between 37% and 46% of blacks in the United States have dyslipidemia. The statistics are worse for women than for men, especially after age 50. This means that more than 100 million American adults have total blood cholesterol values of 200 mg/dL and higher, and 37.7 million American adults have levels of 240 or greater.
  - Relative dyslipidemia with changes in the vascular wall is common in children in the United States.
  - 1 in 500 people has identifiable heterozygous or homozygous familial hypercholesterolemia.
  - There is a high incidence of dyslipidemia in people with diabetes and hypertension.
  - The causes of dyslipidemia include the following: (1) common (polygenic) hypercholesterolemia; (2) familial hypercholesterolemia; (3) a diet high in saturated fats and/or cholesterol; (4) diabetes (metabolic syndrome and insulin resistance states); (5) renal failure; (6) drugs (thiazides, steroids); (7) smoking; and (8) hypothyroidism.

- Atherosclerosis.
  - Atherosclerotic cardiovascular disease (including coronary artery disease and stroke) is the leading cause of death in the United States.
  - *Genetics:* More than 25 candidate genes for atherosclerotic disease have been identified, including those that contribute to dyslipidemia, hypertension, homocystinemia, thrombosis, fibrinolysis, platelet function, and endothelial inflammation.
  - **Conventional or major risk factors** for atherosclerosis that are nonmodifiable include (1) advanced age, (2) male gender or women after menopause, and, (3) family history (genetics). Modifiable major risks include (1) dyslipidemia, (2) cigarette smoking, (3) hypertension, (4) diabetes and insulin resistance, (5) obesity, (6) sedentary life-style and (7) atherogenic diet.
    1. *Dyslipidemia*—contributes to endothelial cell injury and atherosclerotic plaque formation (see following).
       a. An increased serum concentration of LDL is a strong indicator of atherosclerotic risk. Serum levels of LDL are normally controlled by hepatic receptors for LDL that bind LDL and limit liver synthesis of this lipoprotein. Increased dietary intake of cholesterol and fats, often in combination with a genetic predisposition to accumulations of LDL in the serum (e.g., dysfunction of the hepatic LDL receptor), results in high levels of LDL in the bloodstream. The term LDL actually describes several types of LDL molecules, and the "small dense" LDL particles are the most atherogenic (measurement of LDL-C is recommended).
       b. A decreased serum concentration of HDL cholesterol is an even stronger indicator of atherosclerotic risk, and high levels of HDL may be more protective for the development of atherosclerosis than low levels of LDL. HDL is responsible for "reverse cholesterol transport" and participates in endothelial repair, modulates vessel tone, and decreases thrombosis. It can be fractionated into several particle sizes that have different effects on vascular function.
       c. Other lipoproteins associated with increased cardiovascular risk include elevated serum VLDL (triglycerides) and increased lipoprotein (a) (Lp[a]). Elevated triglycerides are associated with an increased risk for atherosclerosis especially in combination with other risk factors such as diabetes. Lipoprotein (a) is a genetically determined molecular complex between LDL and a serum glycoprotein called apolipoprotein A that has been shown to be an important risk factor for atherosclerosis especially in women and in diabetics.
    2. *Cigarette smoking*—associated with an increase in LDL, a decrease in HDL, and induction of a prothrombotic state. Also associated with increases in inflammatory markers of atherosclerosis such as C-reactive protein and fibrinogen (see following).
    3. *Hypertension*—contributes to endothelial injury and is associated with numerous neurohumoral changes (e.g., increased angiotensin II, decreased nitric oxide, and insulin resistance) that predispose the individual to atherosclerotic plaque formation.
    4. *Diabetes* (insulin resistance)—associated with a two- to sixfold increase in the risk for atherosclerotic disease. Diabetes and insulin resistance have multiple effects on the cardiovascular system through the production of toxic reactive metabolites that alter vascular cell function. These effects can include endothelial damage, thickening of the vessel wall, increased inflammation and leukocyte adhesion, increased thrombosis, glycation of vascular proteins, and decreased production of endothelial-derived vasodilators such as nitric oxide. Diabetes is also associated with dyslipidemia (by altering hepatic lipoprotein synthesis) and increased LDL oxidation.
    5. *Obesity/sedentary life-style*—65% of the U.S. adult population is overweight and an estimated 47 million adults have a combination of obesity, dyslipidemia, and hypertension called the "metabolic syndrome." Abdominal obesity has the strongest link with increased atherosclerotic risk and is related to insulin resistance, decreased HDL, increased blood pressure, and decreased levels of a

recently described cardioprotective protein called adiponectin. Adiponectin has protective actions in the initiation and progression of atherosclerosis through anti-inflammatory and antiatherogenic effects. A sedentary life-style not only increases the risk of obesity, but also has an independent effect on increasing CAD risk.

- **Nontraditional or novel risk factors** for CAD include (1) increased serum markers for inflammation, autoimmunity and thrombosis, (2) hyperhomocystinemia, and (3) infection. The amount of risk conferred by these relatively newly-identified factors is still being explored.

  1. *Markers of inflammation, autoimmunity, and thrombosis*—clinically utilized risk factors include C-reactive protein (CRP), fibrinogen, protein C, and plasminogen activator inhibitor. CRP is an indirect measure of atherosclerotic plaque–related inflammation and is an important indicator of risk for coronary artery disease. Elevated levels of C-reactive protein are associated with numerous other atherosclerotic risk factors including smoking, obesity, and diabetes. Other markers of inflammation and autoimmunity that have been associated with atherosclerosis include the erythrocyte sedimentation rate, von Willebrand factor concentration, autoantibodies to oxidized LDL, interleukin-6, interleukin-18, tumor necrosis factor, and CD 40 ligand.

  2. *Hyperhomocystinemia*—results from a genetic lack of the enzyme that breaks down homocysteine (an amino acid) or because of a nutritional deficiency of folate, cobalamin (vitamin B_{12}), or pyridoxine (vitamin B_6). It is associated with increased LDL, decreased endogenous vasodilators, and thrombosis. Routine serum measurement of homocysteine is not currently recommended, and prevention and management are focused on increasing the dietary intake of folate and B vitamins.

  3. *Infection*—several studies have found that microorganisms, especially *Chlamydia pneumoniae* and *Helicobacter pylori*, are frequently present in atherosclerotic lesions. Serum antibodies to microorganisms have been linked to an increased risk for atherosclerosis, as has the presence of periodontal disease. However, the role of infection in the pathogenesis of atherosclerosis remains controversial.

PATHOPHYSIOLOGY

- Atherosclerosis begins with endothelial injury (Figure 2-1).
  - The above-described effects of genes, dyslipidemia, smoking, hypertension, diabetes, obesity, inflammation, autoimmunity, homocystinemia, and infection all negatively affect endothelial cell structure and function.
  - Aging of the vessel wall also contributes to decreased vessel compliance with increased shear forces and increased vulnerability to endothelial injury.
- Injured endothelial cells.
  - Secrete monocyte chemotactic factors and express inducible cell surface adhesion molecules to which monocytes and lymphocytes bind and promote the recruitment of macrophages to the area of injury.
  - Release inflammatory cytokines (and inflammatory markers such as CRP).
  - Secrete less of the vasodilator nitric oxide and secrete increased vasoconstrictors such as vascular endothelial growth factor (VGEF), platelet-derived growth factor, and endothelin-1.
- Macrophages adhere to injured endothelium via adhesion molecules such as vascular cell adhesion molecule–1 (VCAM-1) and release enzymes and toxic oxygen radicals that create oxidative stress, oxidize LDL, and further injure the vessel wall.
- Oxidation of LDL.
  - Inflammation with oxidative stress and activation of macrophages is the primary mechanism of LDL oxidation. Diabetes, smoking, hypertension, increased lipoxygenase levels, and increased toxic oxygen radical levels contribute to increased LDL oxidation. Interestingly, increased levels of angiotensin II are linked to LDL oxidation through stimulation of the AT_1 receptor.

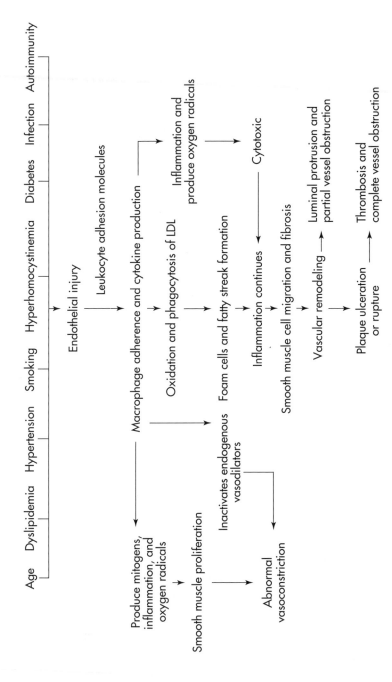

FIGURE **2-1** Pathogenesis of Atherosclerosis.

- - Oxidized LDL activates Toll-like receptor 4 (TLR4) on macrophages, which is a part of the innate immune system and activates numerous inflammatory and immune responses.
  - Oxidized LDL is toxic to endothelial cells (via LOX-1 receptor), promotes superoxide anion production that degrades nitric oxide, facilitates macrophage adhesion to endothelial cells through induction of adhesion molecules, and causes smooth muscle cell proliferation.
- Oxidized LDL penetrates into the intima of the arterial wall and is engulfed by macrophages. Macrophages filled with oxidized LDL are called foam cells. Accumulations of these cells form a pathologic lesion called a fatty streak that induces further immunologic and inflammatory changes that result in progressive vessel damage and vasoconstriction. These macrophages also produce growth factors and mitogens that stimulate smooth muscle cell proliferation.
- Smooth muscle cells proliferate, produce collagen, and migrate over the fatty streak forming a fibrous plaque—this is mediated by a large number of inflammatory cytokines including growth factors such as transforming growth factor beta (TGF-β).
- The fibrous plaque may become calcified, protrude into the vessel lumen, and obstruct blood flow to distal tissues, especially during exercise which may cause symptoms (e.g., angina or intermittent claudication).
- Some plaques, even if they are small and do not extend into the lumen of the vessel, can ulcerate or rupture due to (1) mechanical shear forces, (2) macrophage-derived collagenases, elastases, matrix metalloproteinases and the cathepsins, and (3) apoptosis of cells at the edges of the plaque. The amount of collagen and elastin deposition in the cap (made by smooth muscle cells and fibroblasts) and the amount of LDL in the core determine its stability and vulnerability to rupture. In addition, T lymphocytes produce interferon gamma that decreases collagen production and weakens the plaque (autoimmunity).
- Atherosclerotic plaques can be classified according to their structure, which gives insight into their stability and proneness to rupture. Plaques that have ruptured are called complicated plaques.
- Platelets aggregate and adhere to the surface of the ruptured plaque due to decreased endothelial anticoagulants and exposure of platelet glycoprotein IIb/IIIa surface receptors. The coagulation cascade is initiated and a thrombus forms over the lesion that may completely obstruct the lumen of the vessel. The release of thromboxane A from the vessel wall with resultant vasoconstriction further narrows the vessel lumen.
- The overall result is an artery that is narrowed and vulnerable to vasoconstriction and thrombosis.
- Life-style and pharmacologic interventions are possible at every step in this cascade of events that may prevent or reverse the process (see Pathophysiology → Clinical Link).

PATIENT PRESENTATION

- Dyslipidemia and atherosclerosis are often asymptomatic and the decision to assess a patient is based on a history of risk factors.
- If the patient does present with symptoms, the symptoms are most often the result of atherosclerotic obstruction of major vessels with ischemia of target organs such as the heart, the kidneys, the brain, or the extremities.

History

High-fat diet; weight gain; sedentary life-style; age; gender; race; postmenopausal; smoking; diabetes; hypertension; family history; past medical history of high blood pressure or cardiac, cerebrovascular, or peripheral vascular disease.

Symptoms

Chest pain; shortness of breath; transient or permanent neurologic deficits; intermittent claudication (pain in leg with walking, relieved with rest); hair loss and skin ulcers on extremities; worsening headaches, dizziness, or epistaxis.

Examination

Corneal arcus; xanthomas; increased blood pressure; abdominal bruits; bruits and decreased pulses in extremity arteries; obesity; evidence of congestive heart failure; focal neurologic deficits.

DIFFERENTIAL DIAGNOSIS

- Familial dyslipidemia versus common polygenic dyslipidemia versus secondary dyslipidemia (renal failure, diabetes, drug-induced, hypothyroidism).
- Hypertension (primary as a risk factor, secondary due to renal vascular disease as a target organ effect).
- Ischemic heart disease.
- Cerebrovascular disease.
- Peripheral vascular disease.

KEYS TO ASSESSMENT

- The goals are to identify modifiable risk factors and to assess for target organ effects.
- Remember, if one arterial system is diseased, it is likely that others are too.
- Blood pressure, body mass index, waist circumference, and pulse should be recorded at every visit.
- Lipid profile.
    - Current NCEP recommendations include a screening of total cholesterol, LDL, HDL, and triglycerides in all adults older than 20 years every 5 years. If dyslipidemia is present, LDL-C should also be measured.
    - The patient should be seated for 30 minutes, after fasting for 12 hours, and have had no recent major changes in weight, exercise, smoking, or blood pressure.
    - Fasting lipid profile should be obtained every 2 years in those with other risk factors such as diabetes and hypertension.
- High sensitivity CRP (hs-CRP).
- Lp(a) is a genetically determined risk factor especially in women and diabetics; a test should be ordered if there is advanced atherosclerosis without the conventional risk factors.
- Fasting blood glucose or glycosylated hemoglobin.
- Serum electrolytes and blood urea nitrogen (BUN) and creatinine (Cr).
- Thyroid-stimulating hormone (TSH).
- Liver function tests (aspartate aminotransferase [AST], alanine aminotransferase [ALT], alkaline phosphatase, lactate dehydrogenase [LDH]).
- Electrocardiogram (ECG).
- Doppler ultrasound evaluation of selected arterial systems (popliteal, femoral, carotid) is done if the physical examination and history suggest involvement.
- Radiographic techniques such as intravascular ultrasound, computed tomography, and magnetic resonance imaging (MRI) allow for identification of unstable plaques at high risk for rupture and thrombosis.
- Evaluation for evidence of coronary artery disease (see Chapter 3) or cerebrovascular disease (see Chapter 19).

KEYS TO MANAGEMENT

- Prevention.
    - There is increasing evidence that atherosclerosis begins in childhood. Good diet habits and exercise with weight control should begin in childhood and continue throughout life.
    - Smoking cessation and exercise are associated with increased HDL.
    - Aggressive recognition and management of risk factors such as familial dyslipidemia, obesity, hypertension, and diabetes is crucial (considered AHA Coronary Heart Disease Risk Equivalents).

TABLE **2-1** National Cholesterol Education Program III Treatment Decisions

	Goal	Life-style Changes	Drug Therapy
Coronary heart disease or risk equivalents (10 year risk >20%)	<100 mg/dL	≥100 mg/dL	≥130 mg/dL
2+ Risk factors (10-year risk ≤20%)	<130 mg/dL	≥130 mg/dL	10-year risk 10%-20%: ≥130 mg/dL 10-year risk <10%: ≥160 mg/dL
0-1 Risk factors	<160 mg/dL	≥160 mg/dL	≥190 mg/dL

From Executive Summary of the Third Report of the National Cholesterol Education Program (NCEP) Expert Panel on Detection, Evaluation, and Treatment of High Blood Cholesterol in Adults (Adult Treatment Panel III). (2001). *Journal of the American Medical Association*, 285, 2486-2497.

- The decision to use diet therapy alone or in combination with pharmacologic therapy is based on the level of dyslipidemia and the presence or absence of other risk factors (Table 2-1).
- Diet therapy.
  - A stepwise approach as recommended by NCEP III (Table 2-2).
  - Evidence suggests that a modest increase in the percentage of monounsaturated and ω-3 and ω-6 polyunsaturated fats is as important as reducing total saturated fats.
  - Intake of *trans*-fatty acids should be eliminated or reduced.
  - Increased folate intake that lowers homocysteine levels and has been associated with decreased risk of atherosclerotic disease.
  - Moderate alcohol intake raises HDL, decreases platelet aggregation, and may improve insulin sensitivity.
  - Soy protein, oat fiber, fish oils, and garlic have all been found to reduce cholesterol.
- Pharmacologic intervention.
  - Lipid lowering.
    1. *HMG-CoA reductase inhibitors* ("statins") (pravastatin, lovastatin, atorvastatin, etc.) lower serum total cholesterol and LDL and raise HDL with few side effects (myopathy and increase in liver enzymes). Their long-term safety and efficacy are well established (cause regression of atherosclerotic lesions, reduce the risk of ischemic heart disease) and should be first-line drug therapy. They have been found to be anti-inflammatory, antithrombotic, and to improve endothelial function in addition to their lipid-modifying properties.

TABLE **2-2** National Cholesterol Education Program III: Nutrient Composition of the Therapeutic Life-Style Changes (TLC) Diet

Nutrient	Recommended Intake
Saturated fat*	<7% of total calories
Polyunsaturated fat	Up to 10% of total calories
Monounsaturated fat	Up to 20% of total calories
Total fat	25%-35% of total calories
Carbohydrate†	50%-60% of total calories
Fiber	20-30 g/day
Protein	Approximately 15% of total calories
Cholesterol	<200 mg/day
Total calories‡	Balance energy intake and expenditure to maintain desirable body weight/prevent weight gain

From Executive Summary of the Third Report of the National Cholesterol Education Program (NCEP) Expert Panel on Detection, Evaluation, and Treatment of High Blood Cholesterol in Adults (Adult Treatment Panel III). (2001). *Journal of the American Medical Association*, 285, 2486-2497.
Trans fatty acids are another LDL-raising fat that should be kept at low intake.
†Carbohydrates should be derived predominantly from foods rich in complex carbohydrates including grains, especially whole grains, fruits, and vegetables.
‡Daily energy expenditure should include at least moderate physical activity (consuming approximately 200 kcal/day).

2. *Ezetimibe*—blocks the absorption of cholesterol in the intestines. Lowers LDL, especially when used in combination with statins. The only indication for monotherapy with ezetimibe is intolerance to statins.

3. *Fibric acid derivatives* (gemfibrozil) decrease cholesterol slowly but are more effective than HMG-CoA reductase inhibitors in decreasing triglycerides. They have considerable gastrointestinal side effects (dyspepsia, gallstones).

4. *Nicotinic acid* (also called niacin) reduces total cholesterol, triglycerides, and LDL; raises HDL; and reduces ischemic heart disease events, but is associated with flushing, gastrointestinal upset, and can impair glucose tolerance in prediabetic patients (diabetes is a relative contraindication for this medication).

5. *Bile acid sequestrants* (cholestyramine and colestipol) decrease LDL slowly but increase triglycerides and have significant gastrointestinal side effects.

- **Antithrombosis** may be indicated to prevent thrombus formation on established plaques. Low-dose aspirin has been shown to be effective in reducing the risk of thrombotic complications of atherosclerosis. In coronary disease, aspirin plus clopidogrel is superior to aspirin alone, especially in those undergoing invasive therapies. Other choices include dipyridamole and ticlopidine. The antiplatelet GPIIb/IIIa receptor antibodies (abciximab, eptifibatide, tirofiban, etc.) or the anticoagulants warfarin and heparin are options for selected patients, most often those with acute complications of atherosclerosis.

- Other agents.
  1. Vasodilators such as calcium channel blockers and nitrates are used to reduce vasospasm-induced ischemia.
  2. Angiotensin-converting enzyme (ACE) inhibitors increase endogenous vasodilators, reduce smooth muscle hypertrophy, and decrease fibrosis in arterial walls and reduce the risk of coronary events in hypertension and should be considered for patients with hypertension and atherosclerotic disease. ACE inhibitors also have beneficial effects on vascular remodeling and have anti-inflammatory and antithrombotic effects. Angiotensin receptor blockers (ARBs) have many of the same beneficial effects as ACE inhibitors but have not yet been definitively shown to reduce the risk of myocardial infarction or to prolong survival in individuals with hypertension.
  3. Oral estrogens have been shown to have a beneficial effect on lipid profiles; however, prospective studies using estrogen and progesterone in combination (HRT) documented an increase in coronary events, especially in the first year of use. HRT increases some measures of inflammation (including CRP) and promotes thrombosis. Estrogen used alone (without progesterone) has no effect on coronary risk. Raloxifene and other selective estrogen receptor modulators (SERMS) are being evaluated.
  4. Anti-inflammatories—aspirin and statins have anti-inflammatory effects that may reduce atherosclerotic risk; however, COX-2 inhibitors are associated with increased thrombosis and coronary events. This is hypothesized to be the result of an imbalance between the synthesis of vasodilatory prostaglandins and vasoconstrictive and prothrombotic thromboxanes. The potential role for anti-inflammatories in the prevention and treatment of atherosclerosis is controversial and continues to be explored.
  5. Antibiotics—conflicting results have been obtained from multiple studies, mostly evaluating macrolide antibiotics. More studies are pending.

PATHOPHYSIOLOGY $\longrightarrow$	CLINICAL LINK
What is going on in the disease process that influences how the patient presents and how he or she should be managed?	*What should you do now that you understand the underlying pathophysiology?*
There is a high incidence of dyslipidemia in the U.S. population, including children. $\longrightarrow$	Life-style changes should begin in childhood, and screening should begin by age 20 with repeated measurements at least every 5 years.
Serum plasma lipoprotein levels are determined by many factors including genetics, diet, drugs, gender, age, and other diseases such as diabetes. $\longrightarrow$	A careful history with attention to modifiable risk factors can improve the lipoprotein profile, and patients should be evaluated for diet therapy, exercise, and lipid-lowering drugs when appropriate.
Endothelial injury begins the whole process of atherosclerosis. $\longrightarrow$	Risk factor modification may prevent the initiation of atherosclerosis.
Macrophages and leukocytes are involved in inflammatory and immune processes that promote the atherosclerotic lesion, especially via the production of toxic oxygen radicals. $\longrightarrow$	Anti-inflammatories may provide future therapies for the prevention and treatment of atherosclerosis; however, recent experience with COX-2 inhibitors suggests that new modalities be evaluated carefully.
Abnormal smooth muscle proliferation and inactivation of endogenous vasodilators result in vasoconstriction, which is an important contributor to arterial ischemic syndromes. $\longrightarrow$	Treatment with vasodilators is often indicated in the management of atherosclerotic diseases.
Oxidation of LDL is a vital step in atherogenesis and results in the formation of the fatty streak as well as promotes further inflammation and plaque generation. $\longrightarrow$	Reduction in LDL, decreased smoking, and treatment of diabetes and hypertension reduce oxidation of LDL and atherogenesis and can result in regression of established lesions.
Some plaques are "unstable" and can rupture leading to rapid thrombosis and sudden tissue ischemia. $\longrightarrow$	The ability to identify unstable plaques through the use of intravascular ultrasound, MRI, and other new modalities may improve the rapidity of appropriate intervention.
Endothelial dysfunction due to injury and plaque formation results in super-imposed thrombosis, which is the major cause of complete vessel obstruction and infarction of distal tissues. $\longrightarrow$	Antithrombotic drugs help prevent the adhesion of platelets to the injured endothelium, thus preventing thrombus formation and reducing the risk of infarction.

SUGGESTED READINGS

Ahmed, N. (2005). Advanced glycation endproducts—role in pathology of diabetic complications. *Diabetes Research & Clinical Practice, 67*, 3-21.

Ambrose, J. A. & Barua, R. S. (2004). The pathophysiology of cigarette smoking and cardiovascular disease: an update. *Journal of the American College of Cardiology, 43*, 1731-1737.

Arnal, J. F., Gourdy, P., Elhage, R., Garmy-Susini, B., Delmas, E., Brouchet, L., Castano, C., Barreira, Y., Couloumiers, J. C., Prats, H., Prats, A. C., & Bayard, F. (2004). Estrogens and atherosclerosis. *European Journal of Endocrinology, 150*, 113-117.

Ballantyne, C. M., Blazing, M. A., Hunninghake, D. B., Davidson, M. H., Yuan, Z., DeLucca, P., Ramsey, K. E., Hustad, C.M., & Palmisano, J. (2003). Effect of exetimibe coadministered with atorvastatin in 628 patients with primary hypercholesterolemia. *Circulation, 107*, 2409-2415.

Barbato, J. E. & Tzeng, E. (2004). Nitric oxide and arterial disease. *Journal of Vascular Surgery, 40*, 187-193.

Berenson, G. S., Srinivasan, S. R., Bao, W., Newman, W. P. III, Tracy, R. E., & Wattigney, W. A. (1998). Association between multiple cardiovascular risk factors and atherosclerosis in children and young adults: the Bogalusa Heart Study. *New England Journal of Medicine, 338*, 1650-1656.

Bonetti, P. O., Lerman, L. O., & Lerman, A. (2003). Endothelial dysfunction: a marker of atherosclerotic risk. *Arteriosclerosis, Thrombosis & Vascular Biology, 23*, 168-175.

Boyle, J. J. (2005). Macrophage activation in atherosclerosis: pathogenesis of plaque rupture. *Current Vascular Pharmacology, 3*, 63-68.

Brewer, H. B. & Santamarina-Fojo, S. (2003). Clinical significance of high-density lipoproteins and the development of atherosclerosis. *American Journal of Cardiology, 92*(suppl), 10k-16k.

Brewer, H.B., Jr. (2004). Increasing HDL cholesterol levels. *New England Journal of Medicine, 350*, 1491-1494.

Ceriello, A. (2004). Impaired glucose tolerance and cardiovascular disease: the possible role of post-prandial hyperglycemia. *American Heart Journal, 147*, 803-807.

Chiong, J. R. & Miller, A. B. (2003). Agents that stabilize atherosclerotic plaque. *Expert Opinion on Investigational Drugs, 12*(10),1681-1692.

Correia, M. L. & Haynes, W. G. (2004). Leptin, obesity and cardiovascular disease. *Current Opinion in Nephrology & Hypertension, 13*, 215-223.

Cunningham, K. S. & Gotlieb, A. I. (2005). The role of shear stress in the pathogenesis of atherosclerosis. *Laboratory Investigation, 85*, 9-23.

Danesh, J., Wheeler, J. G., Hirschfield, G. M., Eda, S., Eiriksdottir, G., Rumley, A., Lowe, G. D., Pepys, M.B., & Gudnason. V. (2004). C reactive protein and other circulating markers of inflammation in the prediction of coronary heart disease. *New England Journal of Medicine, 350*, 1387-1397.

Dansinger, M. L., Gleason, J. A., Griffith, J. L., Selker, H. P., & Schaefer, E. J. (2005). Comparison of the Atkins, Ornish, Weight Watchers, and Zone diets for weight loss and heart disease risk reduction: a randomized trial. *Journal of the American Medical Association, 293*(1), 43-53.

Davidson, J. & Rotondo, D. (2003). Lipid metabolism: inflammatory-immune responses in atherosclerosis. *Current Opinion in Lipidology, 14*(3), 337-339.

Davidson, M. H. (2004). Emerging therapeutic strategies for the management of dyslipidemia in patients with the metabolic syndrome. *American Journal of Cardiology, 93*, 3C-11C.

Duvall, W. L. (2005). Endothelial dysfunction and antioxidants. *Mount Sinai Journal of Medicine, 72*(2), 71-80.

Eckel, R. H., Wassef, M., Chait, A., Sobel, B., Barrett, E., King, G., Lopes-Virella, M., Reusch, J., Ruderman, N., Steiner, G., & Vlassara, H. (2002). Prevention conference VI: diabetes and cardiovascular disease: pathogenesis of atherosclerosis in diabetes. *Circulation, 105*, e138.

Expert panel on detection, evaluation, and treatment of high blood cholesterol in adults. (2001). Executive Summary of the Third Report of the National Cholesterol Education Program (NCEP) Expert Panel on Detection, Evaluation, and Treatment of High Blood Cholesterol in Adults (Adult Treatment Panel III). *Journal of the American Medical Association, 285*, 2486-2497.

Ferrario, C. M., Richmond, R. S., Smith, R., Levy, P., Strawn, W. B., & Kivlighn, S. (2004). Renin-angiotensin system as a therapeutic target in managing atherosclerosis. *American Journal of Therapeutics, 11*, 44-53.

Fichtlscherer, S., Heeschen, C., & Zeiher, A. M. (2004). Inflammatory markers and coronary artery disease. *Current Opinion in Pharmacology, 4*, 124-131.

Golden, S. H. & Chong, R. (2004). Are there specific components of the insulin resistance syndrome that predict the increased atherosclerosis seen in type 2 diabetes mellitus? *Current Diabetes Reports, 4*, 26-30.

Gotto, A. M., Jr. & Brinton, E. A. (2004). Assessing low levels of high-density lipoprotein cholesterol as a risk factor in coronary heart disease: a working group report and update. *Journal of American College of Cardiology, 43*, 717-724.

Hackam, D. G. & Anand, S. S. (2003). Emerging risk factors for atherosclerotic vascular disease: a critical review of the evidence. *Journal of the American Medical Association, 290*(7), 932-940.

Haffner, S. M. (2003). Insulin resistance, inflammation, and the prediabetic state. *American Journal of Cardiology, 92*(supp), 18J-26J.

Hamilton, C. A., Miller, W. H., Al Benna, S., Brosnan, M. J., Drummond, R. D., McBride, M. W., & Dominiczak, A. F. (2004). Strategies to reduce oxidative stress in cardiovascular disease. *Clinical Science, 106*, 219-234.

Hansson, G. K. (2005). Inflammation, atherosclerosis, and coronary artery disease. *New England Journal of Medicine, 352*, 1685-1695.

Hayden, M., Pignone, M., Phillips, C., & Mulrow, C. (2002). Aspirin for the primary prevention of cardiovascular events: a summary of the evidence for the US Preventive Services Task Force. *Annals of Internal Medicine, 136*, 161-172.

Heeschen, C., Dimmeler, S., Hamm, C. W., van den Brand, M. J., Boersma, E., Zeiher, A. M., & Simoons, M. L. (2003). Soluble CD40 ligand in acute coronary syndromes. *New England Journal of Medicine, 348*, 1104-1111.

Higgins, J. P. (2003). *Chlamydia pneumoniae* and coronary artery disease: the antibiotic trials. *Mayo Clinic Proceedings, 78*, 321-332.

Hingorani, A. D. (2004). Diet, the endothelium and atherosclerosis. *Clinical Science, 106*, 447-448.

Ho, W. K., Hankey, G. J., & Eikelboom, J. W. (2004). Prevention of coronary heart disease with aspirin and clopidogrel: efficacy, safety, costs and cost-effectiveness. *Expert Opinion on Pharmacotherapy, 5*, 493-503.

Huo, Y. & Ley, K. F. (2004). Role of platelets in the development of atherosclerosis. *Trends in Cardiovascular Medicine, 14*, 18-22.

Ieven, M. M. & Hoymans, V. Y. (2005). Involvement of *Chlamydia pneumoniae* in atherosclerosis: more evidence for lack of evidence. *Journal of Clinical Microbiology, 43*, 19-24.

Ignarro, L. J. & Napoli, C. (2005). Novel features of nitric oxide, endothelial nitric oxide synthase, and atherosclerosis. *Current Diabetes Reports*, 5, 17-23.

Jacoby, D. S. & Rader, D. J. (2003). Renin-angiotensin system and atherothrombotic disease: from genes to treatment. *Archives of Internal Medicine*, 163, 1155-1164.

John, S. & Schmieder, R. E. (2000). Impaired endothelial function in arterial hypertension and hypercholesterolemia: potential mechanisms. *Journal of Hypertension*, 18(4), 363-374.

Kiechl, S., Lorenz, E., Reindl, M., Wiedermann, C. J., Oberhollenzer, F., Bonora, E., Willeit, J., & Schwartz, D. A. (2002). Toll-like receptor 4 polymorphisms and atherogenesis. *New England Journal of Medicine*, 347, 185-192.

Knopp, R. H., Retzlaff, B., Aikawa, K., & Kahn, S. E. (2003). Management of patients with diabetic hyperlipidemia. *American Journal of Cardiology*, 91, 24E-28E.

Kougias, P., Chai, H., Lin, P. H., Yao, Q., Lumsden, A. B., & Chen, C. (2005). Defensins and cathelicidins: neutrophil peptides with roles in inflammation, hyperlipidemia and atherosclerosis. *Journal of Cellular & Molecular Medicine*, 9, 3-10.

Kraus, W. E., Houmard, J. A., Duscha, B. D., Knetzger, K. J., Wharton, M. B., McCartney, J. S., Bales, C. W., Henes, S., Samsa, G. P., Otvos, J. D., Kulkarni, K. R., & Slentz, C. A. (2002). Effects of the amount and intensity of exercise on plasma lipoproteins. *New England Journal of Medicine*, 347, 1483-1492.

Kullo, I. J. & Ballantyne, C. M. (2005). Conditional risk factors for atherosclerosis. *Mayo Clinic Proceedings*, 80, 219-230.

Landmesser, U., Hornig, B., & Drexler, H. (2004). Endothelial function: a critical determinant in atherosclerosis? *Circulation*, 109, II27-II33.

Langheinrich, A. C. & Bohle, R. M. (2005). Atherosclerosis: humoral and cellular factors of inflammation. *Virchows Archiv*, 446, 101-111.

Lee, Y. H. & Pratley, R. E. (2005). The evolving role of inflammation in obesity and the metabolic syndrome. *Current Diabetes Reports*, 5, 70-75.

Libby, P. (2000). Changing concepts of atherogenesis. *Journal of Internal Medicine*, 247(3), 349-358.

Libby, P., Ridker, P., & Maseri, A. (2002). Inflammation and atherosclerosis. *Circulation*, 105, 1135-1143.

Libby, P. & Ridker, P. M. (2004). Inflammation and atherosclerosis: role of C-reactive protein in risk assessment. *American Journal of Medicine*, 116(suppl), 6A, 9S-16S.

Libby, P. (2003). Vascular biology of atherosclerosis: overview and state of the art. *American Journal of Cardiology*, 91, 3A-6A.

Linsel-Nitschke, P. & Tall, A. R. (2005). HDL as a target in the treatment of atherosclerotic cardiovascular disease. *Nature Reviews, Drug Discovery*, 4, 193-205.

Lip, G. Y. & Blann, A. D. (2004). Thrombogenesis, atherogenesis and angiogenesis in vascular disease: a new "vascular triad." *Annals of Medicine*, 36, 119-125.

Maki, K. C. (2004). Dietary factors in the prevention of diabetes mellitus and coronary artery disease associated with the metabolic syndrome. *American Journal of Cardiology*, 93, 12C-17C.

Maksimowicz-McKinnon, K., Bhatt, D. L., & Calabrese, L. H. (2004). Recent advances in vascular inflammation: C-reactive protein and other inflammatory biomarkers. *Current Opinion in Rheumatology*, 16, 18-24.

McKenney, J. (2004). New perspectives on the use of niacin in the treatment of lipid disorders. *Archives of Internal Medicine*, 164, 697-705.

Monaco, C. & Paleolog, E. (2004). Nuclear factor kappaB: a potential therapeutic target in atherosclerosis and thrombosis. *Cardiovascular Research*, 61, 671-682.

Moyna, N. M. & Thompson, P. D. (2004). The effect of physical activity on endothelial function in man. *Acta Physiologica Scandinavica*, 180, 113-123.

Newby, A. C. (2005). Dual role of matrix metalloproteinases (matrixins) in intimal thickening and atherosclerotic plaque rupture. *Physiological Reviews*, 85(1),1-31.

Nissen, S. E., Tuzcu, E. M., Schoenhagen, P., Brown, B. G., Ganz, P., Vogel, R. A., Crowe, T., Howard, G., Cooper, C. J., Brodie, B., Grines, C. L., & DeMaria, A. N. REVERSAL Investigators. (2004). Effect of intensive compared with moderate lipid-lowering therapy on progression of coronary atherosclerosis: a randomized controlled trial. *Journal of the American Medical Association*, 291(9), 1071-1080.

Nissen, S. E., Tuzcu, E. M., Schoenhagen, P., Crowe, T., Sasiela, W. J., Tsai, J., Orazem, J., Magorien, R. D., O'Shaughnessy, C., & Ganz, P. Reversal of atherosclerosis with aggressive lipid lowering (REVERSAL) investigators. (2005). Statin therapy, LDL cholesterol, C-reactive protein, and coronary artery disease. *New England Journal of Medicine*, 352(1), 29-38.

O'Connor, C. M., Dunne, M. W., Pfeffer, M. A., Muhlestein, J. B., Yao, L., Gupta, S., Benner, R. J., Fisher, M. R., & Cook, T. D., for the investigators in the WIZARD study. (2003). Azithromycin for the secondary prevention of coronary heart disease events: the WIZARD study: a randomized controlled trial. *Journal of the American Medical Association*, 290,1459-1466.

O'Keefe, J. H., Jr., Cordain, L., Harris, W. H., Moe, R. M., & Vogel, R. (2004). Optimal low-density lipoprotein is 50 to 70 mg/dl: better and physiologically normal. *Journal of the American College of Cardiology*, 43, 2142-2146.

Patrono, C., Bachmann, F., Baigent, C., Bode, C., De Caterina, R., Charbonnier, B., Fitzgerald, D., Hirsh, J., Husted, S., Kvasnicka, J., Montalescot, G., Garcia Rodriguez, L. A., Verheugt, F., Vermylen, J., & Wallentin, L., Grupo de Trabajo sobre el uso de agentes antiplaquetarios en pacientes con enfermedad cardiovascular aterosclerotica de la Sociedad Europea de Cardiologia. (2004). [Expert consensus document on the use of antiplatelet agents.] The task force on the use of antiplatelet agents in patients with atherosclerotic cardiovascular disease of the European society of cardiology. *European Heart Journal*, 25, 166-181.

Peppa, M., Uribarri, J., & Vlassara, H. (2004). The role of advanced glycation end products in the development of atherosclerosis. *Current Diabetes Reports*, 4, 31-36.

Pischon, T., Girman, C. J., Hotamisligil, G. S., Rifai, N., Hu, F. B., & Rimm, E. B. (2004). Plasma adiponectin levels and risk of myocardial infarction in men. *Journal of the American Medical Association*, 291, 1730-1737.

Prasad, A., Zhu, J., Halcox, J. P., Waclawiw, M. A., Epstein, S. E., & Quyyumi, A. A. (2002). Predisposition to atherosclerosis by infections: role of endothelial dysfunction. *Circulation*, 106(2), 184-190.

Rader, D. J. (2003). High density lipoproteins as an emerging therapeutic target for atherosclerosis. *Journal of the American Medical Association*, 290, 2322-2324.

Ridker, P. M. & Morrow, D. A. (2003). C-reactive protein, inflammation, and coronary risk. *Cardiology Clinics*, 21(3), 315-325.

Ridker, P. (2003). High sensitivity C-reactive protein and cardiovascular risk: rationale for screening and primary prevention. *American Journal of Cardiology*, 92(Suppl), 17K-22K.

Rosenson, R. S. (2004). Statins in atherosclerosis: lipid-lowering agents with antioxidant capabilities. *Atherosclerosis*, 173, 1-12.

Ross, R. (1999). Mechanisms of disease: Atherosclerosis—an inflammatory disease. *New England Journal of Medicine*, 340, 115-126.

Rubbo, H. & O'Donnell, V. (2005). Nitric oxide, peroxynitrite and lipoxygenase in atherogenesis: mechanistic insights. *Toxicology,* 208, 305-317.

Scannapieco, F. A., Bush, R. B., & Paju, S. (2003). Associations between periodontal disease and risk for atherosclerosis, cardiovascular disease, and stroke. A systematic review. *Annals of Periodontology,* 8(1), 38-53.

Scanu, A. (2003). Lipoprotein (a) and the atherothrombotic process: mechanistic insights and clinical applications. *Current Atherosclerosis Reports,* 56, 106-113.

Schonbeck, U. & Libby, P. (2004). Inflammation, immunity, and HMG-CoA reductase inhibitors: statins as antiinflammatory agents? *Circulation,* 109, II18-II26.

Schroecksnadel, K., Frick, B., Wirleitner, B., Winkler, C., Schennach, H., & Fuchs, D. (2004). Moderate hyperhomocysteinemia and immune activation. *Current Pharmaceutical Biotechnology,* 5, 107-118.

Sheikine, Y. & Hansson, G. K. (2004). Chemokines and atherosclerosis. *Annals of Medicine,* 36, 98-118.

Shinozaki, K., Kashiwagi, A., Masada, M., & Okamura, T. (2004). Molecular mechanisms of impaired endothelial function associated with insulin resistance. *Current Drug Targets—Cardiovascular & Haematological Disorders,* 4, 1-11.

Sjoholm, A. & Nystrom, T. (2005). Endothelial inflammation in insulin resistance. *Lancet,* 365, 610-612.

Smeglin, A. & Frishman, W. H. (2004). Elastinolytic matrix metalloproteinases and their inhibitors as therapeutic targets in atherosclerotic plaque instability. *Cardiology in Review,* 12, 141-150.

Spieker, L. E., Ruschitzka, F., Luscher, T. F., & Noll, G. (2004). HDL and inflammation in atherosclerosis. *Current Drug Targets—Immune Endocrine & Metabolic Disorders,* 4, 51-57.

Stary, H. C. (2000). Natural and historical classification of atherosclerotic lesions: an update. *Arteriosclerosis, Thrombosis & Vascular Biology,* 20, 1177–1178.

Stephens, J. W., Sozen, M. M., Whittall, R. A., Caslake, M. J., Bedford, D., Acharya, J., Hurel, S. J., & Humphries, S. E. (2005). Three novel mutations in the apolipoprotein E gene in a sample of individuals with type 2 diabetes mellitus. *Clinical Chemistry,* 51(1), 119-124.

The Homocysteine Studies Collaboration. (2002). Homocysteine and risk of ischemic heart disease and stroke; a meta-analysis. *Journal of the American Medical Association,* 288, 2015-2022.

Thomas, W. G. (2005). Double trouble for type 1 angiotensin receptors in atherosclerosis. *New England Journal of Medicine,* 352(5), 506-508.

Toole, J. F., Girman, C. J., Hotamisligil, G. S., Rifai, N., Hu, F. B., Rimm, E.B. (2004). Lowering homocysteine in patients with ischemic stroke to prevent recurrent stroke, myocardial infarction and death. *Journal of the American Medical Association,* 291, 565-575.

Toth, P. P. (2004). High-density lipoprotein and cardiovascular risk. *Circulation,* 109, 1809-1812.

Trujillo, M. E. & Scherer, P. E. (2005). Adiponectin—journey from an adipocyte secretory protein to biomarker of the metabolic syndrome. *Journal of Internal Medicine,* 257, 167-175.

Viles-Gonzalez, J. F., Anand, S. X., Valdiviezo, C., Zafar, M. U., Hutter, R., Sanz, J., Rius, T., Poon, M., Fuster, V., & Badimon, J. J. (2004). Update in atherothrombotic disease. *Mount Sinai Journal of Medicine,* 71, 197-208.

von Eckardstein, A., Hersberger, M., & Rohrer, L. (2005). Current understanding of the metabolism and biological actions of HDL. *Current Opinion in Clinical Nutrition & Metabolic Care,* 8, 147-152.

Wick, G., Knoflach, M., & Xu, Q. (2004). Autoimmune and inflammatory mechanisms in atherosclerosis. *Annual Review of Immunology,* 22, 361-403.

Yeh, E. T. (2004). CRP as a mediator of disease. *Circulation,* 109, II11-II14.

Zhou, X. & Hansson, G. K. (2004). Immunomodulation and vaccination for atherosclerosis. *Expert Opinion on Biological Therapy,* 4, 599-612.

Dyslipidemia and Atherosclerosis

INITIAL HISTORY

- 69-year-old white male.
- Complains of excruciating left leg pain.
- Reports sudden onset 45 minutes ago while sitting on a bench at the shopping mall, unrelieved with massage/rest, pain is nonradiating.
- Reports has previously had occasional left leg aching discomfort when walking long distances.

Question 1.   *What other questions would you like to ask about his medical, family, and social history?*

ADDITIONAL HISTORY AND HOME MEDICATIONS

- Denies any history of chest pain or focal neurologic symptoms.
- No significant previous medical history; does not think he has ever been told he has hypertension, diabetes, or dyslipidemia.
- 75 pack/year smoking history (continues to smoke).
- Uses alcohol occasionally.
- Not on any medications and has no known allergies.

FAMILY AND SOCIAL HISTORY

- Father died of myocardial infarction at age 78; mother is alive and suffers from hypertension and cerebrovascular disease; 1 brother, age 62, 1 sister, age 58—both alive and well.
- Lives with wife of 45 years, is a retired civil engineer (retired 4 years ago), and enjoys gardening and travel.
- Feels healthy overall, does not seek regular medical care.

INITIAL PHYSICAL FINDINGS

- Left leg is mottled and cyanotic, distal to the knee, cool to touch.
- Right leg is pink and warm.
- Doppler of the left dorsalis pedis (DP) and posterior tibialis (PT) pulses reveals decreased pulses with faint bruits heard.
- Right DP and PT pulses are palpable.

□ **Kathryn B. Reid, PhD, RN, CCRN, APRN-BC contributed this case study.**

Question 2.   *What is your initial diagnosis?*

Question 3.   *What are the possible causes of this patient's problem?*

Question 4.   *What are the potential general sequelae if this problem is not resolved?*

PHYSICAL EXAMINATION

- T = 36.9 PO; BP = 160/90 mm Hg left arm, 166/92 mm Hg right arm (sitting); P = 96 bpm, regular rate; RR = 20 breaths/minute, unlabored.
- Slightly obese man complaining of left lower leg and calf aching/throbbing pain, 8 on a scale of 1 to 10.

HEENT, Neck, Lungs, Cardiac

- Unremarkable, fundi without lesions.
- Supple, no adenopathy or thyromegaly, no bruits.
- Bilateral and symmetric chest expansion with clear breath sounds.
- S_1 S_2 clear; no rub, gallop, or murmur; regular rate.

Abdomen, Neurologic

- Abdomen with positive bowel sounds throughout, nontender, nondistended.
- Alert and oriented, appropriately anxious; cranial nerves X to XII intact; strength 5/5 throughout, DTRs 2+ and symmetric, sensation intact.

Skin, Extremities
- Skin intact, warm, pink except for left leg (cool and mottled distal to knee).
- Peripheral pulses all palpable except for left DP and PT.
- Faint bruits by Doppler.
- No edema.

Question 5.   *What are the immediate therapeutic alternatives for restoring perfusion to this man's leg, and which do you feel would be most appropriate in this case?*

Question 6.   *What studies would you initiate at this time?*

LABORATORY RESULTS

- Glucose = 225; urine myoglobin = negative.
- Triglycerides = 315; cholesterol = 353; HDL = 40; LDL = 165.
- All other bloodwork within normal limits; 12-lead ECG is normal.
- Rectal examination normal; stool guaiac negative.

Question 7.   *What risk factors for atherosclerotic peripheral vascular disease do you identify for this man?*

PATIENT UPDATE

- Patient is admitted to the hospital, is anticoagulated, and undergoes urokinase therapy. Resolution of his blood clot is noted on fluoroscopy, as well as improved distal pulses. Two hours later, however, his status changes as follows:
  - Left DP is absent by Doppler; left PT is unchanged.
  - Left leg is increasingly mottled.
  - Left leg demonstrates increased calf size, edema, and tightness.
  - Urine is positive for myoglobin.
  - Patient reports numbness and tingling in his left leg and foot.

Question 8. *Based on these new findings, what complications is this patient exhibiting and what precautions must be taken?*

ADDITIONAL PATIENT UPDATE

- Left calf fasciotomy is performed with the following results:
  - Left DP pulse improves to present pulsatile flow by Doppler; left PT pulse also is present by Doppler.
  - Patient reports resolving numbness and tingling.
  - Mottled appearance of the left leg begins to disappear.

PATIENT COURSE

- Patient's left femoral artery clot is successfully dissolved with urokinase therapy, and normal perfusion is restored to his left leg. The fasciotomy site is sutured and closed 2 days later.
- Angiographically documented severe distal femoral artery stenosis is successfully opened through percutaneous transluminal angioplasty.
- Patient's diastolic blood pressure remains 88 to 98 mm Hg and his blood glucose levels remain 150 to 270 during his hospital course.

Question 9. *What are the immediate priorities for medical aspects of care now that this patient's acute problem has been resolved?*

Question 10. *For what other diseases should this patient be screened given his current status and health conditions?*

Question 11. *What essential information and education do you need to provide this patient before discharge?*

Ischemic Heart Disease

DEFINITION

- Ischemic heart disease (IHD) develops if the supply of coronary blood cannot meet the demand of the myocardium for oxygen and nutrients.
- Can be categorized as:
    - Transient ischemic syndromes.
        1. Stable angina.
        2. Silent ischemia.
        3. Prinzmetal angina.
    - Acute coronary syndromes.
        1. Unstable angina.
        2. Non–ST-segment elevation myocardial infarction (non-STEMI).
        3. ST-segment elevation myocardial infarction (STEMI).
    - Most commonly caused by obstruction of coronary flow by atherosclerotic disease of the coronary vessels, especially when accompanied by an increase in myocardial demand for perfusion and/or thrombus formation on a ruptured atherosclerotic plaque.

EPIDEMIOLOGY

- In 2005, the American Heart Association estimated that more than 13 million Americans have coronary artery disease, and that 2600 people die each day from cardiovascular disease in the United States. The economic effect of this disease in 2005 was estimated to be $393.5 billion.
- Cardiovascular deaths have decreased 50% in the past three decades; this rate of decline is greatest in white males and lowest in black females.
- Risk factors are the same as those for atherosclerosis (see Chapter 2):
    - Conventional: Nonmodifiable risks include: (1) advanced age, (2) male gender or women after menopause, and, (3) family history (genetics). Modifiable major risks include (1) dyslipidemia, (2) cigarette smoking, (3) hypertension, (4) diabetes and insulin resistance, (5) obesity, (6) sedentary life-style, and (7) atherogenic diet.
    - Nontraditional: (1) increased serum markers for inflammation, autoimmunity and thrombosis (C-reactive protein [CRP], fibrinogen) and (2) hyperhomocystinemia.

PATHOPHYSIOLOGY

- Atherosclerotic plaques form in coronary vessels (see Chapter 2). Further evolution of the plaque determines the progression of myocardial ischemia. Figure 3-1 provides an overview of the basic steps in the development of ischemic heart disease.

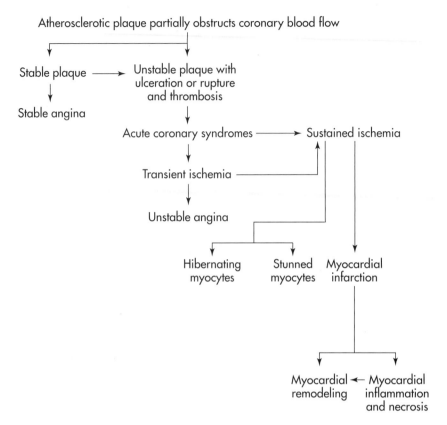

FIGURE **3-1 Pathogenesis of Ischemic Heart Disease.**

Transient Coronary Ischemic Syndromes

- Stable angina.
    - The atherosclerotic lesion partially obstructs flow. Stenoses of proximal "conduit" vessels results in autoregulation of distal "resistive" vessels to maintain flow. If stenoses exceed the resistance of the distal bed (60% to 75% occlusion), then autoregulation can no longer compensate.
    - Slowly increasing atherosclerotic coronary obstructions allow for collateral perfusion such that there is little risk of infarction and overall prognosis is fairly good; however, risk of MI and death increases as the number of affected vessels and the severity of the obstructions increase.
    - Transient ischemia occurs when there is increased myocardial demand for coronary flow.
        1. Anaerobic metabolism leads to lactic acid inhibition of myocardial contractility, resulting in transient decreases in ejection fraction with pulmonary congestion and poor peripheral perfusion of tissues.
        2. Lactic acid causes stimulation of sympathetic afferents, giving the sensation of pain in the substernal area; cross-stimulation of other sympathetic afferents results in the "radiation" of pain to the neck, jaw, left shoulder, or left arm.
        3. Although there is no acute infarction of myocardial tissue in stable angina, repetitive ischemia results in ischemic myocardial remodeling and a risk of heart failure.
- Silent ischemia.
    - Silent ischemia is defined as significant transient myocardial ischemia without associated symptoms.

- It is common in older adult and diabetic patients, as well as in a significant number of men ages 45 to 65, especially during episodes of mental stress. The presence of silent ischemia indicates a significant risk for myocardial infarction in patients who also have episodes of chronic stable angina or in asymptomatic patients with a history of recent myocardial infarction or bypass surgery.
- Proposed mechanisms include:
  1. The presence of a global or regional abnormality in left ventricular symptomatic afferent innervation. This abnormality might occur as part of metabolic dysfunction in diabetes mellitus, following surgical denervation during coronary artery bypass grafting (CABG) or cardiac transplantation, or following ischemic local nerve injury by myocardial infarction.
  2. Silent ischemia may be associated with less local inflammation, suggesting that a high level of inflammatory cytokines may be necessary to induce anginal pain.
- Prinzmetal angina.
  - It presents with chest pain attributable to transient ischemia of myocardium that occurs unpredictably and at rest; the pain frequently occurs at night during rapid-eye-movement sleep and may have a cyclic pattern of occurrence.
  - It is caused by vasospasm of one or more major coronary arteries with or without atherosclerosis. It may result from hyperactivity of sympathetic nervous system, increased calcium flux in arterial smooth muscle, or impaired production or release of prostaglandin or thromboxane (imbalance of coronary vasodilators and vasoconstrictors).

Acute Coronary Syndromes

- The acute coronary syndromes result from sudden coronary obstruction due to thrombus formation over an atherosclerotic plaque. Most often, these plaques obstruct less than 70% of the coronary vessel lumen and therefore may not have caused preceding episodes of angina and may not be detected by routine tests for coronary artery disease.
- The American Heart Association Committee on Vascular Lesions provided criteria for subdividing coronary atherosclerotic plaque progression into five phases with different lesion types corresponding to each phase. The basic thrust of this system is that some atherosclerotic lesions are "stable" and progress by gradually occluding the vessel lumen, whereas other lesions are "unstable" and are prone to sudden plaque rupture and thrombus formation, resulting in the acute coronary syndromes of **unstable angina, non–ST elevation myocardial infarction (non-STEMI), ST elevation myocardial infarction (STEMI),** and even sudden death.
- Plaques that are unstable and prone to rupture are those with a core that is especially rich in deposited oxidized LDL and those with thin fibrous caps (Figure 3-2).
- Plaque disruption (erosions, fissuring, or rupture) occurs due to shear forces, inflammation with release of multiple inflammatory mediators (e.g., interferon, tumor necrosis factor), secretion of macrophage-derived degradative enzymes (metalloproteinases, cystine proteases), and apoptosis of cells at the edges of the lesions.
- Clinical "triggers" for plaque rupture include circadian variation (increased risk in the morning), seasonal variation (increased risk in the winter), physical exertion, and emotional stress.
- Exposure of the plaque substrate activates the clotting cascade and exposes platelet glycoprotein IIb/IIIa surface receptors. Platelet activation results in the release of additional coagulants resulting in further platelet aggregation and adherence.
- The resulting thrombus can form very quickly to completely obstruct the vessel.
- Vessel obstruction is further exacerbated by the release of vasoconstrictors such as thromboxane A_2 from the vessel wall.
- The thrombus may break up before permanent myocyte damage has occurred (unstable angina) or it may cause prolonged ischemia with infarction of the heart muscle (myocardial infarction).

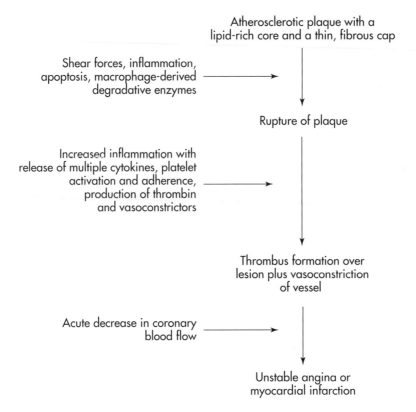

FIGURE **3-2 Pathogenesis of the Plaque Rupture.**

- Unstable angina.
    - Plaque rupture or erosion leads to transient episodes of thrombotic vessel occlusion and vasoconstriction at the site of plaque damage.
    - The thrombus is labile and occludes the vessel for no more than 10 to 20 minutes, with return of perfusion before significant myocardial necrosis occurs.
    - Unstable angina presents as new-onset angina, angina that is occurring at rest, or angina that is increasing in severity or frequency. Patients may experience increased dyspnea, diaphoresis, and anxiety as the angina worsens.
    - Unstable angina indicates a markedly increased risk of myocardial infarction or death— approximately 20% of individuals with unstable angina will progress to myocardial infarction or death within 30 days.
- Myocardial infarction (MI).
    - Plaque rupture occurs at the edge of the lesion in rest MI, or at an area of cap thinning in exertional MI, resulting in rapid thrombus formation and complete vessel occlusion.
    - Prolonged ischemia results in permanent damage to myocardial cells, with loss of contractility and release of cellular enzymes.
    - If the thrombus breaks up before complete distal tissue necrosis has occurred, the infarction will involve only the myocardium directly beneath the endocardium. This type of myocardial infarction most often presents with no elevation of the ST segment on electrocardiogram (ECG) and therefore is termed non-STEMI. In addition, this form of infarction will not be associated with the classic Q-wave tracing on the ECG (non–Q-wave MI). It is especially important to recognize this form of acute coronary syndrome because recurrent clot formation on the disrupted atherosclerotic plaque is likely, with resultant infarct expansion.
    - If the thrombus lodges more permanently in the vessel, the infarction will extend through the myocardium from endocardium to epicardium, resulting in severe cardiac dysfunction. This usually presents with significant ST-segment elevation on

ECG (STEMI). Often a characteristic Q wave will develop on ECG some hours later (Q-wave MI). STEMI requires rapid intervention to prevent serious complications and sequelae.

- Ischemic damage results in necrosis with infiltration of inflammatory cells and fibroblasts that lay down scar tissue (fibrosis) and result in permanent decreases in myocardial contractility and compliance.
- Myocardial "stunning" may occur in the area around the infarcted tissue, a process in which myocytes lose their normal conductive and contractile function for prolonged periods even after perfusion has been restored. It is mediated by free radical–induced lipid peroxidation, enzyme defects (Na/K pump), and alterations in calcium homeostasis.
- "Hibernating myocardium" is ischemic but not infarcted myocardium in regions near the infarct area that has persistently impaired myocardial function due to reduced coronary blood flow (persistent ischemia).
    1. Myocytes may remain viable for months to years due to down-regulation of biochemical and physiologic activity to prolong myocyte survival (perfusion-contraction matching).
    2. Hibernating myocardium responds to reperfusion/revascularization (percutaneous coronary intervention [PCI] or surgery). Calcium channel blockers may also improve function.
- Myocardial "remodeling" is a process mediated in part by the renin-angiotensin-aldosterone (RAA) system that causes myocyte hypertrophy and abnormal contractile function in the areas surrounding the infarcted area; this process contributes to infarct expansion and the development of chronic congestive heart failure (CHF) (see Chapter 4).
- During the ischemic episode, ventricular function is abnormal and ejection fraction falls, with increases in ventricular end-diastolic volume (VEDV). If the coronary obstruction involves the perfusion to the left ventricle, pulmonary venous congestion ensues; if the right ventricle is ischemic, increases in systemic venous pressures occur.
- In addition to ischemic dysfunction, conductive abnormalities can result in bradycardia and heart block, tachyarrhythmias, ventricular fibrillation, or asystole.
- Cardiogenic shock may occur if contractility is severely compromised, if there is rupture of the septal or ventricular wall, if there is infarction of the chordae tendineae with abrupt regurgitation of the mitral valve, or if there are arrhythmias.

PATIENT PRESENTATION

History

Previous coronary disease; family history of heart disease; hypertension; smoking; dyslipidemia; diabetes; obesity, previous episodes of dyspnea on exertion; light-headed or syncopal episodes.

Symptoms

Substernal pressure/pain or chest tightness with or without radiation to the neck, jaw, left shoulder, or arm; dyspnea; nausea or vomiting; diaphoresis; light-headedness or loss of consciousness; onset of symptoms associated with exercise, cold exposure, or stress; pain relieved with rest versus prolonged and persistent; remember that older adult and diabetic patients may not have any of the classic symptoms and present only with a feeling of unease or dyspnea.

Examination

Between ischemic episodes, the examination may be normal or reveal evidence of underlying risk factors such as hypertension, manifestations of dyslipidemia such as xanthelasma, corneal arcus, or diabetic manifestations such as intertrigo or neuropathy. There may be signs of atherosclerotic disease in the other arteries as evidenced by bruits, decreased pulses, or neurologic findings. Some patients will exhibit the signs of CHF from previous ischemic events (see Chapter 4). During acute ischemic episodes, the patient is usually anxious, tachycardic, and tachypneic, with possible pulmonary rales, S_3, S_4, or murmurs. If there is cardiogenic shock, hypotension with poor tissue perfusion occurs. Finally, acute arrhythmias may manifest with ectopic beats or the absence of a detectable pulse, shock, and loss of consciousness.

DIFFERENTIAL DIAGNOSIS

- Peptic ulcer disease with or without perforation.
- Gastroesophageal reflux.
- Pericarditis.
- Costochondritis.
- Aortic dissection.
- Mitral valve prolapse.
- Pulmonary embolus.
- Other pulmonary disease (e.g., pneumonia, pneumothorax).
- Panic attack.

KEYS TO ASSESSMENT

- Acute chest pain.
    - Rapid assessment is important while initiating supportive care measures.
    - An ECG should be done immediately, and if possible, both with pain and after pain relief. ST-segment elevation indicates STEMI, and appropriate intervention should begin immediately. ST depression can be seen in transient ischemia, but the ECG is neither sensitive (~30% will be nondiagnostic even with ischemia) nor specific. Bundle branch blocks make the interpretation of the ECG for ischemia more difficult and may themselves indicate myocardial damage.
    - Blood should be drawn immediately for complete blood count (CBC), coagulation parameters, electrolytes, creatinine phosphokinase MB (CPK-MB), and troponin I. If the CPK-MB and troponin are elevated, then myocardial infarction has been "ruled in." If these are negative and the ECG is nondiagnostic, the CPK-MB and troponin must be repeated several times over the next 12 hours to rule out MI.
    - Figure 3-3 summarizes the steps in the diagnosis of the acute coronary syndromes.

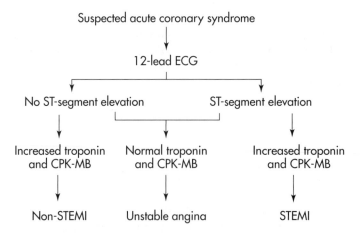

FIGURE **3-3** Diagnosis of Acute Coronary Syndromes.

- Further evaluation of nonacute symptoms or MI ruled out.
  - Evaluation focuses on risk factors and character of the pain to determine likelihood that a history of chest pain was cardiac in origin.
  - If the history is consistent with cardiac pain and the symptoms occurred at rest, were more severe than in the past, or are occurring more frequently, the diagnosis of unstable angina must be considered and the patient should be referred for immediate hospital evaluation.
  - If the history is consistent with cardiac pain but it is predictable, relieved with rest, and of normal severity and duration compared to any previous episodes, this most likely represents stable angina and the patient should undergo one of many possible diagnostic studies to determine the extent of coronary disease and the possible need for invasive therapy. Each of the following tests has been found to be useful in evaluating patients for coronary disease; the choice rests on the local availability of the test:
    1. Stress ECG with thallium—correlates with amount of myocardium at risk.
    2. Single photon emission computed tomography (SPECT) done at rest or with exercise is highly sensitive for coronary disease and has been correlated with prognosis.
    3. Multidetector computed tomography and electron-beam computed tomography—some studies suggest sensitivity and specificity >90% and that this will become the noninvasive modality of choice for the detection of coronary obstruction.
    4. Intravascular ultrasound is being increasingly used due to its ability to not only detect coronary obstruction but also evaluate the intimal structure of plaques (and therefore their stability and likelihood for rupture), even for those plaques that do not yet significantly obstruct the lumen.
    5. Dipyridamole, dobutamine, or arbutamine echocardiography is highly sensitive and specific for detection of coronary disease in some centers.
    6. Coronary angiography should be considered if the noninvasive testing suggests significant coronary obstruction (see following).

KEYS TO MANAGEMENT

- Prevention.
  - Exercise and smoking cessation.
  - NCEP III diet, increased monounsaturated and ω-3 and ω-6 polyunsaturated; intake of *trans*-fatty acids should be eliminated or reduced; increased folate intake that lowers homocysteine levels; moderate alcohol intake (see Chapter 2).
  - Optimization of hypertension and diabetes treatment.
  - Pharmacologic therapy.
    1. Antiplatelet drugs (aspirin and clopidogrel) significantly reduce risk.
    2. Cholesterol-lowering drugs, especially the HMG-CoA reductase inhibitors (statins), greatly reduce risk in patients with dyslipidemias and cause regression of atherosclerotic lesions. They may also reduce risk in those who, according to current guidelines, have "normal" lipids (see Chapter 2). Niacin and ezetimibe are alternatives for specific indications.
    3. Secondary prevention after MI includes β-blockers, aspirin and clopidogrel, and lipid-lowering drugs; in patients with CHF following MI, the use of angiotensin-converting enzyme (ACE) inhibitors, nitrates, and warfarin has been associated with decreased MI recurrence and mortality.
- Stable angina.
  - Risk reduction: weight loss, exercise, diet, treatment for hypertension, diabetes, and dyslipidemia; smoking cessation.
  - Antithrombotic medications: aspirin + clopidogrel if no contraindications.
  - β-blockers are indicated for all patients with stable angina without contraindications, especially if tachycardic or hypertensive.

- ACE inhibitors are indicated for all patients with coronary artery disease who also have diabetes and/or left ventricular systolic dysfunction.
- Sublingual or spray nitrates as needed for episodes of pain. Calcium channel blockers can be considered for continued symptoms.
- Coronary angiography with percutaneous coronary intervention (PCI) or coronary artery bypass grafting (CABG) is indicated if noninvasive testing reveals significant coronary disease, angina is refractory despite optimal treatment, the individual survives a serious arrhythmia, or has congestive heart failure.
- If angina is refractory, consider percutaneous myocardial revascularization (PMR), transmyocardial laser revascularization (TMR), enhanced external counterpulsation, or biorevascularization.
- Unstable angina and non-STEMI.
  - Aspirin is given immediately on admission; plus clopidogrel unless CABG is anticipated. GPIIb/IIIa antagonists should be given to all patients with continuing ischemia or when PCI is anticipated.
  - Pain control: morphine and nitrates.
  - Low-molecular-weight heparin (LMWH), unfractionated heparin, or direct thrombin inhibitors (hirudin, bivalirudin) should be given to all patients without contraindications.
  - Oral β-blockers should be given to all individuals without contraindications.
  - ACE inhibitors should be given to all individuals with decreased cardiac output or hypertension. Angiotensin receptor blockers (ARBs) should be used only in individuals intolerant of ACE inhibitors.
  - Consideration should be given for early PCI versus thrombolytics. PCI has better outcomes in most studies.
  - High-dose statins should be administered before discharge and continued with close follow-up.
- STEMI.
  - Oxygen, intravenous (IV) access, support ventilation, and circulation.
  - Morphine and nitrates given as needed for pain control.
  - Immediate administration of antithrombotic aspirin and clopidogrel and/or GPIIb/IIIa receptor blockers.
  - Emergent catheterization with percutaneous transluminal coronary intervention (PCI) with or without coronary artery stenting and plus GPIIb/IIIa blockade plus clopidogrel. PCI is preferred if a skilled interventionist is rapidly available and for those in cardiogenic shock.

  OR

  - Immediate administration of thrombolytics (alteplase or reteplase) plus heparin, GPIIb/IIIa inhibitor or bivalirudin in patients without contraindications. STEMI patients presenting to a facility without the capability for expert, prompt intervention with primary PCI within 90 minutes of first medical contact should undergo thrombolysis unless contraindicated.
  - Emergency CABG is indicated in those that fail or have contraindications to PCI or thrombolysis and have continuing ischemia.
  - An insulin infusion to normalize blood glucose is recommended for patients with STEMI and complicated courses.
  - Oral β-blocker administered to all without contraindications. If not tolerated, calcium channel blockers are an alternative.
  - ACE inhibitors should be given to all individuals with decreased cardiac output or hypertension. Angiotensin receptor blockers (ARBs) should be used only in individuals intolerant of ACE inhibitors.
  - New cardioprotective drugs such as the sodium-hydrogen exchange inhibitor agent cariporide (reduces calcium influx into ischemic cells) and the potassium/ATP channel openers such as nicorandil are being investigated.
  - In those individuals with arrhythmias, antiarrhythmics or implantable cardiac defibrillator placement should be considered.

- For patients with severe left ventricular dysfunction, ventricular assist devices may provide a bridge to transplantation. Investigational therapies with stem cell transplantation are ongoing.
- Discharged patients should continue antithrombotic medications and statins.
- Patient teaching before discharge is vital to recovery and risk reduction.
- After discharge, patients should be enrolled in a cardiac rehabilitation program.

PATHOPHYSIOLOGY ⟶	CLINICAL LINK
What is going on in the disease process that influences how the patient presents and how he or she should be managed?	*What should you do now that you understand the underlying pathophysiology?*
The spectrum of ischemic heart disease includes all of the stages in the pathogenesis of atherosclerosis and has the same risk factors, with superimposed threat of thrombosis. ⟶	Prevention of coronary artery disease rests on the reduction in risk factors for atherosclerosis plus antiplatelet drugs and/or anticoagulant drugs.
Ischemic myocardium produces lactic acid that stimulates the sympathetic nervous system. ⟶	Older adult patients and those with diabetes may not have pain with myocardial ischemia. The examiner must have a high index of suspicion in patients with risk factors.
Myocardial ischemia can be transient or prolonged with necrosis of heart muscle; myocyte death results in the release of the cardiac enzymes CPK-MB and troponin I. ⟶	Measurement of serum cardiac enzymes differentiates angina or noncardiac pain from true MI, but the serum levels of these markers may take hours to rise, thus delaying the definitive diagnosis.
Cardiac ischemia results in decreased LV contractility with increased LVEDV and pulmonary venous congestion. ⟶	Dyspnea and transient or persistent CHF and pulmonary edema are common features of MI and carry a negative effect on prognosis.
Transient ischemia with exercise or stress occurs when there is a fixed but partial coronary obstruction such that demand exceeds supply for coronary perfusion. ⟶	Stable angina has predictable precipitating factors and is relieved with rest; life-style modification can reduce anginal symptoms.
MI occurs when a coronary atherosclerotic plaque ruptures and thrombus forms. ⟶	In patients without contraindications, the rapid administration of antiplatelet or thrombolytic drugs or rapid PCI can restore perfusion, limit infarct size, and reduce mortality.
Unstable angina occurs when a coronary atherosclerotic plaque is beginning to crack and platelets begin sticking to the lesion. ⟶	Unstable angina is essentially one step from MI in its pathophysiology and must be treated aggressively to avoid MI.
Some of the effects of myocardial ischemia include remodeling and stunning; these have deleterious effects on LV function. ⟶	Treatment of ischemic disease with ACE inhibitors and β-blockers may prevent future CHF.

SUGGESTED READINGS

ACC/AHA 2002 guideline update for the management of patients with chronic stable angina. *Journal of the American College of Cardiology,* 41, 59-168.

ACC/AHA 2002 guideline update for the management of patients with unstable angina and non-ST-segment elevation myocardial infarction. (2002). *Journal of the American College of Cardiology,* 40, 1366-1374.

ACC/AHA 2004 Guideline Update for Coronary Artery Bypass Graft Surgery (2004). *Journal of the American College of Cardiology,* 44(5),1146-54, e213-310.

ACC/AHA guidelines for the management of patients with ST-elevation myocardial infarction. (2004). *Journal of the American College of Cardiology,* 44(3), 671-719.

Akhtar, S. & Silverman, D. G. (2004). Assessment and management of patients with ischemic heart disease. *Critical Care Medicine,* 32, S126-S136.

Alam, S. E., Nasser, S. S., Fernainy, K. E., Habib, A. A., & Badr, K. F. (2004). Cytokine imbalance in acute coronary syndrome. *Current Opinion in Pharmacology,* 4, 166-170.

Almeda, F. Q., Kason, T. T., Nathan, S., & Kavinsky, C. J. (2004). Silent myocardial ischemia: concepts and controversies. *American Journal of Medicine,* 116, 112-118.

Alpert, J. S., Thygesen, K., Antman, E., & Bass, J. P. (2000). Myocardial infarction redefined—a consensus document of The Joint European Society of Cardiology/American College of Cardiology Committee for the redefinition of myocardial infarction. *Journal of the American College of Cardiology,* 36, 959-969.

American Heart Association Committee on Vascular Lesions. (1995). A definition of advanced types of atherosclerotic lesions and a histological classification of atherosclerosis. *Arteriosclerosis, Thrombosis, and Vascular Biology,* 15, 1512-1531.

American Heart Association. Heart Disease and Stroke Statistics—2004 update. Dallas: American Heart Association, 2003.

Atwater, B. D., Roe, M. T., & Mahaffey, K. W. (2005). Platelet glycoprotein IIb/IIIa receptor antagonists in non-ST segment elevation acute coronary syndromes: a review and guide to patient selection. *Drugs,* 65, 313-324.

Bello, N. & Mosca, L. (2004). Epidemiology of coronary heart disease in women. *Progress in Cardiovascular Diseases,* 46, 287-295.

Betriu, A. & Masotti, M. (2005). Comparison of mortality rates in acute myocardial infarction treated by percutaneous coronary intervention versus fibrinolysis. *American Journal of Cardiology,* 95, 100-101.

Blake, G. J. & Ridker, P. M. (2003). C-reactive protein and other inflammatory risk markers in acute coronary syndromes. *Journal of the American College of Cardiology,* 41, 37S-42S.

Boersma, E., Mercado, N., Poldermans, D., Gardien, M., Vos, J., & Simoons, M. L. (2003). Acute myocardial infarction. *Lancet,* 361, 847-858.

Boyle, J. J. (2005). Macrophage activation in atherosclerosis: pathogenesis and pharmacology of plaque rupture. *Current Vascular Pharmacology,* 3, 63-68.

Brieger, D. (2004). Optimizing adjunctive antithrombotic therapy in the treatment of acute myocardial infarction: a role for low-molecular-weight heparin. *Clinical Cardiology,* 27, 3-8.

Brilakis, E. S., Reeder, G. S., & Gersh, B. J. (2003). Modern management of acute myocardial infarction. *Current Problems in Cardiology,* 28, 7-127.

Brown, W. V. (2003). Benefits of statin therapy in patients with special risks: coronary bypass surgery, stable coronary disease, and acute coronary syndromes. *Clinical Cardiology,* 26, III13-III18.

Budoff, M. J. (2005). Noninvasive coronary angiography using computed tomography. *Expert Review of Cardiovascular Therapy,* 3, 123-132.

Cannon, C. P., Braunwald, E., McCabe, C. H., Rouleau, J. L., Belder, R., Joyal, S. V., Pfeffer, M. A., & Skene, A. M. Pravastatin or Atorvastatin Evaluation and Infection Therapy—Thrombolysis Myocardial Infarction 22 Investigators. (2004). Intensive versus moderate lipid lowering with statins after acute coronary syndromes. *New England Journal of Medicine,* 350(15), 1495-1504.

Canty, J. M., Jr. & Fallavollita, J. A. (2005). Hibernating myocardium. *Journal of Nuclear Cardiology,* 12, 104-119.

Carnethon, M. R., Gidding, S. S., Nehgme, R., Sidney, S., Jacobs, D. R., Jr., & Liu, K. (2003). Cardiorespiratory fitness in young adulthood and the development of cardiovascular disease risk factors. *Journal of the American Medical Association,* 290, 3092-3100.

Cavusoglu, E., Cheng, J., Bhatt, R., Kunamneni, P. B., Marmur, J. D., & Eng, C. (2003). Clopidogrel in the management of ischemic heart disease. *Heart Disease,* 5, 144-152.

Chiong, J. R. & Miller, A. B. (2003). Agents that stabilize atherosclerotic plaque. *Expert Opinion on Investigational Drugs,* 12(10), 1681-1692.

Cohen, M. (2003). The role of low-molecular-weight heparin in the management of acute coronary syndromes. *Journal of the American College of Cardiology,* 41, 55S-61S.

Collinson, P. O., Stubbs, P. J., & Kessler, A. C., Multicentre Evaluation of Routine Immunoassay of Troponin T Study. (2003). Multicentre evaluation of the diagnostic value of cardiac troponin T, CK-MB mass, and myoglobin for assessing patients with suspected acute coronary syndromes in routine clinical practice. *Heart,* 89, 280-286.

Corti, R., Fuster, V., & Badimon, J. J. (2003). Pathogenetic concepts of acute coronary syndromes. *Journal of the American College of Cardiology,* 41, 7S-14S.

Crossman, D. C. (2004). The pathophysiology of myocardial ischaemia. *Heart (British Cardiac Society),* 90, 576-580.

Crouch, M. A., Nappi, J. M., & Cheang, K. I. (2003). Glycoprotein IIb/IIIa receptor inhibitors in percutaneous coronary intervention and acute coronary syndrome. *Annals of Pharmacotherapy,* 37, 860-875.

Dalal, H., Evans, P. H., & Campbell, J. L. (2004). Recent developments in secondary prevention and cardiac rehabilitation after acute myocardial infarction. *British Medical Journal,* 328, 693-697.

Danesh, J., Wheeler, J. G., Hirschfield, G. M., Eda, S., Eiriksdottir, G., Rumley, A., Lowe, G. D., Pepys, M. B., & Gudnason, V. (2004). C reactive protein and other circulating markers of inflammation in the prediction of coronary heart disease. *New England Journal of Medicine,* 350, 1387-1397.

DeJongste, M. J., Tio, R. A., & Foreman, R. D. (2004). Chronic therapeutically refractory angina pectoris. *Heart (British Cardiac Society),* 90, 225-230.

Dembo, L. G., Shifrin, R. Y., & Wolff, S. D. (2004). MR imaging in ischemic heart disease. *Radiologic Clinics of North America,* 42, 651-673.

Dimmeler, S., Zeiher, A. M., & Schneider, M. D. (2005). Unchain my heart: the scientific foundations of cardiac repair. *Journal of Clinical Investigation,* 115, 572-583.

Eikelboom, J., White, H., & Yusuf, S. (2003). The evolving role of direct thrombin inhibitors in acute coronary syndromes. *Journal of the American College of Cardiology,* 41, 70S-78S.

Epstein, B. J. & Gums, J. G. (2005). Angiotensin receptor blockers versus ACE inhibitors: prevention of death and myocardial infarction in high-risk populations. *Annals of Pharmacotherapy,* 39, 470-480.

Expert Panel on Detection, Evaluation, and Treatment of High Blood Cholesterol in Adults. (2001). Executive Summary of the Third Report of the National Cholesterol Education Program (NCEP) Expert Panel on Detection, Evaluation, and Treatment of High Blood Cholesterol in Adults (Adult Treatment Panel III). *Journal of the American Medical Association*, 285, 2486-2497.

Freed, D. H., Cunnington, R. H., Dangerfield, A. L., Sutton, J. S., & Dixon, I. M. (2005). Emerging evidence for the role of cardiotrophin-1 in cardiac repair in the infarcted heart. *Cardiovascular Research*, 65, 782-792.

French, J. K., Edmond, J. J., Gao, W., White, H. D., & Eikelboom, J. W. (2004). Adjunctive use of direct thrombin inhibitors in patients receiving fibrinolytic therapy for acute myocardial infarction. *American Journal of Cardiovascular Drugs*, 4, 107-115.

Galinanes, M. & Fowler, A. G. (2004). Role of clinical pathologies in myocardial injury following ischaemia and reperfusion. *Cardiovascular Research*, 61, 512-521.

Gersh, B. J., Stone, G. W., White, H. D., & Holmes, D. R., Jr. (2005). Pharmacological facilitation of primary percutaneous coronary intervention for acute myocardial infarction: is the slope of the curve the shape of the future? *Journal of the American Medical Association*, 293, 979-986.

Gluckman, T. J., Sachdev, M., Schulman, S. P., & Blumenthal, R. S. (2005). A simplified approach to the management of non-ST-segment elevation acute coronary syndromes. *Journal of the American Medical Association*, 293, 349-357.

Goldberg, R. F., Fass, A. E., & Frishman, W. H. (2005). Transmyocardial revascularization: defining its role. *Cardiology in Review*, 13, 52-55.

Grech, E. D. & Ramsdale, D. R. (2003). Acute coronary syndrome: ST segment elevation myocardial infarction. *British Medical Journal*, 326, 1379-1381.

Greenland, J., Abrams, G. P. Aurigemma, M. G., Bond, L. T., Clark, M. H, Criqui, J. R., Crouse, III, L., Friedman, V., Fuster, D. M., Herrington et al., (2000). AHA Conference Proceedings: Prevention Conference V. Beyond secondary prevention: identifying the high-risk patient for primary prevention. Noninvasive tests of atherosclerotic burden. *Circulation,* 101, 111-116.

Gregg, E . (2003). Relationship of changes in physical activity and mortality among older women. *Journal of the American Medical Association,* 289, 2379-2386.

Grines, C., Patel, A., Zijlstra, F., Weaver, W. D., Granger, C., Simes, R. J., & PCAT Collaborators. (2003). Percutaneous transluminal coronary angioplasty. Primary coronary angioplasty compared with intravenous thrombolytic therapy for acute myocardial infarction: six-month follow up and analysis of individual patient data from randomized trials. *American Heart Journal*, 145, 47-57.

Grobbee, D. E. & Bots, M. L. (2003). Statin treatment and progression of atherosclerotic plaque burden. *Drugs*, 63, 893-911.

Hansson, G. K. (2005). Inflammation, atherosclerosis, and coronary artery disease. *New England Journal of Medicine*, 352, 1685-1695.

Hayden, M., Pignone, M., Phillips, C., & Mulrow, C. (2002). Aspirin for the primary prevention of cardiovascular events: a summary of the evidence for the US Preventive Services Task Force. *Annals of Internal Medicine, 136,* 161-172.

Heart Protection Study Collaborative Group. (2002). MRC/BHF Heart Protection Study of cholesterol lowering with simvastatin in 20,536 high-risk individual: a randomized placebo-controlled trial. *Lancet,* 360, 7-22.

Heusch, G., Schulz, R., & Rahimtoola, S. H. (2005). Myocardial hibernation: a delicate balance. *American Journal of Physiology—Heart & Circulatory Physiology,* 288, H984-H999.

Hohnloser, S. H. & Gersh, B. J. (2003). Changing late prognosis of acute myocardial infarction: impact on management of ventricular arrhythmias in the era of reperfusion and the implantable cardioverter-defibrillator. *Circulation,* 107, 941-946.

Holmes, D. R., Jr. (2003). State of the art in coronary intervention. *American Journal of Cardiology*, 91, 50A-53A.

Houslay, E. S. & Uren, N. G. (2005). Intravascular ultrasound: defining plaque regression. *Hospital Medicine (London)*, 66, 27-31.

Hull, S. K., Collins, L. J., & Saseen, J. J. (2005). Clinical inquiries. How useful is high-sensitivity CRP as a risk factor for coronary artery disease? *Journal of Family Practice,* 54, 271-272.

Jabbour, S., Young-Xu, Y., Graboys, T. B., Blatt, C. M., Goldberg, R. J., Bedell, S. E., Bilchik, B. Z., Lown, B., & Ravid, S. (2004). Long-term outcomes of optimized medical management of outpatients with stable coronary artery disease. *American Journal of Cardiology*, 93, 294-299.

Jeremias, A. & Gibson, C. M. (2005). Narrative review: alternative causes for elevated cardiac troponin levels when acute coronary syndromes are excluded. *Annals of Internal Medicine,* 142, 786-791.

Jneid, H., Bhatt, D. L., Corti, R., Badimon, J. J., Fuster, V., & Francis, G. S. (2003). Aspirin and clopidogrel in acute coronary syndromes: therapeutic insights from the CURE study. *Archives of Internal Medicine,* 163, 1145-1153.

Kalus, J. S. & Moser, L. R. (2005). Evolving role of low-molecular-weight heparins in ST-elevation myocardial infarction. *Annals of Pharmacotherapy*, 39, 481-491.

Kandzari, D. E., Hasselblad, V., Tcheng, J. E., Stone, G. W., Califf, R. M., Kastrati, A., Neumann, F. J., Brener, S. J., Montalescot, G., Kong, D. F., & Harrington, R. A. (2004). Improved clinical outcomes with abciximab therapy in acute myocardial infarction: a systematic overview of randomized clinical trials. *American Heart Journal*, 147, 457-462.

Kaplan, R. C., Strickler, H. D., Rohan, T. E., Muzumdar, R., & Brown, D. L. (2005). Insulin-like growth factors and coronary heart disease. *Cardiology in Review*, 13, 35-39.

Kaul, S. & Ito, H. (2004). Microvasculature in acute myocardial ischemia: part II: evolving concepts in pathophysiology, diagnosis, and treatment. *Circulation*, 109, 310-315.

Keeley, E. C., Boura, J. A., & Grines, C. L. (2003). Primary angioplasty versus intravenous thrombolytic therapy for acute myocardial infarction: a quantitative review of 23 randomised trials. *Lancet*, 361, 13-20.

Keely, E. & Grines, C. (2004). Primary coronary intervention for acute myocardial infarction. *Journal of the American Medical Association*, 291, 736-739.

Khot, U. N., Khot, M. B., Bajzer, C. T., Sapp, S. K., Ohman, E. M., Brener, S. J., Ellis, S. G., Lincoff, A. M., & Topol, E. J. (2003). Prevalence of conventional risk factors in patients with coronary heart disease. *Journal of the American Medical Association*, 290, 898-904.

Lee, M. S., Lill, M., & Makkar, R. R. (2004). Stem cell transplantation in myocardial infarction. *Reviews in Cardiovascular Medicine*, 5, 82-98.

Linton, M. F. & Fazio, S. (2003). National Cholesterol Education Program (NCEP)—the Third Adult Treatment Panel (ATP III). A practical approach to risk assessment to prevent coronary artery disease and its complications. *American Journal of Cardiology*, 92(suppl), 19i-26i.

Luss, H., Schafers, M., Neumann, J., Hammel, D., Vahlhaus, C., Baba, H. A., Janssen, F., Scheld, H. H., Schober, O., Breithardt, G., Schmitz, W., & Wichter, T. (2002). Biochemical mechanisms of hibernation and stunning in the human heart. *Cardiovascular Research*, 56(3), 411-421.

Lutgens, E., van Suylen, R. J., Faber, B.C., Gijbels, M. J., Eurlings, P. M., Bijnens, A. P., Cleutjens, K. B.,

Heeneman, S., & Daemen, M. J.A.P. (2003). Atherosclerotic plaque rupture: local or systemic process? *Arteriosclerosis, Thrombosis & Vascular Biology,* 23(12), 2123-2130.

Markkanen, J. E., Rissanen, T. T., Kivela, A., & Yla-Herttuala, S. (2005). Growth factor-induced therapeutic angiogenesis and arteriogenesis in the heart—gene therapy. *Cardiovascular Research,* 65, 656-664.

Maytin, M., & Colucci, W. S. Molecular and cellular mechanisms of myocardial remodeling. (2002). *Journal of Nuclear Cardiology,* 9(3), 319-327.

McClelland, A. J., Owens, C. G., Walsh, S., & Adgey, A. A. (2004). Acute coronary syndromes. *Clinical Medicine,* 4, 27-31.

Mehta, R. H., Sadiq, I., Goldberg, R. J., Gore, J. M., Avezum, A., Spencer, F., Kline-Rogers, E., Allegrone, J., Pieper, K., Fox, K. A., & Eagle, K. A. GRACE Investigators. (2004). Effectiveness of primary percutaneous coronary intervention compared with that of thrombolytic therapy in elderly patients with acute myocardial infarction. *American Heart Journal,* 147(2), 253-259.

Mehta, S. R. & Yusuf, S. (2003). Short- and long-term oral antiplatelet therapy in acute coronary syndromes and percutaneous coronary intervention. *Journal of the American College of Cardiology,* 41, 79S-88S.

Monroe, V. S., Kerensky, R. A., Rivera, E., Smith, K. M., & Pepine, C. J. (2003). Pharmacologic plaque passivation for the reduction of recurrent cardiac events in acute coronary syndromes. *Journal of the American College of Cardiology,* 41, 23S-30S.

Nabel, E. G. (2003). Cardiovascular disease. *New England Journal of Medicine,* 349, 60-72.

Newby, L. K., Goldmann, B. U., & Ohman, E. M. (2003). Troponin: an important prognostic marker and risk-stratification tool in non-ST-segment elevation acute coronary syndromes. *Journal of the American College of Cardiology,* 41, 31S-36S.

Nissen, S. E., Tuzcu, E. M., Schoenhagen, P., Brown, B. G., Ganz, P., Vogel, R. A., Crowe, T., Howard, G., Cooper, C. J., Brodie, B., Grines, C. L., DeMaria, A. N., & REVERSAL Investigators. (2004). Effect of intensive compared with moderate lipid-lowering therapy on progression of coronary atherosclerosis: a randomized controlled trial. *Journal of the American Medical Association,* 291(9), 1071-1080.

O'Toole, L. & Grech, E. D. (2003). Chronic stable angina: treatment options. *British Medical Journal,* 326, 1185-1188.

Papaioannou, G. I. & Heller, G. V. (2003). Risk assessment by myocardial perfusion imaging for coronary revascularization, medical therapy, and noncardiac surgery. *Cardiology in Review,* 11, 60-72.

Penttila, H. J., Lepojarvi, M. V., Kaukoranta, P. K., Kiviluoma, K. T., Ylitalo, K. V., & Peuhkurinen, K. J. (2003). Ischemic preconditioning does not improve myocardial preservation during off-pump multivessel coronary operation. *Annals of Thoracic Surgery,* 75(4), 1246-1252; discussion 1252-1253.

Petersen, J. L., Mahaffey, K. W., Hasselblad, V., Antman, E. M., Cohen, M., Goodman, S. G., Langer, A., Blazing, M. A., Moigne-Amrani, A., de Lemos, J. A., Nessel, C. C., Harrington, R. A., Ferguson, J. J., Braunwald, E., & Califf, R. M. (2004). Efficacy and bleeding complications among patients randomized to enoxaparin or unfractionated heparin for antithrombin therapy in non-ST-Segment elevation acute coronary syndromes: a systematic overview. *Journal of the American Medical Association,* 292, 89-96.

Piper, H. M., Abdallah, Y., & Schafer, C. (2004). The first minutes of reperfusion: a window of opportunity for cardioprotection. *Cardiovascular Research,* 61, 365-371.

Pischon, T., Girman, C. J., Hotamisligil, G. S., Rifai, N., Hu, F. B., & Rimm, E. B. (2004). Plasma adiponectin levels and risk of myocardial infarction in men. *Journal of the American Medical Association,* 291, 1730-1737.

Pope, J. H. & Selker, H. P. (2003). Diagnosis of acute cardiac ischemia. *Emergency Medicine Clinics of North America,* 21, 27-59.

Raggi, P. & Berman, D. S. (2005). Computed tomography coronary calcium screening and myocardial perfusion imaging. *Journal of Nuclear Cardiology,* 12, 96-103.

Rebeiz, A. G., Roe, M. T., Alexander, J. H., Mahaffey, K. W., Granger, C. B., Peterson, E. D., Califf, R. M., & Harrington, R. A. (2004). Integrating antithrombin and antiplatelet therapies with early invasive management for non-ST-segment elevation acute coronary syndromes. *American Journal of Medicine,* 116, 119-129.

Ridker, P. (2003). High sensitivity C-reactive protein and cardiovascular risk: Rationale for screening and primary prevention. *American Journal of Cardiology,* 92(suppl), 17K-22K.

Rosenson, R. S. & Koenig, W. (2003). Utility of inflammatory markers in the management of coronary artery disease. *American Journal of Cardiology,* 92(1A),10i-8i.

Saririan, M. & Eisenberg, M. J. (2003). Myocardial laser revascularization for the treatment of end-stage coronary artery disease. *Journal of the American College of Cardiology,* 41, 173-183.

Scanu, A. (2003). Lipoprotein (a) and the atherothrombotic process: mechanistic insights and clinical applications. *Current Atherosclerosis Reports,* 56, 106-113.

Schinkel, A. F., Bax, J. J., Geleijnse, M. L., Boersma, E., Elhendy, A., Roelandt, J. R., & Poldermans, D. (2003). Noninvasive evaluation of ischaemic heart disease: myocardial perfusion imaging or stress echocardiography? *European Heart Journal,* 24, 789-800.

See, F., Kompa, A., Martin, J., Lewis, D. A., & Krum, H. (2005). Fibrosis as a therapeutic target post-myocardial infarction. *Current Pharmaceutical Design,* 11, 477-487.

Selwyn, A. P. (2003). Prothrombotic and antithrombotic pathways in acute coronary syndromes. *American Journal of Cardiology,* 91, 3H-11H.

Shah, P. K. (2003). Mechanisms of plaque vulnerability and rupture. *Journal of the American College of Cardiology,* 41, 15S-22S.

Sharpe, N. (2004). Cardiac remodeling in coronary artery disease. *American Journal of Cardiology,* 93, 17B-20B.

Smeglin, A. & Frishman, W. H. (2004). Elastolytic matrix metalloproteinases and their inhibitors as therapeutic targets in atherosclerotic plaque instability. *Cardiology in Review,* 12, 141-150.

Tan, K. T. & Lip, G. Y. (2005). Fondaparinux. *Current Pharmaceutical Design,* 11, 415-419.

Thomas, G. S. (2005). Should we screen asymptomatic individuals for coronary artery disease or implement universal lipid-lowering therapy? *Cardiology in Review,* 13, 40-45.

Tousoulis, D., Davies, G., Stefanadis, C., Toutouzas, P., & Ambrose, J. A. (2003). Inflammatory and thrombotic mechanisms in coronary atherosclerosis. *Heart,* 89, 993-997.

Wehrmacher, W. H., & Bellows, R. (2004). Unstable angina. *Comprehensive Therapy,* 30, 6-9.

Wong, G. C., Giugliano, R. P., & Antman, E. M. (2003). Use of low-molecular-weight heparins in the management of acute coronary artery syndromes and percutaneous coronary intervention. *Journal of the American Medical Association,* 289, 331-342.

Zarich, S. W. (2005). The role of intensive glycemic control in the management of patients who have acute myocardial infarction. *Cardiology Clinics,* 23, 109-117.

Zimetbaum, P. J. & Josephson, M. E. (2003). Use of the electrocardiogram in acute myocardial infarction. *New England Journal of Medicine,* 348, 933-940.

Ischemic Heart Disease

INITIAL HISTORY

- 40-year-old male complaining of substernal chest pain that began approximately 30 minutes before he came to the emergency department
- Pain has eased slightly but is still present; was 8/10 in severity, now 5/10.

Question 1. *Based on this history alone, what is your differential diagnosis?*

Question 2. *What other symptoms would you like to ask him about?*

ADDITIONAL HISTORY

- Also feels pain in his left shoulder.
- Feels short of breath and somewhat sick to his stomach, but has not vomited.
- Denies coughing, fever, or change in the nature of the pain with deep breathing.

Question 3. *What risk factors would you like to ask him about?*

MORE HISTORY AND FAMILY HISTORY

- 40 pack/year history of smoking.
- Blood pressure has been a little elevated (148/92) on his last two visits to his nurse practitioner.
- Eats a lot of fatty foods but says his total cholesterol doesn't change no matter what he eats; it was 242 mg/dL last month.
- Father has angina that began at age 53.
- Denies diabetes.
- Exercises regularly and has not gained weight.

Question 4.   *What else would you like to know about his past medical history?*

MEDICAL HISTORY

- Says he has had a couple of episodes of shortness of breath while jogging but attributed it to "growing old."
- Has never been hospitalized except for one case of influenza complicated by pneumonia 3 years ago.
- Perceives himself as very healthy, is on no medications, and has no known allergies.

Question 5.   *Based on the history, now what is your differential diagnosis?*

PHYSICAL EXAMINATION

- Alert, moderately anxious man in mild distress.
- T = 37 orally; P = 100 with occasional premature beat; RR = 24; BP = 160/98 in both arms (sitting).

HEENT, Skin, Neck

- Skin warm and diaphoretic without cyanosis.
- PERRLA, fundi benign, pharynx clear.
- Neck supple without thyromegaly, adenopathy, or bruits.
- <2 cm jugular venous distention.

Lungs

- Tachypneic, mild use of accessory muscles of respiration.
- No tenderness upon palpation of the chest wall.
- No dullness to percussion.
- Slight inspiratory crackles (rales) heard at both bases without egophony.
- No rubs.

Cardiac

- Tachycardia with occasional premature beat.
- Apical pulse at 5th intercostal space just lateral to the midclavicular line.
- Soft S_3, no S_4, no murmurs.
- No rubs.

Abdomen, Extremities, Neurologic

- Abdomen with bowel sounds heard throughout; no organomegaly or tenderness; no bruits; rectal guaiac negative.
- Extremities with full and symmetric pulses; slight bruit over left femoral artery; no pedal edema.
- Alert and oriented; neurologic examination intact to cognition, strength, sensation, gait, and deep tendon reflexes.

Question 6.   *What are the pertinent positives and negatives on the examination and what might they mean?*

Question 7.   *What diagnostics would you like to obtain now?*

INITIAL DIAGNOSTIC RESULTS

- ECG shows 4-mm ST elevation with T-wave inversion in the anterior precordial leads with occasional premature ventricular contraction.
- Oximetry shows oxygen saturation of 95%.
- Chest radiograph with borderline cardiomegaly and mild pulmonary congestion without acute infiltrates or pleural disease and no widening of the mediastinum.

Question 8. *What do these initial diagnostic results indicate?*

Question 9. *What therapeutic interventions would you like to initiate while obtaining additional diagnostic data?*

INITIAL MANAGEMENT

- Patient is placed on nasal cannula and an IV D$_5$W at KVO is started.
- He is given aspirin and clopidogrel.
- He receives morphine, IV furosemide, and topical nitrates.
- He is reassured and kept up-to-date with his diagnosis and care.

ADDITIONAL DIAGNOSTIC RESULTS

- Electrolytes and CBC normal.
- PT and PTT normal.
- CPK-MB normal.
- Troponin I normal.

Question 10.   *What now?*

PATIENT UPDATE

- Pain is now 2/10 in severity, dyspnea is better.
- P = 98; RR = 20; BP = 148/92.
- Lungs are now clear.
- Cardiac with continued occasional PCV, S_3 is gone, no new murmurs.
- Repeat ECG with ST elevation now down to 2 mm and new Q waves in anterior leads.

Question 11.   *What interventions should be considered now?*

FURTHER MANAGEMENT

- Patient is given 2 mg morphine and the amount of topical nitrate is increased.
- Echocardiogram reveals wall motion abnormality of the anterior left ventricle; ejection fraction is now 50%.
- History reveals no contraindications to thrombolysis.

Question 12.   *What medications should be given now?*

ADDITIONAL MANAGEMENT

- Patient receives thrombolytic therapy followed by heparin.
- He receives oral β-blockers.
- His blood pressure normalizes and he has no more pain.
- His ECG normalized over time except for small Q waves anteriorly.
- He is admitted to the floor.

HOSPITAL COURSE

- Patient continues to do well without recurrence of chest pain or dyspnea.
- Telemetry reveals no more ectopy.
- Patient is started on an ACE inhibitor on day 3 post-MI.
- He undergoes SPECT evaluation and is found to have no additional myocardium at risk consistent with single-vessel disease and completed infarction.
- He is gradually ambulated and is ready for discharge by day 6.

Question 13. *What should this patient be told and what medications should he be given before he is discharged?*

Heart Failure

DEFINITION

- Heart failure, commonly known as congestive heart failure (CHF), is a clinical syndrome that can result from any functional or structural cardiac disorder that impairs the ability of the heart to fill with or eject blood. It is the pathophysiologic condition in which there is inadequate perfusion of tissues due to a decreased cardiac output (systolic failure) and/or an increase in pulmonary capillary pressures due to increased diastolic filling pressure (diastolic failure).
- Heart failure can refer to dysfunction of either the right or the left ventricle, but the term CHF refers to primary dysfunction of the left ventricle.
- Primary dysfunction of the right ventricle is associated most commonly with pulmonary disease (see Chapter 6) and is not considered congestive heart failure.

EPIDEMIOLOGY

- The American Heart Association Statistics published in 2005 states that in the United States 2.3% of adults were diagnosed with CHF, with 550,000 new cases occurring each year. In those over 65 years of age, the incidence of heart failure is nearly 10%. In 2005 the estimated cost of CHF in the United States was $27.9 billion.
- It is estimated that more than 20% of the population have some diastolic ventricular dysfunction, and 6% have systolic ventricular dysfunction indicating increased risk for the development of CHF.
- The most common risk factor for the development of heart failure is age. More than 75% of individuals with CHF have a history of hypertension. Approximately 22% of males and 46% of females who suffer a myocardial infarction will be disabled from CHF within 6 years. Diabetes is the greatest risk factor for CHF in individuals with known coronary heart disease. Other risk factors for CHF include inherited cardiomyopathies (e.g., familial dilated cardiomyopathy), acquired cardiomyopathies (e.g., hyper- or hypothyroidism, hemochromatosis, myocarditis, systemic lupus erythematosus, alcohol and drug abuse, amyloidosis), arrhythmias, renal failure, and valvular heart disease.
- 80% of men and 75% of women with CHF before the age of 65 will die within 8 years; for women that translates into one in five women with CHF will die within the next year. Between 1992 and 2002, death rates for CHF increased nearly 8%.

PATHOPHYSIOLOGY

- CHF results from a complex interaction between factors that affect the contractility, afterload, preload, or lusitropic function of the heart, and the subsequent neurohumoral and hemodynamic responses that seek to create circulatory compensation.

- *Genes:* Numerous genetic polymorphisms have been identified in association with CHF including those for the inherited cardiomyopathies, for myocardial cell contractility, for neurohumoral receptors, for cardiac conduction, and for the risk factors for CHF such as those associated with coronary artery disease, hypertension, and diabetes.
- Although the hemodynamic consequences of heart failure respond to standard pharmacologic interventions, there are critical neurohumoral interactions whose combined effect is to exacerbate and perpetuate the syndrome.
  - Renin-angiotensin-aldosterone (RAA) system.
    1. Angiotensin II and aldosterone increase peripheral resistance and circulating blood volume, thus contributing to the workload of the heart.
    2. Angiotensin II (both systemic and tissue synthesized) and aldosterone also cause myocardial remodeling in response to ischemia and hypertension. They contribute to sarcomere death, loss of the normal collagen matrix, and interstitial fibrosis.
    3. These changes result in myocyte and sarcomere slippage, heart dilation, and scar formation with loss of normal myocardial compliance and contribute to the hemodynamic and symptomatic features of CHF.
    4. Aldosterone also contributes to endothelial dysfunction, prothrombotic effects, ventricular arrhythmias, autonomic dysfunction, and electrolyte disturbances (sodium retention and potassium and magnesium loss).
  - Sympathetic nervous system (SNS).
    1. Catecholamines (epinephrine and norepinephrine) cause increased peripheral resistance with increased work for the heart, tachycardia (decreased ventricular filling time and increased oxygen consumption by the myocardium), and an increased risk for arrhythmias.
    2. The catecholamines also contribute to ventricular remodeling through direct toxicity to myocytes, the induction of myocyte apoptosis, and increased autoimmune responses.
    3. Finally the SNS has prothrombotic and inflammatory effects and further promotes activity of the RAA.
  - *Natriuretic peptides:* Atrial natriuretic peptide (ANP) and brain natriuretic peptide (BNP) are vasodilatory and promote salt and water excretion (see Chapter 1). In addition, these hormones have been shown to decrease SNS and RAA activity and limit myocardial remodeling. These compensatory mechanisms are inadequate in CHF.
  - *Immune and inflammatory cytokines:* Tumor necrosis factor alpha (TNF-α) and interleukin-6 (IL-6) contribute to ventricular remodeling with myocyte apoptosis, ventricular dilation, and decreased contractility. Furthermore, they have been implicated in systemic effects such as weight loss and weakness seen in severe CHF (cardiac cachexia).
- The initial etiologic event influences the early responses of the myocardium (e.g., MI or hypertension), but as the syndrome progresses, common mechanisms emerge such that patients with advanced CHF share similar symptomatic presentations and respond to similar pharmacologic interventions irrespective of the initial cause of their CHF.
- Although many patients have both systolic and diastolic left ventricular dysfunction, these categories are best considered separately in order to understand their effects on circulatory homeostasis and their responses to various interventions.
  - Systolic left ventricular dysfunction—diminished cardiac output due to decreased contractility, increased afterload, or increased preload results in a decreased ejection fraction and an increased left ventricular end-diastolic volume (LVEDV). This increases the left ventricular end-diastolic pressure (LVEDP) and causes pulmonary venous congestion and pulmonary edema.
    1. *Decreased contractility (inotropy)* results from inadequate or uncoordinated myocardial function such that the LV cannot eject more than 60% of its end-diastolic volume (LVEDV). This causes a gradual increase in LVEDV (also called preload), resulting in an increase in LVEDP and pulmonary venous congestion.

The most common cause of decreased contractility is ischemic heart disease, which not only results in necrosis of myocardial tissue, but also causes ischemic ventricular remodeling. Ischemic remodeling is a process mediated in part by angiotensin II and aldosterone that causes scarring and sarcomere dysfunction in the heart muscle surrounding the area of ischemic injury. Cardiac arrhythmias and primary cardiomyopathies such as those caused by alcohol, infection, hemochromatosis, hyper- or hypothyroidism, drug toxicity, and amyloidosis also cause decreased contractility. Decreased cardiac output leads to underperfusion of the systemic circulation and activation of the sympathetic nervous system and the RAA system, causing increased peripheral resistance and increased afterload.

2. *Increased afterload* means there is increased resistance to LV ejection. This is usually due to the increased peripheral vascular resistance commonly seen in hypertension. It may also be due to aortic valvular stenosis. The LV responds to this increased work with myocardial hypertrophy, a response that increases LV muscle mass but at the same time increases LV demand for coronary perfusion. An energy-starved state is created that, in concert with angiotensin II, aldosterone, and other neuroendocrine responses, causes deleterious changes in the myocytes such as fewer mitochondria for energy production, altered gene expression with production of abnormal contractile proteins (actin, myosin, and tropomyosin), interstitial fibrosis, and decreased myocyte survival. Over time, contractility begins to decline with decreased cardiac output and ejection fraction, increased LVEDV, and pulmonary congestion.

3. *Increased preload* means increased LVEDV, which can be caused directly by excess intravascular volume such as that seen with excessive infusion of intravenous fluids or with renal failure. In addition, decreased ejection fraction caused by changes in contractility or afterload result in increased LVEDV and thus increased preload. As LVEDV increases, it stretches the heart, putting the sarcomeres at a mechanical disadvantage and thus decreasing contractility. This decreased contractility, resulting in a decreased ejection fraction, contributes further to the increased LVEDV, thus creating a vicious cycle of worsening heart failure.

4. Thus a patient can enter this cycle of decreased contractility, increased afterload, and increased preload for a number of reasons (e.g., myocardial infarction [MI], hypertension, fluid overload) and will eventually develop all of the hemodynamic and neurohumoral features of CHF as one mechanism leads to the other (Figure 4-1).

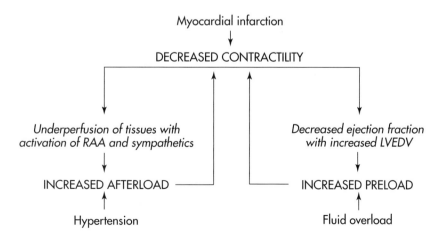

FIGURE **4-1 The Self-Perpetuating Cycle of CHF.**

- Diastolic left ventricular dysfunction.
  1. Diastolic heart failure is often termed "heart failure with preserved systolic function" and is defined as a condition with classic findings of congestive failure with abnormal diastolic but normal systolic function. Pure diastolic dysfunction is characterized by resistance to ventricular filling with an increase in LVEDP without an increase in LVEDV or a decrease in cardiac output.
  2. This type of heart failure is especially common in older women and in those with a history of untreated hypertension. Obesity and diabetes are important risks also.
  3. The resistance to left ventricular filling results from abnormal relaxation (lusitropy) of the LV and can be caused by any condition that stiffens the ventricular myocardium such as ischemic remodeling, scarring, hypertension (hypertrophic cardiomyopathy), restrictive cardiomyopathy, valvular disease, or pericardial disease.
  4. Structural and functional defects in myocytes and myocardial architecture lead to abnormal relaxation and decreased compliance.
      a. Abnormal myosin and actin.
      b. Dilated cardiomyocyte skeleton.
      c. Destruction of the extracellular matrix.
  5. Increases in heart rate allow less time for diastolic filling and exacerbate the symptoms of diastolic dysfunction. Therefore exercise intolerance is common.
  6. Abnormal lusitropy often results in the presence of an S_4 on examination; other classic features of CHF clinical presentation (see following) may be absent.
  7. Because treatment would require actually changing myocardial compliance, the effectiveness of currently available drugs is limited. Acute symptoms should be managed with diuretics. Chronic management is aimed at reversing underlying conditions. Nitrates and calcium channel blockers have been shown to improve symptoms. β-blockers improve lusitropic function, decrease heart rate, and improve symptoms. Angiotensin-converting enzyme (ACE) inhibitors can help reverse hypertrophy and structural changes at the tissue level in patients with ischemic remodeling or hypertension. Inotropic agents should be avoided.

PATIENT PRESENTATION

Patients with CHF will usually present in one of three ways: (1) a syndrome of decreased exercise tolerance; (2) a syndrome of fluid retention; and/or (3) no symptoms or symptoms of another cardiac or noncardiac disorder.

History

Previous myocardial infarction; risk factors for ischemic heart disease (smoking, hyperlipidemia, diabetes); hypertension; valvular disease; cardiomyopathy (familial, metabolic, toxic, inflammatory); renal failure; excessive intravenous; recent high intake of salt.

Symptoms

Dyspnea especially on exertion; orthopnea; paroxysmal nocturnal dyspnea; cough; pedal edema; decreased urine output; fatigue; weight gain; chest pain; palpitations.

Examination

Weight gain; tachypnea; tachycardia; murmurs; cyanosis; inspiratory crackles (rales); frothy sputum production; edema; cold, clammy skin; weak peripheral pulses; jugular venous distention; hepatojugular reflux, hepatosplenomegaly; muscle wasting; **systolic dysfunction:** S_3, shift of apical pulse, hypotension during episodes of pulmonary edema; **diastolic dysfunction:** S_4, strong but nondisplaced apical pulse, hypertension during episodes of pulmonary edema.

DIFFERENTIAL DIAGNOSIS

- CHF must be differentiated from the following:
    - Noncardiogenic pulmonary edema (acute respiratory distress syndrome [ARDS]).
    - Chronic obstructive pulmonary disease (COPD).
    - Pneumonia.
    - Asthma.
    - Interstitial pulmonary fibrosis.
    - Other primary lung diseases.
- The underlying cause of the CHF must be established from the following:
    - Myocardial ischemia/infarction.
    - Hypertensive hypertrophic cardiomyopathy.
    - Valvular heart disease.
    - Primary cardiomyopathy (inherited, idiopathic, alcohol, metabolic, postinfectious, amyloidosis, restrictive).
    - Fluid overload (iatrogenic vs. renal failure).

KEYS TO ASSESSMENT

- CHF is a manifestation of an underlying cardiac insult; begin immediately to assess for the cause of LV dysfunction.
- A quick physical examination can often establish the diagnosis of CHF; therapeutic intervention can begin even as assessment progresses.
- Early electrocardiographic (ECG) monitoring for ischemia or arrhythmias is vital.
- If there is evidence of significant respiratory distress, obtain arterial blood gases immediately, then begin oxygen, monitor oximetry.
- Obtain serum electrolytes, glucose, blood urea nitrogen (BUN) and creatinine (Cr); liver function tests, complete blood count (CBC); and TSH.
- Serum brain natriuretic peptide (BNP) levels are correlated with the severity of CHF, but their role in diagnosis is less clear. A BNP level >100 pg/mL supports the diagnosis of abnormal cardiac function consistent with CHF, but is not specific. They are helpful in differentiating between pulmonary and cardiac causes of dyspnea, but the role of BNP levels in the diagnosis of CHF requires further investigation.
- A chest radiograph may show cardiomegaly, pulmonary edema, and pleural effusions; the diagnosis of pericardial or valvular disease can often be made on the chest radiograph.
- Echocardiography can estimate ejection fraction and therefore cardiac output, demonstrate LV wall motion abnormalities consistent with ischemia, show hypertrophic cardiomyopathy, or diagnose valvular and pericardial disease.
- Emergent cardiac catheterization may be indicated in patients suspected of acute coronary artery disease and thrombosis.
- Hemodynamic monitoring (central venous catheter) remains controversial; current indications include uncertainty about diagnosis, deteriorating course, lack of expected response to interventions, and when high-dose intravenous nitrates or inotropics are indicated.
- Clinical classification of CHF can help determine appropriate therapy and prognosis. There are two widely used classification schemes: the American Heart Association/American College of Cardiology (AHA/ACC) Classification of Heart Failure system, and the New York Heart Association CHF Classification system. The AHA/ACC system is emerging as the most widely used classification scheme:
    Stage A: Many risk factors for CHF but no apparent structural abnormality of the heart.
    Stage B: Structural abnormality of the heart but have never had symptoms of heart failure.
    Stage C: Structural abnormality of the heart and current or previous symptoms of heart failure.
    Stage D: End-stage symptoms of heart failure that are refractory to treatment.

KEYS TO MANAGEMENT

- Prevention.
  - Manage hypertension appropriately.
  - Treat lipid disorders.
  - Treat atherosclerotic coronary disease and ischemic heart disease.
  - Avoid behaviors that may increase the risk of HF (e.g., smoking, excessive alcohol consumption, and illicit drug use).
  - Control the ventricular rate (or restore sinus rhythm in patients with supraventricular tachyarrhythmias).
  - Treat thyroid disorders.
  - ACE inhibitors or ARBs should be considered for high-risk individuals who have a history of atherosclerotic vascular disease, diabetes mellitus, or hypertension with associated cardiovascular risk factors.
- Acute CHF.
  - Let the patient sit up if he/she is not hypotensive.
  - Oxygen—get arterial blood gas on room air quickly, then put on a mask at 60%; intubate if there is ventilatory failure or if the patient is progressively cyanotic and has decreasing mental status.
  - Treat myocardial ischemia if indicated (see Chapter 3).
  - Administer morphine, nitroglycerin, and IV diuretic (furosemide) if no significant hypotension. Several studies suggest that continuous furosemide infusion is more effective than bolus administration.
  - Consider intravenous (IV) inotropics (dobutamine, dopamine)—use them early if hypotensive.
  - If persistently hypertensive, consider IV nitrates to reduce peripheral vascular resistance. Nitroglycerin is safer than nitroprusside.
  - Nesiritide (human recombinant BNP) given IV for acute decompensated CHF enhances sodium excretion and arteriolar and venous dilation, and decreases SNS and RAA activity. It has been shown to have more rapid hemodynamic improvement with fewer adverse effects than IV nitroglycerin in several studies, but its overall safety has been questioned (evidence for increased renal dysfunction and short-term mortality).
  - An intra-aortic balloon pump is indicated if there is refractory hypotension (cardiogenic shock), refractory ischemia in preparation for emergency coronary bypass grafting (CABG), or acute mitral regurgitation in preparation for operative valvular repair or replacement.
  - Emergent coronary catheterization and percutaneous coronary intervention (PCI) or CABG is used in selected patients with ischemia.
  - Discharge can be considered when weight, renal function, fluid balance, and symptoms have returned to baseline and the individual has been stable without needed medication changes for 24 hours. Patients should be prescribed diet modifications and a carefully described medication regimen and return to clinic within 5 to 10 days.
- Chronic CHF.
  - For all individuals, definitive management of underlying cause is optimal. Reduction of risk factors, life-style modification with salt restriction, exercise, and education about monitoring symptoms (daily weights, dyspnea, edema, chest pain) are recommended.
  - The current treatment recommendations were established by the 2005 AHA/ACC task force on practice guidelines and are based on CHF stage (Table 4-1).
    1. *Diuretics:* These drugs reduce fluid volume and improve symptoms.
       a. Loop diuretics are recommended (more effective than thiazides). Furosemide remains the most commonly used diuretic along with bumetanide or torsemide. Diuretics clearly improve exercise intolerance and edema, but electrolyte imbalance and adverse effects on serum lipids and glucose must be watched.
       b. Aldosterone-blocking diuretics such as spironolactone and eplerenone have been shown to reduce mortality in severe CHF. They should be avoided in individuals with hyperkalemia or renal dysfunction (Cr ≥2.5 mg/dL).

TABLE **4-1** ACC/AHA 2005 Guidelines for the Treatment of Heart Failure

Stage			
Stage A	**Stage B**	**Stage C**	**Stage D**
GOALS	GOALS	GOALS	GOALS
Treat hypertension Encourage smoking cessation Treat lipid disorders Encourage regular exercise Discourage alcohol intake, illicit drug use Control metabolic syndrome DRUGS ACEI or ARB in appropriate patients (e.g., vascular disease or diabetes)	All measures under Stage A DRUGS ACEI or ARB in appropriate patients β-blockers in appropriate patients	All measures under Stages A and B Dietary salt restriction DRUGS FOR ROUTINE USE Diuretics for fluid retention ACEI β-blockers DRUGS IN SELECTED PATIENTS Aldosterone antagonist ARBs Digitalis Hydralazine/nitrates DEVICES IN SELECTED PATIENTS Biventricular pacing Implantable defibrillators	Appropriate measures under Stages A, B, C Decision re: appropriate level of care OPTIONS Compassionate end-of-life care/hospice Extraordinary measures: • Heart transplant • Chronic inotropes • Permanent mechanical support • Experimental surgery or drugs

From Hunt, S.A., Abraham, W.T., Chin, M.H., Feldman, A.M., Francis, G.S., Ganiats, T.G., Jessup, M., Konstam, M.A., Mancini, D.M., Michl, K., Oates, J.A., Rahko, P.S., Silver, M.A., Stevenson, L.W., Yancy, C.W. ACC/AHA 2005 guideline update for the diagnosis and management of chronic heart failure in the adult: a report of the American College of Cardiology/American Heart Association Task Force on Practice Guidelines (Writing Committee to Update the 2001 Guidelines for the Evaluation and Management of Heart Failure). American College of Cardiology web wite. Available at: http://www.acc.org/clinical/guidelines/failure/index.pdf.

2. *ACE inhibitors:* These drugs affect the hemodynamic and neurohumoral manifestations of CHF with improvements in symptoms and survival.
   a. They should be used in Stage A CHF for individuals with hypertension, coronary disease, and diabetes. They should be used for all individuals in all other stages of CHF unless there is a contraindication or if they are not tolerated.
   b. Primary adverse reactions include hypotension, worsening renal function, cough, angioedema, and hyperkalemia.
   c. These drugs should be started slowly and are usually combined with diuretics and β-blockers in symptomatic CHF.
   d. Angiotensin-receptor blockers (ARBs) should be used in those individuals who do not tolerate ACE inhibitors. Although their effects on long-term outcomes in CHF are not well established, combination therapy with ACE inhibitors and ARBs is being investigated.
3. *β-blockers* (carvedilol, metoprolol, labetalol) increase ejection fraction, decrease sympathetic tone with vasodilation and decreased myocardial oxygen consumption, and decrease ventricular remodeling. They reduce symptoms, improve functional status, and reduce the risk of death.
   a. Carvedilol is emerging as the drug of choice with significant decreases in mortality and improvement symptoms.
   b. These drugs should be started slowly (may cause fluid retention, fatigue, bradycardia, and heart block) and are usually combined with diuretics and ACE inhibitors in symptomatic CHF.

    4. *Inotropics.*

        a. Digoxin is indicated to improve symptoms and clinical status in those individuals who do not respond optimally to diuretics, ACE inhibitors and β-blockers. It is used routinely in individuals with CHF who also have atrial fibrillation. Digoxin improves exercise tolerance, increases cardiac output, slows the progression of CHF, decreases sympathetic and RAA activity, and improves quality of life in selected patients. It may decrease mortality when used with ACE inhibitors, however mortality may be increased in patients for whom digoxin is subsequently discontinued. It is important to follow blood levels and avoid hypokalemia (arrhythmias).

        b. Levosimendan is a calcium sensitizer that improves contractility and was found to significantly decrease mortality in severe left ventricular (LV) dysfunction when compared to adrenergic agonists. It is not yet approved in the United States, but studies are promising.

        c. Adrenergic agonists (continuous IV dobutamine or xamoterol) have short-term benefits, but may cause increased mortality; phosphodiesterase inhibitors have also shown similar short-term improvements in cardiac function but are associated with an increase in mortality.

- Other agents.
  1. Hydralazine and isosorbide dinitrate reduce mortality and improve symptoms when compared with placebo, but are not as effective as ACE inhibitors and β-blockers for most individuals.
  2. Vasopeptide inhibitors (e.g., omapatrilat) are under investigation and in small studies have been shown to be superior to ACE inhibitors.
  3. Cytokine blockers (e.g., etanercept [blocks TNF]) are being evaluated but have not demonstrated significant improvements in outcomes in early studies.
  4. Anticoagulants are indicated if there is atrial fibrillation, valvular disease, or a known intraventricular thrombus.
- Calcium channel blockers, most antiarrhythmic drugs, and nonsteroidal anti-inflammatory agents should be avoided.
- Synchronized biventricular pacing has been shown to improve exercise tolerance.
- Implantable cardioverter defibrillators are indicated for patients at risk for life-threatening arrhythmias.
- Ventricular assist devices can improve symptoms and serve as a bridge to heart transplant.
- Cardiomyoplasty, passive containment, and other surgical techniques have shown promise in some studies but cannot yet be recommended.
- Heart transplantation is currently the only established surgical approach to refractory heart failure. Indications include severe functional impairment or continued dependence on intravenous inotropic medications.
- Stem cell transplantation to restore viable myocardium is being explored.

PATHOPHYSIOLOGY $\longrightarrow$	CLINICAL LINK
What is going on in the disease process that influences how the patient presents and how he or she should be managed?	*What should you do now that you understand the underlying pathophysiology?*
CHF is a common syndrome and age is the greatest risk factor along with underlying coronary or hypertensive heart disease.	A careful history and physical are important when evaluating elderly patients and those at risk for heart disease.
Acute congestive heart failure is a common complication of acute myocardial infarction, severe valvular disease, underlying fluid overload, and hypertensive crisis.	The management of acute CHF must include evaluation and therapy for the initiating process, not just for CHF.
Both hemodynamic and neurohumoral mechanisms contribute to the pathophysiology of CHF and to both acute and chronic symptoms.	These mechanisms contribute to the progression of CHF resulting in a significant mortality for patients with this syndrome. Treatment aimed at reversing these mechanisms provides not only short-term relief of symptoms, but also improvements in morbidity and mortality over time.
Brain natriuretic peptide (BNP) is an important compensatory hormone that is elevated in CHF in an effort to increase renal salt and water excretion.	Serum levels of BNP can be used to monitor for response to treatment in CHF and may be useful for diagnosis in certain situations. Nesiritide (human recombinant BNP) provides rapid and effective diuresis in acute CHF, but increases in mortality and renal dysfunction have been reported.
Systolic LV dysfunction results in a vicious cycle of decreased contractility, increased afterload, and increased preload.	Once the full picture of CHF is established, many patients with systolic dysfunction will require inotropics, diuretics, and vasodilators.
Diastolic LV dysfunction is common and results from decreased LV compliance and abnormal lusitropy, most commonly from the effects of hypertension and the RAA system.	Diastolic function should be suspected in symptomatic patients with normal ejection fraction; current treatment and prevention includes β-blockers and ACE inhibitors.
CHF morbidity and mortality remain very high despite marked advances in therapy including the use of ACE inhibitors, β-blockers, aldosterone antagonists, diuretics, and inotropic agents.	Management of advanced CHF may require biventricular pacing, new surgical techniques, ventricular assist devices, and heart transplant. New inotropic agents are being tested (e.g., levosimendan).

SUGGESTED READINGS

Ahmed, A. (2004). Management of diastolic heart failure in older adults. *British Medical Journal, 328,* 1114.

Anker, S. D. & von Haehling, S. (2004). Inflammatory mediators in chronic heart failure: an overview. *Heart (British Cardiac Society), 90*(4), 464-470.

Banerjee, P., Clark, A. L., & Cleland, J. G. (2004). Diastolic heart failure: a difficult problem in the elderly. *American Journal of Geriatric Cardiology, 13,* 16-21.

Barnes, B. J. & Howard, P. A. (2005). Eplerenone: a selective aldosterone receptor antagonist for patients with heart failure. *Annals of Pharmacotherapy, 39,* 68-76.

Benjamin, I. J. & Schneider, M. D. (2005). Learning from failure: congestive heart failure in the postgenomic age. *Journal of Clinical Investigation, 115,* 495-499.

Bhatia, G., Sosin, M., Leahy, J. F., Connolly, D. L., Davis, R. C., & Lip, G. Y. (2005). Hibernating myocardium in heart failure. *Expert Review of Cardiovascular Therapy, 3,* 111-122.

Brown, R. D., Ambler, S. K., Mitchell, M. D., & Long, C. S. (2005). The cardiac fibroblast: therapeutic target in myocardial remodeling and failure. *Annual Review Pharmacology & Toxicology, 45,* 657-687.

Bukhari, F., MacGillivray, T., del Monte, F., & Hajjar, R. J. (2005). Genetic maneuvers to ameliorate ventricular function in heart failure: therapeutic potential and future implications. *Expert Review of Cardiovascular Therapy, 3,* 85-97.

Burger, A. J. (2005). A review of the renal and neurohormonal effects of B-type natriuretic peptide. *Congestive Heart Failure, 11,* 30-38.

Camici, P. G. (2004). Myocardial hibernation and heart failure: introduction. *Heart, 90,* 136.

Cheng, J. W. (2005). Tezosentan in the management of decompensated heart failure. *Cardiology in Review, 13,* 28-34.

Cleland, J. G., Nikitin, N., & McGowan, J. (2004). Levosimendan: first in a new class of inodilator for acute and chronic severe heart failure. *Expert Review of Cardiovascular Therapy, 2*(1), 9-19.

Dawson, A., Davies, J. I., & Struthers, A. D. (2004). The role of aldosterone in heart failure and the clinical benefits of aldosterone blockade. *Expert Review of Cardiovascular Therapy, 2,* 29-36.

Dec, G. W. (2003). Digoxin remains useful in the management of chronic heart failure. *Medical Clinics of North America, 87*(2), 317-37.

de Denus, S., Pharand, C., & Williamson, D. R. (2004). Brain natriuretic peptide in the management of heart failure: the versatile neurohormone. *Chest, 125,* 652-668.

DiDomenico, R. J., Park, H. Y., Southworth, M. R., Eyrich, H. M., Lewis, R. K., Finley, J. M., & Schumock, G. T. (2004). Guidelines for acute decompensated heart failure treatment. *Annals of Pharmacotherapy, 38,* 649-660.

Doust, J. A., Pietrzak, E., Dobson, A., & Glasziou, P. (2005). How well does B-type natriuretic peptide predict death and cardiac events in patients with heart failure: systematic review. *British Medical Journal, 330,* 625.

Epstein, A. E. (2004). An update on implantable cardioverter-defibrillator guidelines. *Current Opinion in Cardiology, 19,* 23-25.

Epstein, B. J. & Gums, J. G. (2005). Angiotensin receptor blockers versus ACE inhibitors: prevention of death and myocardial infarction in high-risk populations. *Annals of Pharmacotherapy, 39,* 470-480.

Ferrario, C., Abdelhamed, A. I., & Moore, M. (2004). AII antagonists in hypertension, heart failure, and diabetic nephropathy: focus on losartan. *Current Medical Research & Opinion, 20,* 279-293.

Fonarow, G. C. (2004). Managing the patient with diabetes mellitus and heart failure: issues and considerations. *American Journal of Medicine, 116*(suppl), 5A, 76S-88S.

Fonarow, G. C. (2004). Role of in-hospital initiation of carvedilol to improve treatment rates and clinical outcomes. *American Journal of Cardiology, 93,* 77B-81B.

Garry, D. J., Masino, A. M., Naseem, R. H., & Martin, C. M. (2005). Ponce de Leon's Fountain: stem cells and the regenerating heart. *American Journal of the Medical Sciences, 329,* 190-201.

Goodlin, S. J. (2005). Heart failure in the elderly. *Expert Review Cardiovascular, 3,* 99-106.

Gorman, R. C., Jackson, B. M., & Gorman, J. H. (2004). The potential role of ventricular compressive therapy. *Surgical Clinics of North America, 84,* 45-59.

Guyatt, G. H. & Devereaux, P. J. (2004). A review of heart failure treatment. *Mount Sinai Journal of Medicine, 71,* 47-54.

Hauptman, P. J. (2005). Integrating palliative care into heart failure care. *Archives of Internal Medicine, 165,* 374-378.

Hogg, K., Swedberg, K., & McMurray, J. (2004). Heart failure with preserved left ventricular systolic function; epidemiology, clinical characteristics, and prognosis. *Journal of the American College of Cardiology, 43,* 317-327.

Hunt, S. A., Abraham, W. T., Chin, M. H., Feldman, A. M., Francis, G. S., Ganiats, T. G., Jessup, M., Konstam, M. A., Mancini, D. M., Michl, K., Oates, J. A., Rahko, P. S., Silver, M. A., Stevenson, L. W., & Yancy, C. W. (2005). ACC/AHA 2005 guideline update for the diagnosis and management of chronic heart failure in the adult: a report of the American College of Cardiology/American Heart Association Task Force on Practice Guidelines (Writing Committee to Update the 2001 Guidelines for the Evaluation and Management of Heart Failure). American College of Cardiology Web Site. Available at: http://www.acc.org/clinical/guidelines/failure/index.pdf.

Iyengar, S., Feldman, D. S., Trupp, R., & Abraham, W. T. (2004). Nesiritide for the treatment of congestive heart failure. *Expert Opinion on Pharmacotherapy, 5,* 901-907.

Jessup, M. & Brozena, S. (2003). Heart failure. *New England Journal of Medicine, 348,* 2007-2018.

Kamath, S. A., Laskar, S. R., & Yancy, C. W. (2005). Novel therapies for heart failure: vasopressin and aldosterone antagonists. *Congestive Heart Failure, 11,* 21-29.

Khan, N. U. & Movahed, A. (2004). The role of aldosterone and aldosterone-receptor antagonists in heart failure. *Reviews in Cardiovascular Medicine, 5,* 71-81.

Kirchengast, M. & Luz, M. (2005). Endothelin receptor antagonists: clinical realities and future directions. *Journal of Cardiovascular Pharmacology, 45,* 182-191.

Kivikko, M. & Lehtonen, L. (2005). Levosimendan: a new inodilatory drug for the treatment of decompensated heart failure. *Current Pharmaceutical Design, 11,* 435-455.

Lane, R. E., Cowie, M. R., & Chow, A. W. (2005). Prediction and prevention of sudden cardiac death in heart failure. *Heart (British Cardiac Society), 91,* 674-680.

Latini, R., Masson, S., Staszewsky, L., & Maggioni, A. P. (2004). Valsartan for the treatment of heart failure. *Expert Opinions in Pharmacotherapeutics, 5*(1), 181-193.

Lee, M. S. (2004). Stem-cell transplantation in myocardial infarction: a status report. *Annals of Internal Medicine, 140,* 729-737.

Lowery, S. L., Massaro, R., & Yancy, C. W., Jr. (2004). Advances in the management of acute and chronic decompensated heart failure. *Lippincott's Case Management, 9,* 4-18.

Maisel, A. S. (2003). The diagnosis of acute congestive heart failure: role of BNP measurements. *Heart Failure Reviews, 8*(4), 327-334.

Manohar, P. & Pina, I. L. (2003). Therapeutic role of angiotensin II receptor blockers in the treatment of heart failure. *Mayo Clinic Proceedings, 78*(3), 334-338.

Massad, M. G. (2004). Current trends in heart transplantation. *Cardiology,* 101, 79-92.

Matsumori, A. (2004). Anti-inflammatory therapy for heart failure. *Current Opinion in Pharmacology,* 4, 171-176.

McBride, B. F. & White, C. M. (2005). Critical differences among beta-adrenoreceptor antagonists in myocardial failure: debating the MERIT of COMET. *Journal of Clinical Pharmacology,* 45, 6-24.

McConnell, P. I. & Michler, R. E. (2004). Clinical trials in the surgical management of congestive heart failure. surgical ventricular restoration and autologous skeletal myoblast and stem cell cardiomyoplasty. *Cardiology,* 101, 48-60.

Meier, P., Maillard, M., & Burnier, M. (2005). The future of angiotensin II inhibition in cardiovascular medicine. *Current Drug Targets—Cardiovascular & Haematological Disorders,* 5, 15-30.

Ott, P. (2005). Cardiac resynchronization therapy: a new therapy for advanced congestive heart failure. *American Journal of Geriatric Cardiology,* 14, 31-34.

Piccini, J. P., Klein, L., Gheorghiade, M., & Bonow, R. O. (2004). New insights into diastolic heart failure: role of diabetes mellitus. *American Journal of Medicine,* 116(suppl 5A), 64S-75S.

Prahash, A. & Lynch, T. (2004). B-type natriuretic peptide: a diagnostic, prognostic, and therapeutic tool in heart failure. *American Journal of Critical Care,* 13, 46-53.

Rich, M. W. (2005). Office management of heart failure in the elderly. *American Journal of Medicine,* 118, 342-348.

Ripley, T. L. (2005). Valsartan in heart failure. *Annals of Pharmacotherapy,* 39, 460-469.

Sackner-Bernstein, J. D. & Hart, D. (2004). Neurohormonal antagonism in heart failure: what is the optimal strategy? *Mount Sinai Journal of Medicine,* 71, 115-126.

Soaly, E. & Al Suwaidi, J. (2005). Statin therapy in heart failure. *Expert Review of Cardiovascular Therapy,* 3, 5-7.

Soran, O. (2004). A new treatment modality in heart failure enhanced external counterpulsation (EECP). *Cardiology in Review,* 12, 15-20.

Stroe, A. F. & Gheorghiade, M. (2004). Carvedilol: beta-blockade and beyond. *Reviews in Cardiovascular Medicine,* 5(suppl 1), S18-S27.

Udelson, J. E. (2004). Ventricular remodeling in heart failure and the effect of beta-blockade. *American Journal of Cardiology,* 93, 43B-48B.

Vasan, R. S., Sullivan, L. M., Roubenoff, R., Dinarello, C. A., Harris, T., Benjamin, E. J., Sawyer, D. B., Levy, D., Wilson, P. W., & D'Agostino, R. B. (2003). Framingham Heart Study. Inflammatory markers and risk of heart failure in elderly subjects without prior myocardial infarction: the Framingham Heart Study. *Circulation,* 107(11), 1486-1491.

von Harsdorf, R., Poole-Wilson, P. A., & Dietz, R. (2004). Regenerative capacity of the myocardium: implications for treatment of heart failure. *Lancet,* 363, 1306-1313.

Wasywich, C. A., Whalley, G. A., & Doughty, R. N. (2005). Brain natriuretic peptide in the contemporary management of congestive heart failure. *Expert Review of Cardiovascular Therapy,* 3, 71-84.

Wijetunga, M. & Strickberger, S. A. (2005). Cardiac resynchronization therapy for congestive heart failure. *Expert Review of Cardiovascular Therapy,* 3, 107-110.

Young, J. B. (2004). Management of chronic heart failure: what do recent clinical trials teach us. *Reviews in Cardiovascular Medicine,* 5(suppl 1), S3-S9.

Asthma

DEFINITION

- Asthma is defined by the National Asthma Education and Prevention Program (NAEPP) of the National Heart, Lung, and Blood Institute (NHLBI) as "*a chronic inflammatory disorder* of the airways in which many cells and cellular elements play a role, in particular, mast cells, eosinophils, T lymphocytes, macrophages, neutrophils, and epithelial cells. In susceptible individuals, this inflammation causes *recurrent episodes* of wheezing, breathlessness, chest tightness, and coughing, particularly at night or in the early morning. These episodes are usually associated with widespread but variable *airflow obstruction that is often reversible* either spontaneously or with treatment. The inflammation also causes an associated increase in the existing *bronchial hyperresponsiveness to a variety of stimuli.* Subbasement membrane *fibrosis* may occur in some patients with asthma and these changes contribute to persistent abnormalities in lung function" (www.nhlbi.nih.gov/guidelines/asthma/asthgdln.htm).
- Asthma classification and management in the United States is based on clinical severity (mild intermittent, mild persistent, moderate persistent, and severe persistent) (Table 5-1; updated by the NAEPP in 2002 www.nhlbi.nih.gov/guidelines/asthma/asthupdt.htm).

EPIDEMIOLOGY

- The Global Initiative for Asthma states: "Asthma is one of the most common chronic diseases in the world. It is estimated that around 300 million people in the world currently have asthma." It goes on to say: "The rate of asthma increases as communities adopt western lifestyles and become urbanized. With the projected increase in the proportion of the world's population that is urban from 45% to 59% in 2025, there is likely to be a marked increase in the number of asthmatics worldwide over the next two decades." It is estimated that there may be an additional 100 million persons with asthma by 2025 (www.ginasthma.com).
- Approximately 5% of adults and 8% of children in the United States have asthma. Prevalence is higher in urban areas, and the prevalence of exercise-induced asthma may be as high as 10% to 20%. Asthma incidence and mortality increased from 1980 to 1995 and then stabilized; there is some evidence that both incidence and mortality in the United States are declining slightly in recent years.
- Risk factors.
  - More than 20 genetic abnormalities have been linked to asthma including those for interleukin-4 (IL-4), IgE, *ADAM33* susceptibility gene, interferon gamma (INF-γ), thymus and activation regulated cytokine (TARC), β-adrenergic receptors, 5-lipoxygenase, and leukotrienes.
  - Allergen exposure (even during fetal life via transplacental leakage) increases the risk of asthma in genetically predisposed individuals by shifting the immune system toward humoral (antibody-mediated) immunity. The most common allergens are dust mites, dog or cat dander, and cockroaches as the major causes of year-round symptoms; pollens and grasses for seasonal symptoms.

TABLE **5-1** Asthma Classification

Classify Severity: Clinical Features Before Treatment or Adequate Control			Medications Required to Maintain Long-Term Control
	Symptoms	PEF or FEV₁ PEF Variability	Daily Medications
Step 4: Severe persistent	Day: Continual Night: Frequent	PEF or FEV_1: ≤60% PEF Variability: >30%	**Preferred treatment** High-dose inhaled corticosteroids *and* Long-acting inhaled β_2-agonists *and*, if needed, Corticosteroid tablets or syrup long term (2 mg/kg/day, generally do not exceed 60 mg/day). (Make repeat attempts to reduce systemic corticosteroids and maintain control with high-dose inhaled corticosteroids.)
Step 3: Moderate persistent	Day: Daily Night: more than once/week	PEF or FEV_1: >60% to <80% PEF Variability: >30%	**Preferred treatment** Low- to medium-dose inhaled corticosteroids and long-acting inhaled β_2-agonists *Alternative treatments* (listed alphabetically): Increase inhaled corticosteroids within medium-dose range *or* Low- to medium-dose inhaled corticosteroids and either leukotriene modifier or theophylline
Step 2: Mild persistent	Day: more than twice/ week but less than once/day Night: less than twice/month	PEF or FEV_1: ≥80% PEF Variability: 20% to 30%	**Preferred treatment** Low-dose inhaled corticosteroids *Alternative treatment* (listed alphabetically): cromolyn, leukotriene modifier, nedocromil, *or* sustained-release theophylline to serum concentration of 5 to 15 mcg/mL
Step 1: Mild intermittent	Day: less than twice/week Night: more than twice/month	PEF or FEV_1: ≥80% PEF Variability: <20%	**No daily medication needed** Severe exacerbations may occur, separated by long periods of normal lung function and no symptoms. A course of systemic corticosteroids is recommended

Step down
Review treatment every 1 to 6 months; a gradual stepwise reduction in treatment may be possible

Step up
If control is not maintained, consider step up. First review patient medication technique, adherence, and environmental control

- The "hygiene hypothesis" suggests that allergen exposure shifts the immune system toward the production of antibodies (TH₂ shift; see Chapter 26) and that this effect is normally balanced by exposure to numerous siblings, daycare, farming, endotoxin, and certain organisms (e.g., *Toxoplasma gondii*, hepatitis A, and *Helicobacter pylori*). It is proposed that children exposed to a highly hygienic environment lack adequate exposure to common pathogens and therefore do not achieve a proper balance of their immune systems. This hypothesis has been substantiated by some studies, but challenged by others and further research is underway.
- Urban residence with exposure to ozone, nitrogen and sulfur dioxide, carbon monoxide, tire debris, and particles from the combustion of fuels has been linked to increased asthma risk. Occupational exposures such as dusts, chemicals, and irritants have also been linked to asthma.
- Recurrent respiratory viral infections (especially respiratory syncytial virus [RSV]) in childhood can increase the subsequent risk for asthma in genetically susceptible individuals. Viral infections cause inflammation and injury to lower respiratory airways (exposes sensory nerves) by inducing the release of a wide variety of inflammatory cytokines, and may cause remodeling of the airways in young children. Respiratory viruses are also the most common cause of acute exacerbations of asthma.
- Allergic rhinitis occurs in most individuals with asthma and upper airway inflammation can exacerbate lower airway pathophysiology and asthma symptoms. Treatment of upper airway allergy (antihistamines or nasal steroids) improves asthma symptoms in many individuals.

- Gastroesophageal reflux disease (GERD) has been linked to asthma risk. This relationship remains controversial and may be related to vagal stimulation caused by reflux of acid into the lower esophagus and to microaspiration of acidic proximal esophageal contents. It is estimated that 75% of individuals with asthma have GERD and several studies have found that the administration of proton-pump inhibitors is safe and effective in reducing asthma symptoms in many individuals.

PATHOPHYSIOLOGY

- Inflammatory mechanisms in asthma (Figure 5-1).
  - Allergens are presented to the immune system by macrophages, dendritic cells, and B lymphocytes resulting in the activation of CD4 lymphocytes (T helper lymphocytes).
  - B cell and dendritic cell antigen presentation favors the production of what are called the TH$_2$ cytokines by the T helper cell (in allergic patients the number of dendritic cells in the respiratory mucosa is increased). The primary TH$_2$ cytokines are IL-4, IL-5, IL-8, and IL-13. These cytokines activate other cells of immunity and inflammation including B lymphocytes, eosinophils, and polymorphonucleocytes (PMNs).
  - In allergic individuals, a high level of IL-4 causes B cell proliferation and B cell "isotype switch" from producing IgM to producing large amounts of IgE, which attaches to receptors on the mast cells and results in mast cell degranulation.
  - Mast cell degranulation releases multiple mediators such as histamine, leukotrienes, prostaglandins, and inflammatory cell chemotactants causing intense airway inflammation.

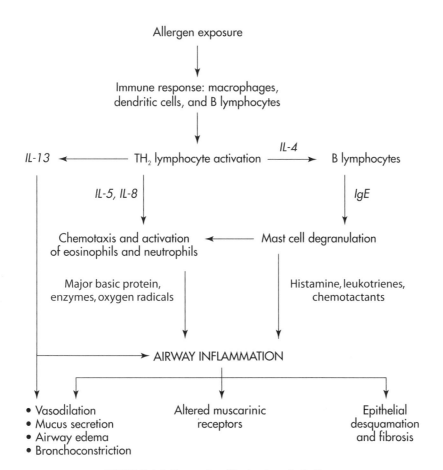

FIGURE **5-1 Inflammatory Mechanisms in Asthma.**

- This inflammation causes bronchoconstriction, mucus secretion, and mucosal edema, resulting in an acute attack.
- High levels of IL-5 stimulate eosinophils, which results in direct tissue injury and release toxic neuropeptides that cause desquamation of the bronchial epithelium leading to increased bronchial hyperresponsiveness. IL-5 and eosinophil-derived cytokines also cause activation of fibroblasts and smooth muscle cells, leading to long-term airway scarring.
- IL-8 activates PMNs and promotes adhesion molecule expression on endothelial and epithelial cells, leading to more migration of inflammatory cells, especially PMNs. Inflammatory cytokines from PMNs lead to a more exaggerated immune response to allergens and contribute to the tissue effects of mast cell mediators.
- IL-13 affects airway cells by causing impaired mucociliary clearance contributing to airway obstruction; inducing the release of TGF-β from epithelial cells, which enhances fibroblast secretion; impairing nitric oxide (NO) production leading to bronchoconstriction; increasing production of the anaphylatoxin complement factor 3 (C3); and impairing β_2-adrenergic receptor–mediated relaxation of airway smooth muscle.
- Airway epithelial cells (AECs) are important components of the allergic response. Irritants stimulate the AECs to produce cytokines that recruit and activate dendritic cells, causing them to present allergens more efficiently. This sensitizes the immune response.
- Inflammatory cytokines also alter muscarinic receptor function leading to increased levels of acetylcholine, which causes bronchial smooth muscle contraction and mucus secretion.
- In allergic disease, there may be a late asthmatic response (LAR)—eosinophils release neuropeptides and lymphocytes are further activated, resulting in a recurrence of bronchoconstriction at 4 to 12 hours after the initial attack.
- Untreated airway inflammation in asthma can lead to long-term desquamation of the bronchial epithelium with increasing bronchial hyperresponsiveness and eventual scarring of the airways with permanent airway obstruction—airway remodeling.
- Pathophysiology of an acute asthma attack.
  - These pathophysiologic events produce airway obstruction that is worse with expiration.
  - Airway obstruction leads to $\dot{V}/\dot{Q}$ mismatch and hypoxemia early.

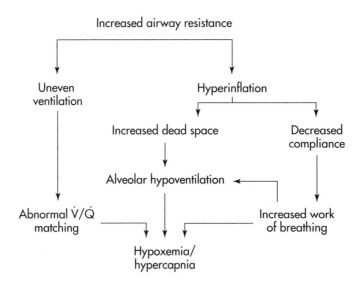

FIGURE **5-2 Pathophysiology of Asthma Attack.**

- Air trapping puts the respiratory muscles at a mechanical disadvantage with increased work of breathing that can eventually result in decreased ventilation and hypercapnia.
- Thus, most patients with acute symptoms start out with rapid respirations, hypoxemia, and a respiratory alkalosis, but persistent airway obstruction leads to shallow inefficient ventilation and respiratory acidosis.
- Infants have greater peripheral airway resistance, fewer collateral channels of ventilation, further extension of airway smooth muscle into the peripheral airways, less elastic recoil, and mechanical disadvantage of the diaphragm. Edematous airways result in relatively greater obstruction to airflow with severe air trapping and hyperinflation, atelectasis, and decreased ventilation. Progression to respiratory failure can be rapid and close monitoring is critical.

PATIENT PRESENTATION

History

Allergic reactions: especially in children; allergic rhinitis and eczematous rashes are particularly common; *recurrent respiratory infections* such as "bronchitis" or "pneumonia" may be complications of asthma, or may represent misdiagnoses of asthma attacks; *episodic dyspnea and chest tightness:* initially may be related to allergic reactions or infections, but careful history can often bring out *exercise limitation; episodic audible wheezing:* worse during expiration but may be inspiratory in severe episodes; *recurrent cough:* airway inflammation may present with cough, especially at night or after exercise; *assess severity:* continuous versus intermittent symptoms; frequency of episodic symptoms; degree of exercise or activity limitation; presence and frequency of nocturnal symptoms.

Symptoms

Intermittent dry cough, wheezing, chest tightness, dyspnea, often after a predictable stimulus (allergen, cold exposure, smoke, etc.); may be associated with rhinitis, postnasal drainage, pharyngitis, sputum production, or viral prodromal symptoms.

Examination

Anxiety, cyanosis, tachypnea, tachycardia, accessory muscle use, chest hyperexpansion; expiratory wheezing with prolonged expiratory phase of breathing; increased pulsus paradoxus.

DIFFERENTIAL DIAGNOSIS

- Bronchitis or bronchiolitis.
- Exacerbation of chronic obstructive pulmonary disease (COPD).
- Pneumonia.
- Allergic rhinitis and sinusitis.
- Pneumonitis.
- Anaphylaxis.
- Foreign body.
- Upper airway obstruction.
- Congestive heart failure.
- Pulmonary embolus.
- Bronchogenic carcinoma.
- Bronchopulmonary aspergillosis.

KEYS TO ASSESSMENT

Assessment Between Attacks (Diagnostic or to Assess Severity [Table 5-1])

- Between attacks, the patient will often have a completely normal examination, or there may be evidence of allergic rhinitis or rashes.
- Peak flow—once the diagnosis of asthma has been established, it is important to determine the "personal best" peak expiratory flow rate (PEFR).
  - Record the PEFR at home two to four times daily for 2 to 3 weeks; best if done in the early afternoon with the same meter each time.

- Used to monitor response to therapy and to help with patient decision making about management.
- Spirometry.
  - A reduction in forced expiratory volume in 1 second (FEV_1) of >20% with acute attack or methacholine challenge.
  - A >12% increase in FEV_1 after short-acting bronchodilator.
- Sputum stain may reveal the presence of eosinophils or mucoid casts.
- Allergy skin testing or radioallergosorbent testing (RAST)—for patients with persistent asthma, recognized initiators for attacks, or other allergic symptoms.

Assessment of Acute Attack

- Level of consciousness, cyanosis.
- Respiratory rate, heart rate, blood pressure, use of accessory muscles of respiration, lung expansion, expiratory phase, wheezing.
- Peak flow is used for monitoring the severity of airflow obstruction and contributes to management decisions; often a peak flow of <50% of predicted indicates the need for hospital admission.
- Pulsus paradoxus—drop in systolic blood pressure with inspiration of >10 mm Hg; a drop of >25 mm Hg is suggestive of a severe asthma attack and the need for immediate hospitalization.
- Oximetry is adequate for assessment of oxygenation in patients who fall into the mild or moderate severity of exacerbation category, but is not adequate in severe cases because it does not test Pa_{CO_2}.
- Arterial blood gases: indicated in severe attacks and when oxygen saturation falls to <91%.
  - Calculate the A-a gradient.
  - Expect respiratory alkalosis and mild hypoxemia.
  - Normalization of arterial pH and carbon dioxide (Pa_{CO_2}) may indicate impending respiratory failure.
- Chest radiograph.
  - Indicated only if pneumothorax, pneumonia, or other complications are suspected.
  - May appear completely normal except for hyperexpansion or mucus plugging, or infiltrates may be visible.
- Sputum—assess for evidence of bacterial infection.
- Complete blood count (CBC) and electrolyte analysis may reveal anemia, evidence of infection, or changes in potassium, magnesium, and phosphate.
- Electrocardiogram (ECG) is indicated in patients older than 50 years of age or any with a history of cardiac disease; patients should be monitored while undergoing emergency treatment.

KEYS TO MANAGEMENT

- Prevention and nonpharmacologic management.
  - Limit allergen or irritant exposure.
  - Home peak flow monitoring and develop action plan to guide care.
  - Consider immunotherapy in the atopic patient.
  - Treat any allergic rhinitis or gastroesophageal reflux disease.
  - Treat infections early.
  - Annual influenza vaccine.
  - Patient education.
- Chronic management is based on the NAEPP guidelines updated in 2002 (see Table 5-1).
  - Management is based on clinical severity.
  - Goals are:
    1. Minimal or no chronic symptoms day or night.
    2. Minimal or no exacerbations.
    3. No limitations on activities; no school/work missed.

4. Maintain (near) normal pulmonary function.
5. Minimal use of short-acting inhaled β_2 agonist.
6. Minimal or no adverse effects from medications.
- The NAEPP guidelines include the following statements:
    1. Treatment should be reviewed every 1 to 6 months and therapy should be "stepped up" or down depending on the response.
    2. The stepwise approach is meant to assist, not replace, the clinical decision making required to meet individual patient needs.
    3. Classify severity: assign patient to most severe step in which any feature occurs.
    4. Gain control as quickly as possible (consider a short course of systemic corticosteroids), then step down to the least medication necessary to maintain control.
    5. Minimize use of short-acting inhaled β_2 agonists. Overreliance on short-acting inhaled β_2 agonists (e.g., use of approximately one canister a month even if not using it every day) indicates inadequate control of asthma and the need to initiate or intensify long-term-control therapy.
    6. Provide education on self-management and controlling environmental factors that make asthma worse (e.g., allergens, irritants).
    7. Refer to an asthma specialist if there are difficulties controlling asthma or if step 4 care is required. Referral may be considered if step 3 care is required.
- In all patients, except those with mild intermittent asthma, daily anti-inflammatories are crucial for preventing long-term airway damage. Inhaled corticosteroids are safe and are the most effective first-line anti-inflammatory agents.
- Recommend starting anti-inflammatory therapy (inhaled corticosteroids) early, even in young children. Latest studies suggest that low-dose inhaled steroids do not retard growth and that they are more effective than cromolyn in children.
- Long-acting β-agonists are effective, but are associated with increased mortality. These medications should be used only as an adjunct to inhaled corticosteroids, and should be discontinued if symptoms worsen or do not improve.
- Leukotriene receptor antagonists may be used as first-line drugs for mild persistent asthma but their efficacy is not as great as inhaled steroids. They can be added to inhaled corticosteroids to enhance symptom control. Nedocromil can also be considered.
- Consider theophylline if symptoms persist.
- Ipratropium bromide may be additive but its use in the treatment of asthma is controversial in the United States.
- Use oral steroids for chronic therapy only as a last resort.
- Omalizumab (monoclonal antibodies to immunoglobulin E [IgE]).
    1. Indications include: IgE level 30 to 700 international units/ml; skin test or serum antibody testing positive for at least one perennial allergen; age more than 12 years; and poor asthma control on low- or moderate-dose inhaled corticosteroids plus long-acting β-agonist.
    2. Given subQ every 2 or 4 weeks; dosage is determined by weight.
    3. Adverse events include headache, injection site reaction, upper respiratory infection (URI), and sinusitis (rates all similar to placebo).
    4. Use of inhaled corticosteroids can be reduced in many individuals.
- Experimental agents.
    1. Phosphodiesterase type 4 (PDE4) inhibitors in phase III clinical trials; cilomilast and roflumilast have demonstrated variable but significant effects on the number of acute asthma exacerbations and on quality of life, with small improvements in pulmonary function.
    2. Specific cytokine blockers—antibodies to IL-4 and IL-5; interleukin production inhibitors (CCR-3); many others being studied.
    3. T cell cytokine modulation using IL-10–secreting regulatory T cells is promising.
- Refer to asthma specialist for moderate to severe asthma.

- *Acute:* β-agonists remain the mainstay of therapy; high-dose oral steroids are crucial for treating the inflammatory process.
    - Recognition of attack severity includes prompt spirometry or peak flow measurement and awareness of risk factors for death in acute attacks such as a history of severe attacks requiring intubation in the past, recent asthma hospitalization, overuse of β-agonists, recent discontinuation of medications (especially oral steroids), and comorbid conditions such as heart disease.
    - Must initiate management promptly without delaying for diagnostic tests.
    - Start oxygen; consider intubation at the first sign of hypercapnia. Intubation should be done semi-electively under controlled circumstances.
    - Administer inhaled short-acting β-agonists by metered dose inhaler (MDI) or continuous nebulizer.
    - Administer prednisone orally (IV steroids indicated only if cannot take orally or life-threatening attack).
    - Consider ipratropium and aminophylline as adjunctive therapy.
    - Magnesium may be considered in status asthmaticus but is controversial.
    - Most acute attacks are caused by viruses. Antibiotics are not recommended unless there is clear evidence of bacterial infection. Macrolide antibiotics have been found to have anti-inflammatory effects, but have not been found to alter the course of nonbacterial acute asthma attacks.
    - Monitoring of oxygenation, ventilation, mental status, and response to bronchodilators is essential; a newer modality of monitoring exhaled nitric oxide may become widely accepted as a way of noninvasively measuring airway inflammation.
    - Monitor need for admission and for late asthmatic response (4 to 12 hours).

PATHOPHYSIOLOGY ———→	CLINICAL LINK
What is going on in the disease process that influences how the patient presents and how he or she should be managed?	*What should you do now that you understand the underlying pathophysiology?*
More than 20 genetic abnormalities have been identified that are associated with asthma. The most frequently cited abnormality is one associated with an increase in IL-4.	A family history of asthma and allergy is important, and potential new therapies are geared toward blocking IL-4, which is a key component of genetic predisposition in asthma.
Allergen exposure is a risk factor for both the development of asthma and for initiating acute attacks.	Obtaining a thorough history of exposures, skin testing, reduction in allergen exposure, and consideration for immunotherapy are all important in asthma assessment and management.
Respiratory viruses play a role in the natural history of asthma.	The role of vaccination and antivirals is being evaluated; use of steroid bursts during acute viral respiratory infections is being explored.
Mast cells release inflammatory mediators that cause bronchoconstriction, edema, and sputum production.	Management must include anti-inflammatories such as steroids and leukotriene receptor blockers as well as bronchodilators.
Eosinophils and neuropeptides cause the late asthmatic response.	Recurrent symptoms can occur after 4 to 8 hours, and the patient must be monitored during this time.
$\dot{V}/\dot{Q}$ mismatch and hypoxemia with hypocapnia are seen early in an acute attack, but increased work of breathing may lead to hypercapnia and sudden respiratory failure.	Arterial blood gases should be monitored carefully in severe attacks, oximetry is *not* adequate alone because it does not measure Pa_{CO_2}.
Inflammatory mediators induce increased acetylcholine release, which is a bronchoconstrictor.	Additive effects of inhaled anticholinergics (ipratropium) may improve β-agonist bronchodilation.
Production of IgE in response to allergen exposure is a key step in both acute and chronic asthma pathophysiology.	A new medication, omalizumab (monoclonal antibodies to IgE), has been released in the United States and has shown effectiveness in selected patients.

SUGGESTED READINGS

Adcock, I. M. & Ito, K. (2004). Steroid resistance in asthma: a major problem requiring novel solutions or a non-issue? *Current Opinion in Pharmacology, 4,* 257-262.

Akbari, O. & Umetsu, D. T. (2005). Role of regulatory dendritic cells in allergy and asthma. *Current Allergy & Asthma Reports, 5,* 56-61.

Amrani, Y., Tliba, O., Deshpande, D. A., Walseth, T. F., Kannan, M. S., & Panettieri, R. A., Jr. (2004). Bronchial hyperresponsiveness: insights into new signaling molecules. *Current Opinion in Pharmacology, 4,* 230-234.

Bang, L. M. & Plosker, G. L. (2004). Omalizumab: a review of its use in the management of allergic asthma. *Treatments in Respiratory Medicine, 3,* 183-199.

Bazan-Socha, S., Bukiej, A., Marcinkiewicz, C., & Musial, J. (2005). Integrins in pulmonary inflammatory diseases. *Current Pharmaceutical Design, 11,* 893-901.

Bielory, L. (2004). Complementary and alternative interventions in asthma, allergy, and immunology. *Annals of Allergy, Asthma, & Immunology, 93,* S45-S54.

Bisset, L. R. & Schmid-Grendelmeier, P. (2005). Chemokines and their receptors in the pathogenesis of allergic asthma: progress and perspective. *Current Opinion in Pulmonary Medicine, 11,* 35-42.

Buhl, R. (2005). Anti-IgE antibodies for the treatment of asthma. *Current Opinion in Pulmonary Medicine, 11,* 27-34.

Carroll, W. (2005). Asthma genetics: pitfalls and triumphs. *Paediatric Respiratory Reviews, 6,* 68-74.

Cates, C. J., Jefferson, T. O., Bara, A. I., & Rowe, B. H. (2004). Vaccines for preventing influenza in people with asthma. [Update of *Cochrane Database of Systematic Reviews* 2000(4):CD000364; PMID: 11034684]. *Cochrane Database of Systematic Reviews* CD000364.

Cazzola, M., Matera, M. G., & Blasi, F. (2004). Macrolide and occult infection in asthma. *Current Opinion in Pulmonary Medicine, 10,* 7-14.

Cohn, L., Elias, J. A., & Chupp, G. L. (2004). Asthma: mechanisms of disease persistence and progression. *Annual Review of Immunology, 22,* 789-815.

Covar, R. A., Macomber, B. A., & Szefler, S. J. (2005). Medications as asthma triggers. *Immunology & Allergy Clinics of North America, 25,* 169-190.

Currie, G. P., Devereux, G. S., Lee, D. K., & Ayres, J. G. (2005). Recent developments in asthma management. *British Medical Journal, 330,* 585-589.

Davydov, L. (2005). Omalizumab (Xolair) for treatment of asthma. *American Family Physician, 71,* 341-342.

Dixon, A. E. & Irvin, C. G. (2005). Early intervention of therapy in asthma. *Current Opinion in Pulmonary Medicine, 11,* 51-55.

Ducharme, F., Schwartz, Z., Hicks, G., & Kakuma, R. (2004). Addition of anti-leukotriene agents to inhaled corticosteroids for chronic asthma. [Update of *Cochrane Database Systematic Reviews* 2002(1):CD003133; PMID: 11869653]. *Cochrane Database of Systematic Reviews* CD003133.

Eneli, I., Sadri, K., Camargo, C., Jr., & Barr, R. G. (2005). Acetaminophen and the risk of asthma: the epidemiologic and pathophysiologic evidence. *Chest, 127,* 604-612.

Erwin, E. A. & Platts-Mills, T. A. (2005). Allergens. *Immunology & Allergy Clinics of North America, 25,* 1-14.

Ferrara, G., Losi, M., Franco, F., Corbetta, L., Fabbri, L. M., & Richeldi, L. (2005). Macrolides in the treatment of asthma and cystic fibrosis. *Respiratory Medicine, 99,* 1-10.

Fuhlbrigge, A. L. (2004). Asthma severity and asthma control: symptoms, pulmonary function, and inflammatory markers. *Current Opinion in Pulmonary Medicine, 10,* 1-6.

Gern, J. E., Rosenthal, L. A., Sorkness, R. L., & Lemanske, R. F., Jr. (2005). Effects of viral respiratory infections on lung development and childhood asthma. *Journal of Allergy & Clinical Immunology, 115,* 668-674.

Gibson, P. G., Henry, R. L., & Coughlan, J. L. (2003). Gastro-oesophageal reflux treatment for asthma in adults and children. *Cochrane Database of Systematic Reviews* CD001496.

Gibson, P. G. & Powell, H. (2004). Written action plans for asthma: an evidence-based review of the key components. *Thorax, 59,* 94-99.

Gotfried, M. H. (2004). Macrolides for the treatment of chronic sinusitis, asthma, and COPD. *Chest, 125,* 52S-60S.

Guerra, S. (2005). Overlap of asthma and chronic obstructive pulmonary disease. *Current Opinion in Pulmonary Medicine, 11,* 7-13.

Halapi, E. & Hakonarson, H. (2004). Recent development in genomic and proteomic research for asthma. *Current Opinion in Pulmonary Medicine, 10,* 22-30.

Harding, S. M. (2005). Gastroesophageal reflux: a potential asthma trigger. *Immunology & Allergy Clinics of North America, 25,* 131-148.

Hawlisch, H., Wills-Karp, M., Karp, C. L., & Kohl, J. (2004). The anaphylatoxins bridge innate and adaptive immune responses in allergic asthma. *Molecular Immunology, 41,* 123-131.

Hawrylowicz, C. M. & O'Garra, A. (2005). Potential role of interleukin-10-secreting regulatory T cells in allergy and asthma. *Nature Reviews, Immunology, 5,* 271-283.

Heaney, L. G. & Robinson, D. S. (2005). Severe asthma treatment: need for characterising patients. *Lancet, 365,* 974-976.

Holgate, S., Casale, T., Wenzel, S., Bousquet, J., Deniz, Y., & Reisner, C. (2005). The anti-inflammatory effects of omalizumab confirm the central role of IgE in allergic inflammation. *Journal of Allergy & Clinical Immunology, 115,* 459-465.

Homer, R. J. & Elias, J. A. (2005). Airway remodeling in asthma: therapeutic implications of mechanisms. *Physiology, 20,* 28-35.

Hospenthal, M. A. & Peters, J. I. (2005). Long-acting beta(2)-agonists in the management of asthma exacerbations. *Current Opinion in Pulmonary Medicine, 11,* 69-73.

Izuhara, K. & Arima, K. (2004). Signal transduction of IL-13 and its role in the pathogenesis of bronchial asthma. *Drug News & Perspectives, 17,* 91-98.

Jackson, C. M. & Lipworth, B. (2004). Benefit-risk assessment of long-acting beta$_2$-agonists in asthma. *Drug Safety, 27,* 243-270.

James, A. (2005). Airway remodeling in asthma. *Current Opinion in Pulmonary Medicine, 11,* 1-6.

Jani, A. L. & Hamilos, D. L. (2005). Current thinking on the relationship between rhinosinusitis and asthma. *Journal of Asthma, 42,* 1-7.

Kaiser, H. B. (2004). Risk factors in allergy/asthma. *Allergy & Asthma Proceedings, 25,* 7-10.

Kallstrom, T. J. (2004). Evidence-based asthma management. *Respiratory Care, 49,* 783-792.

Lawson, J. A. & Senthilselvan, A. (2005). Asthma epidemiology: has the crisis passed? *Current Opinion in Pulmonary Medicine, 11,* 79-84.

Lipworth, B. J. (2005). Phosphodiesterase-4 inhibitors for asthma and chronic obstructive pulmonary disease. *Lancet, 365,* 167-175.

Loza, M. J., Peters, S. P., & Penn, R. B. (2005). Atopy, asthma, and experimental approaches based on the linear model of T cell maturation. *Clinical & Experimental Allergy, 35,* 8-17.

MacDowell, A. L. & Bacharier, L. B. (2005). Infectious triggers of asthma. *Immunology & Allergy Clinics of North America,* 25, 45-66.

Malerba, G. & Pignatti, P. F. (2005). A review of asthma genetics: gene expression studies and recent candidates. *Journal of Applied Genetics,* 46, 93-104.

Marshall, G. D. (2004). Neuroendocrine mechanisms of immune dysregulation: applications to allergy and asthma. *Annals of Allergy, Asthma, & Immunology,* 93, S11-S17.

Masoli, M., Fabian, D., Holt, S., Beasley, R., & Global Initiative for Asthma. (2004). The global burden of asthma: executive summary of the GINA Dissemination Committee report. *Allergy,* 59, 469-478.

McGhan, S. L., Cicutto, L. C., & Befus, A. D. (2005). Advances in development and evaluation of asthma education programs. *Current Opinion in Pulmonary Medicine,* 11, 61-68.

National Asthma Education and Prevention Program Expert Panel Report: guidelines for the diagnosis and management of asthma—update on selected topics 2002. www.nhlbi.nih.gov/guidelines/asthma/asthupdt.htm. January 2006.

National Asthma Education and Prevention Program Expert Panel Report 2: Guidelines for the diagnosis and management of asthma. www.nhlbi.nih.gov/guidelines/asthma/asthgdln.htm. January 2006.

National Asthma Education and Prevention Program: Asthma and Pregnancy Working Group. (2005). NAEPP expert panel report. Managing asthma during pregnancy: recommendations for pharmacologic treatment—2004 update. *Journal of Allergy & Clinical Immunology,* 115, 34-46.

Nelson, H. S. (2005). Advances in upper airway diseases and allergen immunotherapy. *Journal of Allergy & Clinical Immunology,* 115, 676-684.

Ng, D., Salvio, F., & Hicks, G. (2004). Anti-leukotriene agents compared to inhaled corticosteroids in the management of recurrent and/or chronic asthma in adults and children. [Update of *Cochrane Database Systematic Reviews* 2002(3): CD002314; PMID: 12137655]. *Cochrane Database of Systematic Reviews* CD002314.

Norman, P. S. (2004). Immunotherapy: 1999-2004. *Journal of Allergy & Clinical Immunology,* 113, 1013-1023.

O'Byrne, P. M., Inman, M. D., & Adelroth, E. (2004). Reassessing the Th2 cytokine basis of asthma. *Trends in Pharmacological Sciences,* 25, 244-248.

Ostroukhova, M. & Ray, A. (2005). CD25+ T cells and regulation of allergen-induced responses. *Current Allergy & Asthma Reports,* 5, 35-41.

Parnham, M. J. (2005). Immunomodulatory effects of antimicrobials in the therapy of respiratory tract infections. *Current Opinion in Infectious Diseases,* 18, 125-131.

Passalacqua, G., Guerra, L., Pasquali, M., Lombardi, C., & Canonica, G. W. (103). Efficacy and safety of sublingual immunotherapy. *Annals of Allergy, Asthma, & Immunology,* 93, 3-12.

Peden, D. B. (2005). The epidemiology and genetics of asthma risk associated with air pollution. *Journal of Allergy & Clinical Immunology,* 115, 213-219.

Pelaia, G., Cuda, G., Vatrella, A., Gallelli, L., Caraglia, M., Marra, M., Abbruzzese, A., Caputi, M., Maselli, R., Costanzo, F. S., & Marsico, S. A. (2005). Mitogen-activated protein kinases and asthma. *Journal of Cellular Physiology,* 202, 642-653.

Peters-Golden, M. (2004). The alveolar macrophage: the forgotten cell in asthma. *American Journal of Respiratory Cell & Molecular Biology,* 31, 3-7.

Poole, J. A., Matangkasombut, P., & Rosenwasser, L. J. (2005). Targeting the IgE molecule in allergic and asthmatic diseases: review of the IgE molecule and clinical efficacy. *Journal of Allergy & Clinical Immunology,* 115, S376-S385.

Ramsey, C. D. & Celedon, J. C. (2005). The hygiene hypothesis and asthma. *Current Opinion in Pulmonary Medicine,* 11, 14-20.

Remington, T. L. & Digiovine, B. (2005). Long-acting beta-agonists: anti-inflammatory properties and synergy with corticosteroids in asthma. *Current Opinion in Pulmonary Medicine,* 11, 74-78.

Rodrigo, G. J., Rodrigo, C., & Hall, J. B. (2004). Acute asthma in adults: a review. *Chest,* 125, 1081-1102.

Shore, S. A. (2004). Direct effects of TH2 cytokines on airway smooth muscle. *Current Opinion in Pharmacology,* 4, 235-240.

Sin, D. D., Man, J., Sharpe, H., Gan, W. Q., & Man, S. F. (2004). Pharmacological management to reduce exacerbations in adults with asthma: a systematic review and meta-analysis. *Journal of the American Medical Association,* 292, 367-376.

Spergel, J. M. & Fiedler, J. (2005). Food allergy and additives: triggers in asthma. *Immunology & Allergy Clinics of North America,* 25, 149-167.

Staros, E. B. (2005). Innate immunity: new approaches to understanding its clinical significance. *American Journal of Clinical Pathology,* 123, 305-312.

Storms, W. W. (2005). Asthma associated with exercise. *Immunology & Allergy Clinics of North America,* 25, 31-43.

Szefler, S. J. & Apter, A. (2005). Advances in pediatric and adult asthma. *Journal of Allergy & Clinical Immunology,* 115, 470-477.

Tan, W. C. (2005). Viruses in asthma exacerbations. *Current Opinion in Pulmonary Medicine,* 11, 21-26.

Tatum, A. J. & Shapiro, G. G. (2005). The effects of outdoor air pollution and tobacco smoke on asthma. *Immunology & Allergy Clinics of North America,* 25, 15-30.

Tillie-Leblond, I., Gosset, P., & Tonnel, A. B. (2005). Inflammatory events in severe acute asthma. *Allergy,* 60, 23-29.

Trasande, L. & Thurston, G. D. (2005). The role of air pollution in asthma and other pediatric morbidities. *Journal of Allergy & Clinical Immunology,* 115, 689-699.

Ulevitch, R. J. (2004). Therapeutics targeting the innate immune system. *Nature Reviews, Immunology,* 4, 512-520.

van den Toorn, L. M. (658). Clinical implications of airway inflammation in mild intermittent asthma. *Annals of Allergy, Asthma, & Immunology,* 92, 589-594.

Vigo, P. G. & Grayson, M. H. (2005). Occupational exposures as triggers of asthma. *Immunology & Allergy Clinics of North America,* 25, 191-205.

von Mutius, E. (2004). Influences in allergy: epidemiology and the environment. *Journal of Allergy & Clinical Immunology,* 113, 373-379.

White, A. A. & Simon, R. A. (2005). Macrolide antibiotics as anti-inflammatory agents. *Current Allergy & Asthma Reports,* 5, 1-3.

Williams, L. K., Ownby, D. R., Maliarik, M. J., & Johnson, C. C. (2005). The role of endotoxin and its receptors in allergic disease. *Annals of Allergy, Asthma, & Immunology,* 94, 323-332.

Asthma

INITIAL HISTORY

- 17-year-old girl presents to the emergency department complaining of chest tightness and dyspnea.
- She was mowing lawn when these symptoms developed.
- She describes a prodrome of rhinorrhea and tearing that began soon after she went outside, followed by the chest symptoms.
- She felt no better after going inside.
- It is now 1 hour later.

Question 1.   *What is your differential diagnosis based on the information you have now?*

Question 2.   *What other questions would you like to ask now?*

ADDITIONAL HISTORY

- History of asthma since childhood; mother and brother also have asthma.
- Allergic to grass, ragweed, cats.
- She has a cough productive of clear phlegm that comes and goes.
- She has used a "blue" inhaler when needed for the past 6 months, as often as twice a day.
- No other medical history.

Question 3.   *Now what do you think about her history?*

PHYSICAL EXAMINATION

- Alert but anxious teenager; in some respiratory distress; using accessory muscles of respiration.
- T = 37 orally; P = 105 bpm and regular; RR = 30 breaths/minute and labored; BP = 115/68 mm Hg (sitting).

HEENT, Skin, Neck

- Conjunctivae inflamed and edematous, tearing; fundi without lesions; nasal mucosa edematous, clear discharge; pharynx with clear postnasal drainage.
- Skin flushed and pink; diaphoretic; supple.
- No adenopathy; no thyromegaly, no bruits.

Lungs

- Chest expansion somewhat limited; diaphragm percusses low in posterior chest with 2-cm movement bilaterally.
- Prolonged expiratory phase with expiratory wheezes heard throughout all lung fields.
- Scattered coarse crackles; no fine crackles (rales) or egophony.

Cardiac

- Heart sounds distant; tachycardia but regular.
- Slight systolic ejection murmur (SEM) left lower sternal border (LLSB) without radiation; no gallops or clicks.

Abdomen, Extremities, Neurologic

- Abdomen nondistended; bowel sounds present and not hyperactive; liver percusses 2 cm below the right costal margin, but overall size 8 cm; no tenderness or masses.
- Extremities clammy but good capillary refill at 3 seconds; no edema; no clubbing.
- Alert, oriented but anxious; cranial nerves intact; strength 5/5 throughout; DTR 2+ and symmetric; sensory intact to touch.

Question 4.   *What studies would you initiate now while preparing your interventions?*

Question 5.   *What therapies would you initiate immediately while awaiting results of the laboratory studies?*

LABORATORY RESULTS

- Oximetry = 90% oxygen saturation.
- pH = 7.55, PaO_2 = 60, $PaCO_2$ = 30 (RA).
- Peak flow = 200 (<50% of predicted); electrolytes normal.
- HCT = 37%, WBC = 5500, PLTS = 340,000.
- ECG = sinus tachycardia.

Question 6.   *What is her A-a gradient?*

EMERGENCY ROOM COURSE

- The patient becomes increasingly dyspneic despite nebulizer and oxygen.
- She is also becoming more anxious and confused.

PATIENT UPDATE

- P = 110 and regular; RR = 40 and labored; BP = 130/90.
- Lungs with inspiratory and expiratory wheezes; early cyanosis.
- Extremities cold and clammy; no longer alert or oriented.

REPEAT LABORATORY RESULTS

- pH = 7.35; PaO_2 = 45; $PaCO_2$ = 42 (40% mask).
- Peak flow = cannot cooperate.
- Heart monitor = sinus tachycardia.

Question 7.   *What do you think is happening? Why is she more dyspneic? What does her lung examination suggest? Why are her extremities cold? Why is she confused? Has her A-a gradient changed? What do you think about her $PaCO_2$?*

Question 8. *What interventions should be initiated now?*

ADDITIONAL PATIENT UPDATE/REPEAT LABORATORY RESULTS

- Gradual return of respiratory rate to 35, pulse to 100; color improves; more alert.
- Lungs with expiratory wheezes only; peak flow = 180.
- pH = 7.48, PaO_2 = 90, $PaCO_2$ = 32 (60% mask).

Question 9. *Now what should be done and what can the patient expect?*

HOSPITAL COURSE

- Patient does well with normalization of laboratory results.
- Tired but breathing normally after 3 days.
- Discharged on fourth day.

Question 10. *What instructions and medications should this patient go home with? What should the chronic pharmacologic management of her asthma be?*

Question 11. *What steps can she take to prevent future attacks?*

Chronic Obstructive Pulmonary Disease

DEFINITION

- Chronic obstructive pulmonary disease (COPD) has been defined by the Global Initiative for Chronic Obstructive Lung Disease (GOLD) as "a disease state characterized by airflow limitation that is not fully reversible. The airflow limitation is usually both progressive and associated with an abnormal inflammatory response of the lungs to noxious particles or gases."
- Pathologic lung changes in COPD are consistent with emphysema and/or chronic bronchitis.
  - *Emphysema:* Reduced elastic recoil and disintegration of alveolar walls with bulla formation, expiratory airway collapse with air trapping and hyperinflation.
  - *Chronic bronchitis:* Chronic cough productive of phlegm for at least 3 months per year for at least 2 consecutive years.
- Airflow limitation is worse during expiration (as measured by the forced expiratory volume in 1 second [FEV_1]) and does not show major reversibility in response to pharmacologic agents.

EPIDEMIOLOGY

- COPD is the fourth leading cause of death in the United States. It is estimated that more than 10 million people in the United States have physician-diagnosed COPD and that about 24 million adults have evidence of airflow limitation. The estimated annual economic burden of COPD in the United States is $23.9 billion.
- Risk factors.
  - Smoking accounts for more than 90% of the risk for COPD, and approximately 15% to 30% of smokers get COPD. Some smokers are considered "susceptible" and develop very rapid declines in lung function, and most heavy smokers will develop some airflow limitation. Environmental (passive) smoke exposure has been linked to decreased lung function in children and increased respiratory symptoms in adults, but has not been directly linked to COPD.
  - Air pollution and urban living are associated with an increased risk for COPD morbidity. Indoor air pollution is a major risk factor for COPD worldwide and results from heating and cooking in poorly ventilated homes.
  - Occupational dust exposure (gold, cadmium, coal) is an independent risk factor for COPD. This risk is greatly increased when combined with smoking.
  - There is an increased risk for COPD for first-degree relatives who smoke. In less than 1% of people with COPD, there is an inherited α_1-antitrypsin gene defect that causes early onset of emphysema.

PATHOPHYSIOLOGY

- *Genetics:* In addition to the inherited α_1-antitrypsin gene mutation, several other gene polymorphisms have been linked to the development of COPD including those associated with proteases (macrophage elastase, interstitial collagenase, and gelatinase B), tumor necrosis factor, interleukins, endogenous antioxidants, and adrenergic receptors.

- Many patients with COPD have characteristics of both emphysema and chronic bronchitis, with one or the other predominating.
- *Emphysema:* Reduced elastic recoil resulting in expiratory airway collapse and hyperinflation; disintegration of alveolar walls and bulla formation.
    - In the lung, there is a normal balance between proteases that promote lung remodeling (elastases) and antiproteases that inhibit lung remodeling (antielastases such as α_1-antitrypsin) (Figure 6-1).
    - Cigarette smoke results in oxidant stress (production of toxic oxygen radicals) that inhibits the activity of the normal antiproteases and causes inflammation of the respiratory epithelium.
    - Inflammation and the associated activity of T cytotoxic lymphocytes (CD8), macrophages, and polymorphonucleocytes (PMNs), causes release of inflammatory and immune cytokines and results in increased protease (elastase) activity and direct damage to the lung.
    - This imbalance between proteases and antiproteases results in alveolar and bronchial wall damage and increased mucus production.
    - Production of inflammatory cytokines such as tumor necrosis factor-α (TNF-α) also contributes to systemic symptoms such as weight loss and muscle weakness.
    - Intrabronchial mucous exudates, thickening of alveolar walls, and loss of alveolar surface area lead to ventilation/perfusion ($\dot{V}/\dot{Q}$) mismatching with resultant hypoxemia.
    - Airway collapse during expiration with air-trapping leads to hyperexpansion of the lung and an increase in functional residual capacity. This stretches the chest wall, putting the muscles of respiration at a mechanical disadvantage and increasing the work of breathing. Tidal volume falls, with initial ventilatory compensation provided

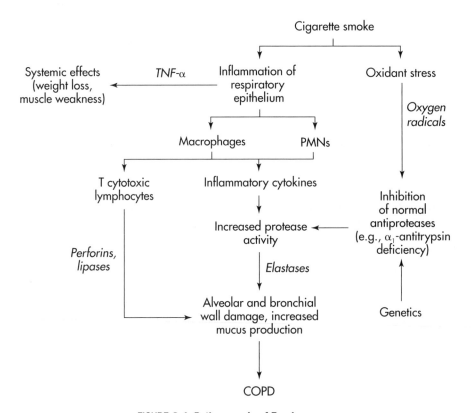

FIGURE **6-1 Pathogenesis of Emphysema.**

by an increase in respiratory rate. As air-trapping and tidal volumes continue to worsen, minute volume falls and hypercapnia with respiratory acidosis begins.
- *Chronic bronchitis:* Chronic cough productive of phlegm for at least 3 months per year for at least 2 consecutive years.
  - Goblet cells in the airway mucosa are increased with hypertrophy and hyperplasia of submucosal glands and production of copious amounts of tenacious sputum. Organisms (especially bacteria) can adhere and grow with persistent colonization of the airways and cause recurrent infectious exacerbations.
  - The associated epithelial inflammation and smooth muscle hypertrophy lead to scarring.
- **Both emphysema and chronic bronchitis.**
  - COPD (both chronic bronchitis and emphysema) results in $\dot{V}/\dot{Q}$ mismatch and expiratory airway obstruction.
    1. $\dot{V}/\dot{Q}$ mismatch leads to hypoxemia.
    2. Expiratory airway obstruction and air-trapping puts the respiratory muscles at a mechanical disadvantage with increased work of breathing.
       a. Shallow rapid breathing is inefficient.
       b. Muscle weakness worsens ventilation.
  - Thus most patients will develop a mixed hypoxemia and hypercapnia.
  - Chronic hypercapnia can lead to decreased sensitivity of the respiratory center such that the individual becomes relatively insensitive to changes in Pa_{CO_2}. This results in dependence on the chemoreception of low Pa_{O_2} as the main stimulus to breathing. Supplemental oxygen may eliminate this stimulus resulting in decreased ventilatory response and additional carbon dioxide retention. Thus individuals with significant hypoxemia may require both oxygenation and ventilation (noninvasive or mechanical).
  - Diffuse pulmonary damage with associated hypoxemia and hypercapnia results in widespread pulmonary arteriolar vasoconstriction and increased pulmonary artery pressures. The right ventricle responds poorly to this increased workload and may dilate and fail, with increased pressures being transmitted to the systemic venous circulation and resultant peripheral edema (cor pulmonale). Over time, remodeling of the pulmonary vessels leads to fixed pulmonary hypertension.
  - Superimposed infection and bronchospasm result in acute exacerbations with worsening gas exchange.

PATIENT PRESENTATION

History

Active or passive smoking history; occupational history; recurrent respiratory infections; progressive exercise limitation; family history (especially if in nonsmoker); weight loss; sputum production.

Symptoms

Progressive dyspnea on exertion; paroxysmal nocturnal dyspnea; pedal edema; productive cough; wheezing, pedal edema, or abdominal fullness (cor pulmonale).

Examination

Decreased level of consciousness and cyanosis during severe exacerbations; tachypnea; increased anteroposterior chest diameter (barrel chest); use of accessory muscles of breathing; low diaphragms on percussion; decreased breath sounds; prolonged expiratory phase of breathing; expiratory wheezing and coarse crackles; clubbing, and pedal edema (advanced disease).

DIFFERENTIAL DIAGNOSIS

- Asthma.
- Acute bronchitis.
- Pneumonia.

- Bronchiectasis.
- Congestive heart failure.
- Pulmonary fibrosis.
- Recurrent pulmonary emboli.

KEYS TO ASSESSMENT

- It is crucial to assess acuteness of onset of symptoms and deviation from "baseline."
- New pedal edema may indicate worsening hypoxemia/hypercapnia and cor pulmonale.
- Spirometry: all results are compared with "predicted" values based on gender, age, and height.
    - Decreased FEV_1 (forced expiratory volume in first second of expiration) to <80% of predicted value.
    - Decrease in FEV_1 greater than any decrease in FVC (forced vital capacity): decreased FEV_1/FVC ratio (<70%).
    - No significant improvement with bronchodilator treatment (<20%).
    - Specialized pulmonary function testing: decreased diffusion capacity (DLCO) and oxygen desaturation with exercise.
- Several classification schemes for COPD can help determine appropriate therapy. The scheme that is gaining worldwide acceptance is the GOLD scheme.

Stage 0: at risk	Normal spirometry; chronic symptoms (cough, sputum)
Stage I: mild	FEV_1/FVC <70%; FEV_1 >80% predicted; with or without chronic symptoms (cough, sputum)
Stage II: moderate	FEV_1/FVC <70%; 50% <FEV_1 < 80% predicted; with or without chronic symptoms (cough, sputum, dyspnea)
Stage III: severe	FEV_1/FVC <70%; 30% <FEV_1 <50% predicted; with or without chronic symptoms (cough, sputum, dyspnea)
Stage IV: very severe	FEV_1/FVC <70%; FEV_1 <30% predicted or FEV_1 <50% predicted with respiratory failure or clinical signs of right heart failure (cor pulmonale).

- High-resolution spiral computed tomography can diagnosis COPD with high sensitivity.
- Arterial blood gases (ABGs) are useful for evaluating the severity of pulmonary dysfunction in both the stable COPD patient (establish baseline values), and during acute exacerbations.
    - Look for both hypercapnia and hypoxemia (oximetry is inadequate for these patients in that it does not indicate the $Paco_2$). Acidosis is a clear indicator of acute hypercapnia.
    - Severe hypoxemia should not be tolerated even in the patient with long-standing advanced COPD. The institution of oxygen therapy requires close monitoring of ABGs for increasing hypercapnia, and ventilation may be required.
- Chest radiograph is often normal until late-stage disease but is useful for documenting infection.
    - Compare with baseline films.
    - Expect flattened diaphragms, increased retrosternal space, enlarged pulmonary arteries, bullae, and scarring in emphysema.
    - Look closely for pneumothorax or acute infiltrates.
- Sputum stain and culture is useful for the diagnosis of chronic bronchitis and for evaluating acute exacerbations of COPD.
    - Look for PMNs and bacteria on Gram stain.
    - The most common organisms include *Haemophilus influenzae, Moraxella catarrhalis,* and *Streptococcus pneumoniae;* in patients with advanced disease, consider *Pseudomonas aeruginosa.*

KEYS TO MANAGEMENT

- Prevention and nonpharmacologic management.
    - Smoking cessation: many modalities, including hypnosis, nicotine replacements (nasal, oral, dermal), buspirone, and support groups.

1. Causes some prompt improvement in pulmonary function.
2. Slows the rate of lung function decline over years.
3. Reduces number of infectious complications and exacerbations.
4. Often associated with an increase in cough and anxiety during first few weeks.
5. Frequent follow-up contacts between the provider and the patient improve the chances for long-term smoking cessation.

- Vaccination: Regular influenza and pneumococcal vaccination.
- Nutrition: Low body weight is correlated with decreased respiratory muscle strength and increased mortality. High protein, high-carbohydrate, calorie-dense, frequent small meals are recommended. Dietary supplements used in combination with anabolic therapy such as recombinant human growth hormone (rhGH) have been shown to improve strength and exercise tolerance and to improve quality of life. Rapid institution of supplemental feeding if hospitalized is crucial.
- Education: Studies show patients instructed about their disease and the implications of treatment can better understand, recognize, and treat the symptoms of their disease.
- Rehabilitation: Some techniques are more effective than others but all are potentially helpful: breathing control techniques, chest physical therapy, exercise training, respiratory muscle training, and occupational therapy. Exercise also increases appetite.
- Psychologic support: Anxiety, depression, and fatigue are common in patients with COPD. Evidence is strong that participation in a rehabilitation program with education, exercise, and relaxation techniques is more effective in reducing anxiety than is psychotherapy.
- Oxygen therapy: In an acute exacerbation with severe hypoxemia, oxygen is vital to sustain life. In patients with severe COPD and sustained hypoxemia, home oxygen therapy improves quality of life, exercise tolerance, cognitive functioning, emotional status, and sleep quality and controls polycythemia. Oxygen should be administered to maintain an oxygen saturation of at least 90% for a minimum of 15 hours per day to affect survival. Oxygen administration should be adjusted for rest, exertion, and sleep to meet the individual patient's needs.
- Ventilation: Noninvasive positive pressure ventilation (NIPPV) is indicated for individuals who have symptoms of nocturnal hypoventilation despite maximum bronchodilator therapy, who cannot tolerate long-term oxygen therapy without becoming increasingly hypercapnic, or who have repeated admissions to the hospital with acute hypercapnic ventilatory failure. NIPPV can improve gas exchange and symptoms but does not affect mortality. Complications include nasal congestion and ulceration, eye irritation, facial skin breakdown, aspiration, and gastric distention.
- Chronic pharmacotherapy.
  - Stepwise therapy for COPD is recommended based on GOLD stage.
    1. Stages 0 to IV: avoidance of risk factors and vaccination; nutrition.
    2. Stages I to IV: short-acting inhaled β-agonist or anticholinergic when needed.
    3. Stages II to IV: Long-acting inhaled β-agonist or long-acting anticholinergic (tiotropium) and pulmonary rehabilitation.
    4. Stages III and IV: combination therapy; consider inhaled steroids or theophylline.
    5. Stage IV: oxygen therapy and consideration for surgery.
  - Inhaled β$_2$-agonists: Short acting drugs (e.g., albuterol) are for immediate symptom relief. Long-acting β-agonists (e.g., formoterol, salmeterol) improve exercise capacity, nocturnal symptoms, dyspnea, and quality of life.
  - Anticholinergics: Ipratropium is used as a short-acting bronchodilator as needed for symptom relief. Long-acting tiotropium improves adherence (once daily) and is equally effective in relieving symptoms and improving quality of life when compared to β-agonists. There is some highly controversial evidence that tiotropium may slow disease progression in COPD.
  - Combinations of long-acting β-agonists with ipratropium and/or inhaled steroids are additive in their effects on lung function.

- Steroids: Inhaled corticosteroids are controversial in the management of COPD but can be considered in individuals with moderate to severe disease who do not respond adequately to bronchodilators. Some studies have shown that these drugs reduce the rate of exacerbations and may slow the rate of decline of FEV_1, however others have shown no change in the rate of disease progression. Oral steroids should be reserved for the management of acute exacerbations.
- Theophylline: This drug has a relatively narrow benefit/risk ratio, but is useful as an adjunct to β-agonists and anticholinergics in selected individuals with moderate to severe COPD. Serum levels and potential drug interactions should be monitored carefully.
- Phosphodiesterase inhibitors (cilomilast and roflumilast) have been shown to cause bronchodilation, decrease inflammation, and decrease airway remodeling in several studies. They are in phase III trials in the United States as of early 2006.
- Surgery: Several techniques are now available for carefully selected patients.
    1. Lung volume reduction surgery—reduces hyperinflation and can be considered in individuals with severe upper-lobe emphysema and reduced exercise tolerance and inadequate response to medical therapy.
    2. Lung transplant (single) can be considered for those with an FEV_1 <25% of predicted, cor pulmonale, and severe hypoxemia/hypercapnia, however it does not improve overall survival.
- Management of acute exacerbation.
  - Rapid assessment of status, obtain IV access.
  - Begin oxygen—give patient enough to relieve significant hypoxemia (goal of PaO_2 ≥55 mm Hg), but watch for increasing hypercapnia (oximetry is not adequate for full assessment and management). Consider noninvasive positive pressure ventilation if pH falls to <7.35 (some studies suggest it should be begun earlier). Mechanical ventilation should be instituted if noninvasive ventilation is contraindicated or ineffective.
  - Begin $β_2$-agonist by dry inhaler, metered dose inhaler with spacer, or continuous nebulizer.
  - Give ipratropium two puffs 5 minutes after first $β_2$-agonist dose.
  - Antibiotics: Most studies suggest that the majority of acute exacerbations are associated with significant lower airway bacterial infection. Macrolides and fluoroquinolones have been effective in several trials.
  - Steroids: Oral prednisone is associated with significant improvements in outcomes in hospitalized patients with acute exacerbations of COPD. The primary complication is hyperglycemia.
  - The use of aminophylline for acute exacerbations is controversial and not generally recommended.

PATHOPHYSIOLOGY ⟶	CLINICAL LINK
What is going on in the disease process that influences how the patient presents and how he or she should be managed?	*What should you do now that you understand the underlying pathophysiology?*
A small minority of patients have a genetic deficiency of the antielastase α₁-antitrypsin as the cause of early onset emphysema.	A careful examination of family history and genetic testing is indicated in patients with early onset COPD symptoms, especially if there is a minimal smoking history.
Cigarette smoke results in bronchial epithelial inflammation and toxic oxygen radical destruction of antielastases, which, in turn, lead to damage to alveoli and bronchi.	Smoking cessation is vital to slow disease progression but will not normalize lung function.
Damage to bronchial mucosa and the elastin in bronchial walls results in expiratory airway obstruction due to either loss of airway elasticity, increased mucus production, or both.	Patients with both emphysema and chronic bronchitis present with dyspnea, prolonged expiration, and wheezing.
Expiratory obstruction with air-trapping, increased work of breathing, and uneven ventilation result in decreased minute volume and $\dot{V}/\dot{Q}$ mismatching, especially during late stage disease and acute exacerbations.	Mixed hypercapnia and hypoxemia are common in COPD. Evaluation of arterial blood gases helps determine the severity of disease at "baseline" and contributes to appropriate management decisions during acute exacerbations.
Chronic hypercapnia results in reliance on hypoxic ventilatory drive to maintain adequate ventilation.	Oxygen therapy is vital, but patients must be monitored for decreased minute volume and hypercapnia—some may need mechanical ventilation.
Symptoms of COPD are chronic and require constant bronchodilators to reduce exacerbations and improve quality of life.	Long-acting β-agonists or anticholinergics are indicated for moderate COPD. Combination therapy and consideration for inhaled corticosteroids should be given if the COPD worsens or there is inadequate response to therapy.
Chronic hypoxemia and hypercapnia in COPD is associated with pulmonary hypertension and cor pulmonale. Muscle wasting and poor nutrition commonly accompany this disease.	Nonpharmacologic therapy should include consideration for oxygen treatment, rehabilitation, patient education, psychologic support, nutrition, and possible referral for surgery.

SUGGESTED READINGS

Andrus, M. R., Holloway, K. P., & Clark, D. B. (2004). Use of beta-blockers in patients with COPD. *Annals of Pharmacotherapy*, 38, 142-145.

Balmes, J. R. (2005). Occupational contribution to the burden of chronic obstructive pulmonary disease. *Journal of Occupational & Environmental Medicine*, 47, 154-160.

Barnes, P. J., Ito, K., & Adcock, I. M. (2004). Corticosteroid resistance in chronic obstructive pulmonary disease: inactivation of histone deacetylase. *Lancet*, 363, 731-733.

Bohadana, A., Teculescu, D., & Martinet, Y. (2004). Mechanisms of chronic airway obstruction in smokers. *Respiratory Medicine*, 98, 139-151.

Calverley, P. M. & Koulouris, N. G. (2005). Flow limitation and dynamic hyperinflation: key concepts in modern respiratory physiology. *European Respiratory Journal*, 25, 186-199.

Campos, M. A. & Wanner, A. (2005). The rationale for pharmacologic therapy in stable chronic obstructive pulmonary disease. *American Journal of the Medical Sciences*, 329, 181-189.

Cazzola, M. & Dahl, R. (2004). Inhaled combination therapy with long-acting beta 2-agonists and corticosteroids in stable COPD. *Chest*, 126, 220-237.

Chapman, K. R. (2004). Chronic obstructive pulmonary disease: are women more susceptible than men? *Clinics in Chest Medicine*, 25, 331-341.

Cooper, C. B. & Tashkin, D. P. (2005). Recent developments in inhaled therapy in stable chronic obstructive pulmonary disease. *British Medical Journal*, 330, 640-644.

Decramer, M., Gosselink, R., Bartsch, P., Lofdahl, C. G., Vincken, W., Dekhuijzen, R., Vestbo, J., Pauwels, R., Naeije, R., & Troosters, T. (2005). Effect of treatments on the progression of COPD: report of a workshop held in Leuven, Belgium, 11-12 March 2004. *Thorax*, 60, 343-349.

Decramer, M., Gosselink, R., Rutten-Van Molken, M., Buffels, J., Van Schayck, O., Gevenois, P. A., Pellegrino, R., Derom, E., & De Backer, W. (2005). Assessment of progression of COPD: report of a workshop held in Leuven, Belgium, 11-12 March 2004. *Thorax*, 60, 335-342.

Dolovich, M. B., Ahrens, R. C., Hess, D. R., Anderson, P., Dhand, R., Rau, J. L., Smaldone, G. C., Guyatt, G., American College of Chest Physicians, & American College of Asthma. (2005). Device selection and outcomes of aerosol therapy: Evidence-based guidelines: American College of Chest Physicians/American College of Asthma, Allergy, and Immunology. *Chest*, 127, 335-371.

Gan, W. Q., Man, S. F., Senthilselvan, A., & Sin, D. D. (2004). Association between chronic obstructive pulmonary disease and systemic inflammation: a systematic review. *Thorax*, 59, 574-580.

Global Initiative for Chronic Obstructive Lung Disease. Global Strategy for the Diagnosis, Management, and Prevention of Chronic Obstructive Pulmonary Disease. Available at: www.goldcopd.com.

Gotfried, M. H. (2004). Macrolides for the treatment of chronic sinusitis, asthma, and COPD. *Chest*, 125, 52S-60S.

Guerra, S. (2005). Overlap of asthma and chronic obstructive pulmonary disease. *Current Opinion in Pulmonary Medicine*, 11, 7-13.

Highland, K. B. (2004). Inhaled corticosteroids in chronic obstructive pulmonary disease: is there a long-term benefit? *Current Opinion in Pulmonary Medicine*, 10, 113-119.

Hill, N. S. (2004). Noninvasive ventilation for chronic obstructive pulmonary disease. *Respiratory Care*, 49, 72-87.

Hogg, J. C. (2004). Pathophysiology of airflow limitation in chronic obstructive pulmonary disease. *Lancet*, 364, 709-721.

Kim, S. & Nadel, J. A. (2004). Role of neutrophils in mucus hypersecretion in COPD and implications for therapy. *Treatments in Respiratory Medicine*, 3, 147-159.

Kutty, K. (2004). Sleep and chronic obstructive pulmonary disease. *Current Opinion in Pulmonary Medicine*, 10, 104-112.

Lipson, D. A. (2004). Redefining treatment in COPD: new directions in bronchodilator therapy [erratum appears in *Treatments in Respiratory Medicine*, 2004;3(3):181]. *Treatments in Respiratory Medicine*, 3, 89-95.

Lipworth, B. J. (2005). Phosphodiesterase-4 inhibitors for asthma and chronic obstructive pulmonary disease. *Lancet*, 365, 167-175.

MacIntyre, N. R. (2004). Chronic obstructive pulmonary disease: emerging medical therapies. *Respiratory Care*, 49, 64-69.

Molfino, N. A. (2004). Genetics of COPD. *Chest*, 125, 1929-1940.

Mulroy, J. (2005). Chronic obstructive pulmonary disease in women. *DCCN—Dimensions of Critical Care Nursing*, 24, 1-18.

Nathan, S. D. (2005). Lung transplantation: disease-specific considerations for referral. *Chest*, 127, 1006-1016.

Parnham, M. J. (2005). Immunomodulatory effects of antimicrobials in the therapy of respiratory tract infections. *Current Opinion in Infectious Diseases*, 18, 125-131.

Pauwels, R. A. & Rabe, K. F. (2004). Burden and clinical features of chronic obstructive pulmonary disease (COPD). *Lancet*, 364, 613-620.

Presberg, K. & Dincer, H. (2003). Pathophysiology of pulmonary hypertension due to lung disease. *Current Opinion in Pulmonary Medicine*, 9, 131-138.

Ram, F. S., Picot, J., Lightowler, J., & Wedzicha, J. A. (2004). Non-invasive positive pressure ventilation for treatment of respiratory failure due to exacerbations of chronic obstructive pulmonary disease. *Cochrane Database of Systematic Reviews*, CD004104.

Ram, F. S., Wedzicha, J. A., Wright, J., & Greenstone, M. (2004). Hospital at home for patients with acute exacerbations of chronic obstructive pulmonary disease: systematic review of evidence. *British Medical Journal*, 329, 315.

Rennard, S. I. (2004). Treatment of stable chronic obstructive pulmonary disease. *Lancet*, 364, 791-802.

Schumaker, G. L. & Epstein, S. K. (2004). Managing acute respiratory failure during exacerbation of chronic obstructive pulmonary disease. *Respiratory Care*, 49, 766-782.

Sethi, S. (2004). New developments in the pathogenesis of acute exacerbations of chronic obstructive pulmonary disease. *Current Opinion in Infectious Diseases*, 17, 113-119.

Sutherland, E. R. & Cherniack, R. M. (2004). Management of chronic obstructive pulmonary disease. *New England Journal of Medicine*, 350, 2689-2697.

Tashkin, D. P. & Cooper, C. B. (2004). The role of long-acting bronchodilators in the management of stable COPD. *Chest*, 125, 249-259.

Tobin, M. J. (2004). Chronic obstructive pulmonary disease, pollution, pulmonary vascular disease, transplantation, pleural disease, and lung cancer in AJRCCM 2003. *American Journal of Respiratory & Critical Care Medicine*, 169, 301-313.

Tomas, L. H. & Varkey, B. (2004). Improving health-related quality of life in chronic obstructive pulmonary disease. *Current Opinion in Pulmonary Medicine*, 10, 120-127.

Tovar, J. M. & Gums, J. G. (2004). Monitoring pulmonary function in asthma and COPD: point-of-care testing. *Annals of Pharmacotherapy*, 38, 126-133.

Trow, T. K. (2004). Lung-volume reduction surgery for severe emphysema: appraisal of its current status. *Current Opinion in Pulmonary Medicine*, 10, 128-132.

Varkey, A. B. (2004). Chronic obstructive pulmonary disease in women: exploring gender differences. *Current Opinion in Pulmonary Medicine*, 10, 98-103.

Vignola, A. M. (2004). PDE4 inhibitors in COPD—a more selective approach to treatment. *Respiratory Medicine*, 98, 495-503.

Wouters, E. F. (2004). Management of severe COPD. *Lancet*, 364, 883-895.

Chronic Obstructive Pulmonary Disease

INITIAL HISTORY

- 62-year-old female presents to the clinic complaining of shortness of breath that has increased slowly for years.
- Symptoms have become worse in recent months, and has become much worse over the last 2 days and now with productive cough.
- Also complaining of new-onset ankle swelling.

Question 1. *What other questions would you like to ask?*

ADDITIONAL HISTORY

- 80 pack/year smoking history; quit 5 years ago.
- Sputum is yellow; no blood.
- No fever, chills, or chest pain.
- Usually brings up only scant white sputum in the morning.
- Denies weight loss.
- Denies history of heart disease.

Question 2. *What would you like to ask about the past medical history?*

MEDICAL HISTORY

- Has been fairly healthy.
- Denies TB or asbestos exposure; no occupational exposures.
- No known allergies.
- Occasional bronchitis treated as an outpatient with antibiotics.
- No history of asthma.
- Family history positive for heart disease (brother in his 50s).

Question 3.   *What is the differential diagnosis at this time?*

PHYSICAL EXAMINATION

- Alert, mild dyspnea with climbing onto the examination table.
- Afebrile.
- P = 95; RR = 28; BP = 135/85, no orthostatic changes.
- No cyanosis.
- No rashes.

HEENT, Neck
- PERRLA, fundi without hemorrhages or exudates.
- Yellowed teeth.
- Nares clear; pharynx clear.
- Pursed-lip breathing.
- Mild jugular venous distention.
- Shotty anterior cervical adenopathy.

Lungs
- Using accessory muscles at rest.
- Barrel chest; decreased diaphragmatic excursion bilaterally.
- Percussion hyperresonant; decreased breath sounds throughout.
- Prolonged expiration with expiratory wheezes with rhonchi in all lung fields.
- No supraclavicular or axillary adenopathy.

Cardiac
- Regular rate rhythm with occasional premature beat.
- Normal S_1, loud S_2, no S_3 or S_4.

Abdomen, Extremities
- Liver palpable, span 12 cm at the right midclavicular line.
- Spleen palpable.
- No masses or tenderness.
- No cyanosis or clubbing.
- 2+ bilateral pitting pedal edema.

Neurologic
- Alert, oriented.
- Cranial nerves intact.
- Strength, sensation, deep tendon reflexes intact and symmetric.
- Gait steady.

Question 4.   *What are the important positive and negative findings on examination and what might they mean?*

Question 5.   *What laboratory tests would you order at this time?*

LABORATORY RESULTS

- Serum chemistries normal except bicarbonate = 38; calcium normal.
- HCT = 49%; WBC = 9000, normal differential.
- Liver function tests normal.
- Sputum = occasional epithelial cell, scattered epithelial cells; numerous PMNs and gram-positive diplococci seen.

Question 6.   *What do these laboratory results tell you?*

ARTERIAL BLOOD GAS RESULTS

- pH = 7.38; $Paco_2$ = 56; Pao_2 = 54 on room air.

Question 7. *What is the A-a gradient?*

SPIROMETRY RESULTS

- Forced expiratory volume in 1 second (FEV_1) = 1.67 L/second (45% of predicted).
- Forced vital capacity (FVC) = 4.10 L (85% of predicted).
- FEV_1/FVC = 37% (predicted = 72%).

Question 8. *What do these spirometry results indicate?*

CHEST RADIOGRAPH AND READING

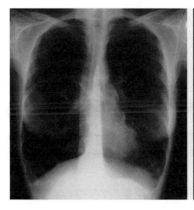 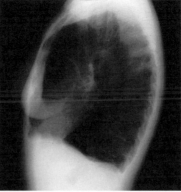

- Hyperinflation with flattened diaphragms.
- Increased anteroposterior diameter and retrosternal space.
- Diffuse scarring and bullae especially in the lower lobes.
- No acute infiltrates.

Question 9.   *What is the pathophysiology behind these chest radiographic findings?*

Question 10.   *What are the key elements of acute management for this patient?*

HOSPITAL COURSE

The patient fully recovers from her acute exacerbation. Repeat spirometry now reveals an FEV_1 of 55% of predicted and an FEV_1/FVC ratio of 58%. Arterial blood gases now reveal pH = 7.39, $Paco_2$ = 50 mm Hg, and Pao_2 = 60 mm Hg.

Question 11.   *How should this patient be managed chronically?*

Pneumonia

DEFINITION

- Although the term "pneumonia" can be used to describe a large number of diseases that cause pulmonary parenchymal consolidation, most commonly it is used to refer to infections of the lower respiratory tract.
- Infectious causes may be viral, bacterial, fungal, protozoal, or parasitic.
- Pneumonia can be categorized as community-acquired (CAP), nursing-home–acquired (NHAP), or nosocomial (hospital acquired).

EPIDEMIOLOGY

- Sixth leading cause of death in the United States—3 to 5.6 million cases annually.
- Increasing prevalence of more severe pneumonia is related in part to the aging population, the increase in iatrogenic immunosuppression (e.g., transplantation and cancer therapy), and HIV. Antimicrobial resistance also plays a role.
- Overall mortality for CAP ranges from 1% to 9% if managed as an outpatient, but increases to 50% for those requiring intensive care unit (ICU) management.
- Advanced age, immunocompromise, reduced forced expiratory volume in 1 second (FEV_1), and high alcohol intake are the greatest risk factors in the general population. Other risk factors include altered consciousness, smoking, underlying lung disease, endotracheal intubation, malnutrition, airway obstruction, and immobilization.
- The most common community-acquired bacterial infections include *Streptococcus pneumoniae*, *Haemophilus influenza*, *Mycoplasma pneumoniae*, *Chlamydia pneumoniae*, *Legionella pneumophila*, and *Moraxella catarrhalis*. *Mycobacterium tuberculosis* prevalence in the United States peaked in 1992 at 26,673 cases, and has since declined by 2% to 7% per year.
- Viral pneumonia is most often caused by influenza, but can also be caused by respiratory syncytial virus (RSV), parainfluenza virus, adenovirus, metapneumovirus, cytomegalovirus, herpesvirus, and the severe acute respiratory syndrome (SARS) virus.
- Fungal pneumonias are most common in immunocompromised individuals and are often caused by *Pneumocystis jiroveci* (formerly *carinii*) and *Candida albicans.*
- NHAP is commonly caused by the same organisms as CAP (unless patient was recently discharged from the hospital), but due to the advanced age of the patients, has a higher mortality rate.
- Nosocomial pneumonia is the second most common nosocomial infection but has the greatest mortality (overall 20% to 50% mortality). It is the most common infection in intensive care units (ICUs) where ventilator-associated pneumonia (VAP) occurs in 9% to 27% of patients. If VAP occurs within the first 48 hours of hospitalization, community-acquired organisms are most common; if late in onset, then *Staphylococcus aureus* and *Pseudomonas aeruginosa* are most common.

PATHOPHYSIOLOGY

- *Genetics:* Host defenses (and susceptibilities) to lung infections are influenced by genetic determinants of innate immunity (inflammation), adaptive immunity, and pulmonary-specific defenses. Genes under study include Toll-like receptor; mannose-binding lectin; immunoglobulin; tumor necrosis factor; interleukin (IL)-1, IL-6, and IL-10; angiotensin-converting enzyme; and surfactant genes.
- Bacterial pneumonia.
  - Aspiration of organisms that colonize the oropharyngeal secretions is the most common route of infection. Other routes of inoculation include inhalation, hematogenous spread from remote sites of infection, and direct extension from contiguous sites of infection.
  - The upper airway is the first line of defense against infection; however, the clearance of organisms by saliva, cough, gag reflex, and secretory IgA can be inhibited by many diseases, immunocompromise, smoking, and endotracheal intubation.
  - The lower airway defenses include mucociliary expulsion, surfactant, macrophage and polymorphonucleocyte (PMN) phagocytosis, and cellular and humoral immunity. These defenses are inhibited by altered consciousness, smoking, abnormal mucus production (e.g., cystic fibrosis or chronic bronchitis), immunocompromise, intubation, and prolonged bed rest.
  - The alveolar macrophage is the primary defender against invasion of the lower respiratory tract and it daily clears the airways of aspirated organisms without initiating significant inflammation.
  - If the number or virulence of the organisms is too great, the macrophage will recruit PMNs and initiate the inflammatory cascade with release of numerous cytokines including leukotrienes, tumor necrosis factor (TNF), interleukins, oxygen radicals, and proteases.
  - This inflammation leads to alveolar filling with ventilation/perfusion mismatching and hypoxemia. Widespread apoptosis of lung cells occurs, which helps to eradicate intracellular organisms such as tuberculosis or chlamydia, but also contributes to lung damage.
  - The infection may remain localized to the lung or may cause bacteremia, resulting in meningitis or endocarditis, the systemic inflammatory response syndrome (SIRS), and/or sepsis.
  - Virulence factors of various organisms can influence the pathophysiology and clinical course of disease. *Streptococcus pneumoniae* (Pneumococcus) provides an example (Figure 7-1).
- Tuberculosis.
  - Mycobacteria are inhaled into the lower respiratory tract and elicit a multifaceted immune response including the recruitment of large numbers of macrophages.
  - Granuloma formation walls off the organism until reactivation occurs, most commonly in response to immunocompromise of the individual. In immunocompromised individuals, diffuse pulmonary and extrapulmonary infection is common.
  - Active pulmonary infection results in widespread inflammation, with inflammatory cell invasion of interstitial and alveolar spaces resulting in dense infiltration of lung parenchyma. Necrosis and lung cavitation are common.
- Influenza pneumonia.
  - Most commonly a complication of influenza in the older adult, patients with cardiopulmonary disease, and pregnant women, but occasionally affects healthy, immunocompetent individuals.
  - Within 1 to 3 days after the onset of symptoms of influenza, airway epithelial cell necrosis and apoptosis begin, with interstitial inflammation.
  - Interstitial inflammation interferes with gas exchange and can lead to significant fibrosis.
- Pneumocystis pneumonia.
  - Fungal cysts, recently renamed *P. jiroveci,* bind to lung alveolar epithelial cells (type I) and proliferate.

Organism is aspirated, inhaled, or spread
hematogenously from another source

↓

Capsular polysaccharide protects organism
from PMNs and diminishes inflammation
until the immune system is activated

↓

Antibodies expose underlying cell wall,
leukocytes are recruited into the lung

↓

Cytokines are produced, alveolar epithelial permeability
is increased, and teichoic acid from the organism
sets off a procoagulant cascade

↓

As organisms are destroyed, bacterial cell wall
components and pneumolysin, which are
cytotoxic to lung cells, are released

↓

Gross pathologic lung changes include
engorgement (fluid exudation into alveoli),
red hepatization (leakage of erythrocytes into alveoli),
and gray hepatization (leukocyte migration into alveoli)

↓

Intense inflammatory response leads to a
clinical "crisis" and subsequent defervescence

↓

Fibrinization with resolution

FIGURE **7-1 Pathogenesis of Pneumococcal Pneumonia.**

- Neutrophilic inflammation is followed by activation of macrophages and T lymphocytes that release inflammatory and immune mediators, including interleukins and tumor necrosis factor.
- Alveolar cell damage, surfactant decreases, and inflammation of the alveolar interstitium lead to interstitial infiltrates that may progress to alveolar consolidation.
- Effects on gas exchange.
  - Infiltration of interstitial and then alveolar air spaces results in consolidation of the lung parenchyma, reducing ventilation to affected segments, lobules, or lobes.

- $\dot{V}/\dot{Q}$ mismatching (shunting) leads to impaired diffusion of oxygen into capillaries leading to hypoxemia.
- Most individuals will present with tachypnea and respiratory alkalosis due to stimulation of pulmonary receptors, but hypercapnia may be seen in individuals with underlying ventilatory compromise or in cases of diffuse overwhelming pulmonary infection.

PATIENT PRESENTATION

History

Age; altered consciousness; immunocompromise; smoking; underlying lung disease; prolonged bed rest; recent hospitalization; and intubation.

Symptoms

Upper respiratory prodrome (headache, rhinitis, postnasal drainage); cough; cough may be dry or associated with sputum production and discoloration; dyspnea; pleuritic chest pain; hemoptysis; fever; rigors; myalgias. Be aware that in the older adult, fewer symptoms or more vague complaints may be noted, including malaise, confusion, anorexia, and falling. In viral pneumonia, rapid progression to fever, tachypnea, tachycardia, cyanosis, and hypotension is common.

Examination

Fever; tachypnea; tachycardia; decreased level of consciousness; cyanosis; use of accessory muscles of respiration; splinting; dullness to percussion; inspiratory crackles (rales); egophony; whispered pectoriloquy; increased tactile fremitus; pleural friction rub; discolored sputum.

DIFFERENTIAL DIAGNOSIS

- Acute or chronic bronchitis.
- Noninfectious pneumonitis.
- Pulmonary embolus.
- Asthma, COPD.
- Congestive heart failure.
- Acute respiratory distress syndrome (ARDS) (pneumonia can cause ARDS).
- Interstitial fibrosis.

KEYS TO ASSESSMENT

- Look for source of infection and assess for septic shock (hypotension, poor tissue perfusion).
- Arterial blood gases.
    - Indicated if the patient is in respiratory distress or has significant underlying lung disease.
    - Expect hypoxemia with respiratory alkalosis in patient without underlying lung disease.
- White blood cell (WBC) count with differential (expect leukocytosis with "left shift" in bacterial pneumonia).
- Electrolytes and liver function tests may be useful in patients with an atypical presentation or severe symptoms (e.g., patients with *Legionella pneumophila*).
- In outpatients, specific identification of the causative organism occurs in as little as 2% to as much as 50% of cases, but does not significantly affect outcome; therefore many studies suggest that examination of sputum, sputum cultures, and blood cultures is not necessary in low-risk patients.
- Sputum.
    - Gram stain is indicated in all inpatients: the presence of numerous PMNs is consistent with bacterial infection. In some cases, the causative organism may be preliminarily identified by staining characteristics and shape.

- Sputum culture is indicated in patients who are hospitalized or have been recently discharged, or who present with severe or unusual symptoms; ventilated patients require lower respiratory cultures (often via bronchoscopy), and semiquantitative or quantitative culture results should be used for management.
- Chest radiograph.
  - Currently recommended in all patients with a history and physical examination suggestive of pneumonia; however, frequently not done in healthy outpatients.
  - Expect lobar, interstitial, or patchy infiltrates; look for air bronchograms.
- Blood cultures are indicated in hospitalized patients.
- Other tests.
  - Urine antigen assay for *S. pneumoniae* (sensitivity 50% to 80%, specificity 90%).
  - Microimmunofluorescence serologic testing for IgG or IgM to *C. pneumoniae.*
  - Urinary antigen assay and polymerase chain reaction assay for *M. pneumoniae.*
  - Throat swab and urinary or serologic antigen tests for *L. pneumophila.*
  - Tuberculosis is diagnosed with a combination of purified protein derivative (PPD) testing, acid-fast staining of the sputum, sputum cultures, and sputum nucleic acid amplification assays.
  - Viral pneumonia: routine sputum stains and cultures negative; antigen detection possible.
  - Sputum induction and staining with silver, monoclonal antibodies, or polymerase chain reaction testing for *P. jiroveci.*
- Bronchoscopy with biopsy may be necessary in high-risk patients and in those unresponsive to empiric therapy.

KEYS TO MANAGEMENT

Prevention

- Vaccination.
  - Pneumococcal vaccine in older adults has been shown to reduce the risk of community-acquired pneumonia and the frequency of severe disease requiring hospitalization.
  - Influenza vaccine reduces the risk for influenza pneumonia by 70% to 90% and can reduce disease severity. Medicare and Medicaid have authorized hospitals to administer and bill for vaccination without a physician's order.
- PPD screening for tuberculosis should be provided for recent close contacts of people with known active tuberculosis and health care workers at facilities where patients with active tuberculosis are treated; foreign-born persons from countries with a high prevalence of tuberculosis; homeless persons; persons living or working in facilities providing long-term care; HIV-infected people; injection drug users; patients receiving immunosuppressive therapy; and patients with end-stage renal disease, silicosis, diabetes mellitus, hematologic malignancies, prior gastrectomy, prior jejunoileal bypass, or severe malnutrition. Treatment for latent infection as evidenced by a positive PPD should include 6 to 9 months of isoniazid (or rifampin).
- Isolation precautions are indicated for immunocompromised patients or if tuberculosis, influenza, or SARS is suspected.
- For individuals with decreased mobility, positioning to prevent aspiration is helpful.
- Noninvasive ventilation should be used whenever possible. If mechanical ventilation is required, careful aseptic maintenance of humidifiers and circuits is vital, and the duration of intubation should be as short as possible. Oral antiseptics and antibiotics can reduce the risk of VAP; orotracheal intubation is preferred over nasotracheal, and continuous subglottic aspiration should be used.
- Prophylaxis against *Pneumocystis* pneumonia in immunocompromised individuals is recommended with trimethoprim-sulfamethoxazole, dapsone, pyrimethamine, pentamidine, or atovaquone.

Management of Acute Infection

- Oxygen and hydration if indicated; respiratory isolation.
- Consider hospitalization.
  - The Pneumonia Severity Index can be used to decide whether an individual needs hospitalization and is based on:
    1. Age older than 50.
    2. Coexistent illness (immunosuppression, COPD, congestive heart failure [CHF], cancer, liver or renal disease).
    3. Altered mental status.
    4. Pulse >125/minute; respiratory rate >30/minute; systolic blood pressure <90 mm Hg.
    5. Temperature <35° C or >40° C.
    6. PaO$_2$ <60 mm Hg or oxygen saturation <90%.
    7. Electrolyte disturbances such as acidosis, hyponatremia, or hyperglycemia.
    8. Uremia.
    9. Anemia.
    10. Pleural effusion on radiograph.
  - Other factors to be considered include living situation, accessibility to follow-up or emergency health care, and ability to tolerate oral medications.
- Antibiotics are indicated for bacterial, parasitic, or fungal pneumonia; antivirals are recommended for some but not all viral pneumonias.
  - Reduced mortality is related to rapid antibiotic administration; it is recommended that the first dose of antibiotics be given within 4 hours of arrival at the hospital.
  - Antimicrobial resistance is a major barrier to effective treatment (up to 25% of *S. pneumoniae* is resistant to three classes of antimicrobials).
  - Most often empiric coverage is used. Choice of empiric antibiotic varies based on outpatient versus inpatient, age, risk factors and coexistent conditions, and clinical presentation; common empiric antibiotic choices are listed in Table 7-1.
- Empiric antibiotic treatment of nosocomial pneumonia is based on whether the pneumonia occurs early in the course of hospitalization (more likely to be a community-acquired organism) or later in the hospitalization (more likely to be *Staphylococcus* or *Pseudomonas* infection, multidrug resistant, and/or highly virulent). These trends do not hold up in individuals who have VAP, have been recently previously hospitalized, or are immunocompromised.
  - In individuals with few risk factors and early onset pneumonia, broad-spectrum cephalosporins, fluoroquinolones, or β-lactam antibiotics are recommended for empiric care.
  - In ventilated or high-risk patients, an antipseudomonal cephalosporin or carbapenem in combination with a fluoroquinolone or an aminoglycoside and linezolid or vancomycin is currently recommended.
- If the etiologic organism is isolated, the choice of antibiotic type and dosage will be determined by antibacterial resistance/susceptibilities.
- Active tuberculosis requires the use of four antimicrobials including combinations of isoniazid, rifampin, pyrazinamide, ethambutol, and rifapentine. Multiple drug resistance is common in HIV infection, often leading to death of the infected individual.
- For influenza pneumonia, amantadine, rimantadine, oseltamivir, or zanamivir is effective if used within 48 hours of the onset of symptoms. Varicella zoster or herpes simplex pneumonia should be treated with intravenous acyclovir. There are no current recommended treatments for respiratory syncytial virus (RSV), parainfluenza, adenovirus metapneumovirus, or SARS (although interferon alfacon-1 plus steroid, or lopinavir/ritonavir or ribavirin plus steroid are being evaluated for SARS).
- *Pneumocystis* pneumonia is usually treated with trimethoprim-sulfamethoxazole, but side effects are common. Primaquine plus clindamycin, atovaquone, or pentamidine are alternative treatments. Antibiotics combined with prednisone improve gas exchange and outcomes.

TABLE **7-1**   Empiric Therapy for Community-Acquired Pneumonia, According to the Infectious Disease Society of America, 2003

Patient Variable	Preferred Treatment Options
Outpatient	
Previously healthy	
No recent antibiotic therapy	A macrolide or doxycycline
Recent antibiotic therapy	A respiratory fluoroquinolone alone, an advanced macrolide plus high-dose amoxicillin, or an advanced macrolide plus high-dose amoxicillin-clavulanate
Comorbidities (COPD, diabetes, renal or congestive heart failure, or malignancy)	
No recent antibiotic therapy	An advanced macrolide or a respiratory fluoroquinolone
Recent antibiotic therapy	A respiratory fluoroquinolone alone or an advanced macrolide plus a β-lactam
Suspected aspiration with infection	Amoxicillin-clavulanate or clindamycin
Influenza with bacterial superinfection	A β-lactam or a respiratory fluoroquinolone
Inpatient	
Medical ward	
No recent antibiotic therapy	A respiratory fluoroquinolone alone or an advanced macrolide plus a β-lactam
Recent antibiotic therapy	An advanced macrolide plus a β-lactam or a respiratory fluoroquinolone alone (regimen selected will depend on nature of recent antibiotic therapy)
ICU	
Pseudomonas infection is not an issue	A β-lactam plus either an advanced macrolide or a respiratory fluoroquinolone
Pseudomonas infection is not an issue but patient has a β-lactam allergy	A respiratory fluoroquinolone, with or without clindamycin
Pseudomonas infection is an issue	Either (1) an antipseudomonal agent plus ciprofloxacin, or (2) an antipseudomonal agent plus an aminoglycoside plus a respiratory fluoroquinolone or a macrolide
Pseudomonas infection is an issue but the patient has a β-lactam allergy	Either (1) aztreonam plus levofloxacin, or (2) aztreonam plus moxifloxacin or gatifloxacin, with or without an aminoglycoside
Nursing Home	
Receiving treatment in nursing home	A respiratory fluoroquinolone alone or amoxicillin-clavulanate plus an advanced macrolide
Hospitalized	Same as for medical ward and ICU

From Mandell, L. A., Bartlett, J. G., & Dowell, S. F. (2003). Update of practice guidelines for the management of community-acquired pneumonia in immunocompetent adults. *Clinical Infectious Diseases*, 37, 1405-1433. © 2003 by the Infectious Disease Society of America.

PATHOPHYSIOLOGY $\longrightarrow$	CLINICAL LINK
What is going on in the disease process that influences how the patient presents and how he or she should be managed?	*What should you do now that you understand the underlying pathophysiology?*
Factors such as smoking, immunocompromise, and recent hospitalization affect the severity of illness, which causative organism is most likely, and the potential for antibiotic resistance.	History of risk factors, underlying health of the patient, and where the infection was acquired are keys to assessment and management.
Aspiration of oropharyngeal secretions is the most common route of inoculation of the lower respiratory tract.	Identify patients at risk with compromised protection of the upper airway such as decreased level of consciousness or tracheal intubation.
Organism virulence factors such as the presence of capsules and toxins can influence the pathophysiology and the clinical manifestations of disease.	Characteristic patient presentations may be suggestive of the causative agent and may influence assessment and management.
Infection can spread via the blood to other organs and can lead to widespread inflammation.	Watch for meningitis, endocarditis, or the onset of sepsis, and systemic inflammatory response syndrome (SIRS).
The etiologic organism determines the patient presentation, clinical course, and management, but can be difficult to identify in an outpatient setting.	Sputum stains should be done in all inpatients with suspected pneumonia, and sputum and blood cultures should be done in hospitalized patients; empiric antibiotic therapy is often necessary.
Inflammation with alveolar filling leads to $\dot{V}/\dot{Q}$ mismatching and resultant hypoxemia.	Patients with significant respiratory distress or underlying lung disease should have arterial blood gas measurement and may require oxygen.
Community-acquired pneumonia (CAP) is commonly caused by *S. pneumoniae* or influenza and has a higher morbidity and mortality in older adults.	Vaccination for disease prevention, and rapid diagnosis and early antibiotic therapy is essential especially in the geriatric population.
Although appropriate support and rapid antibiotic therapy are successful in the majority of patients, there remains significant mortality, especially in older adults.	Patients should be evaluated for admission criteria and be hospitalized if indicated.

SUGGESTED READINGS

Alcon, A., Fabregas, N., & Torres, A. (2005). Pathophysiology of pneumonia. *Clinics in Chest Medicine, 26,* 39-46.

American Thoracic Society; Infectious Diseases Society of America. (2005). Guidelines for the management of adults with hospital-acquired, ventilator-associated, and healthcare-associated pneumonia. *American Journal of Respiratory Critical Care Medicine, 171,* 388-416.

Apisarnthanarak, A. & Mundy, L. M. (2005). Etiology of community-acquired pneumonia. *Clinics in Chest Medicine, 26,* 47-55.

Bartlett, J. G. (2004). Diagnostic test for etiologic agents of community-acquired pneumonia. *Infectious Disease Clinics of North America, 18,* 809-827.

Baughman, R. P. (2005). Microbiologic diagnosis of ventilator-associated pneumonia. *Clinics in Chest Medicine, 26,* 81-86.

Bazan-Socha, S., Bukiej, A., Marcinkiewicz, C., & Musial, J. (2005). Integrins in pulmonary inflammatory diseases. *Current Pharmaceutical Design, 11,* 893-901.

Beutz, M. A. & Abraham, E. (2005). Community-acquired pneumonia and sepsis. *Clinics in Chest Medicine, 26,* 19-28.

Blasi, F. (2004). Atypical pathogens and respiratory tract infections. *European Respiratory Journal, 24,* 171-181.

Bogaert, D., Hermans, P. W., Adrian, P. V., Rumke, H. C., & de Groot, R. (2004). Pneumococcal vaccines: an update on current strategies. *Vaccine, 22,* 2209-2220.

Chakinala, M. M. & Trulock, E. P. (2005). Pneumonia in the solid organ transplant patient. *Clinics in Chest Medicine, 26,* 113-121.

Cheng, V. C., Tang, B. S., Wu, A. K., Chu, C. M., & Yuen, K. Y. (2004). Medical treatment of viral pneumonia including SARS in immunocompetent adult. *Journal of Infection, 49,* 262-273.

Craven, D. E., Palladino, R., & McQuillen, D. P. (2004). Healthcare-associated pneumonia in adults: management principles to improve outcomes. *Infectious Disease Clinics of North America, 18,* 939-962.

Deng, J. C. & Standiford, T. J. (2005). The systemic response to lung infection. *Clinics in Chest Medicine, 26,* 1-9.

de Roux, A., Marcos, M. A., Garcia, E., Mensa, J., Santiago, E., Hartmut, L., & Torres, A. (2004). Viral community-acquired pneumonia in nonimmunocompromised adults. *Chest, 125,* 1343-1351.

Dezfulian, C., Shojania, K., Collard, H. R., Kim, H. M., Matthay, M. A., & Saint, S. (2005). Subglottic secretion drainage for preventing ventilator-associated pneumonia: a meta-analysis. [37 refs]. *American Journal of Medicine, 118,* 11-18.

Dreyfuss, D. & Ricard, J. D. (2005). Acute lung injury and bacterial infection. *Clinics in Chest Medicine, 26,* 105-112.

Fagon, J. Y. & Chastre, J. (2005). Antimicrobial treatment of hospital-acquired pneumonia. *Clinics in Chest Medicine, 26,* 97-104.

Feldman, C. (2005). Pneumonia associated with HIV infection. *Current Opinion in Infectious Diseases, 18,* 165-170.

File, T. M. Jr. (2003). Community-acquired pneumonia. *Lancet, 362,* 1991-2001.

File, T. M. Jr. (2004). Clinical efficacy of newer agents in short-duration therapy for community-acquired pneumonia. *Clinical Infectious Diseases, 39*(suppl 3), S159-S164.

File, T. M. Jr. (2004). *Streptococcus pneumoniae* and community-acquired pneumonia: a cause for concern. *American Journal of Medicine, 117*(suppl 3A), 39S-50S.

File, T. M. Jr. (2005). Community-associated methicillin-resistant *Staphylococcus aureus:* not only a cause of skin infections, also a new cause of pneumonia. *Current Opinion in Infectious Diseases, 18,* 123-124.

File, T. M. Jr. & Niederman, M. S. (2004). Antimicrobial therapy of community-acquired pneumonia. *Infectious Disease Clinics of North America, 18,* 993-1016.

Grap, M. J. & Munro, C. L. (2004). Preventing ventilator-associated pneumonia: evidence-based care. *Critical Care Nursing Clinics of North America, 16,* 349-358.

Hijazi, M. & Al Ansari, M. (2004). Therapy for ventilator-associated pneumonia: what works, what doesn't. *Respiratory Care Clinics of North America, 10,* 341-358.

Hirst, R. A., Kadioglu, A., O'Callaghan, C., & Andrew, P. W. (2004). The role of pneumolysin in pneumococcal pneumonia and meningitis. *Clinical & Experimental Immunology, 138,* 195-201.

Houck, P. M. & Bratzler, D. W. (2005). Administration of first hospital antibiotics for community-acquired pneumonia: does timeliness affect outcomes? *Current Opinion in Infectious Diseases, 18,* 151-156.

Jacobs, M. R. (2004). *Streptococcus pneumoniae:* epidemiology and patterns of resistance. *American Journal of Medicine, 117*(suppl 3A), 3S-15S.

Janssens, J. P. & Krause, K. H. (2004). Pneumonia in the very old. *The Lancet Infectious Diseases, 4,* 112-124.

Kadioglu, A. & Andrew, P. W. (2004). The innate immune response to pneumococcal lung infection: the untold story. *Trends in Immunology, 25,* 143-149.

Kola, A., Eckmanns, T., & Gastmeier, P. (2005). Efficacy of heat and moisture exchangers in preventing ventilator-associated pneumonia: meta-analysis of randomized controlled trials. *Intensive Care Medicine, 31,* 5-11.

Kollef, M. H. (2004). Prevention of hospital-associated pneumonia and ventilator-associated pneumonia. *Critical Care Medicine, 32,* 1396-1405.

Leroy, O. & Soubrier, S. (2004). Hospital-acquired pneumonia: risk factors, clinical features, management, and antibiotic resistance. *Current Opinion in Pulmonary Medicine, 10,* 171-175.

Mandell, L. A. (2004). Epidemiology and etiology of community-acquired pneumonia. *Infectious Disease Clinics of North America, 18,* 761-776.

Mandell, L. A. (2005). Antimicrobial resistance and treatment of community-acquired pneumonia. *Clinics in Chest Medicine, 26,* 57-64.

Mandell, L. A., Bartlett, J. G., & Dowell, S. F. (2003). Update of practice guidelines for the management of community-acquired pneumonia in immunocompetent adults. *Clinical Infectious Diseases, 37,* 1405-1433.

Marrie, T. J. (2004). Empiric treatment of ambulatory community-acquired pneumonia: always include treatment for atypical agents. *Infectious Disease Clinics of North America, 18,* 829-841.

Martin, T. R. (2004). Direct lung injury by bacteria: clarifying the tools of the trade. *Critical Care Medicine, 32,* 2360-2361.

Mason, C. M. & Nelson, S. (2005). Pulmonary host defenses and factors predisposing to lung infection. *Clinics in Chest Medicine, 26,* 11-17.

Metlay, J. P. (2004). Antibacterial drug resistance: implications for the treatment of patients with community-acquired pneumonia. *Infectious Disease Clinics of North America, 18,* 777-790.

Morris, C. G., Safranek, S., & Neher, J. (2005). Clinical inquiries. Is sputum evaluation useful for patients with community-acquired pneumonia? *Journal of Family Practice, 54,* 279-281.

Musher, D. M., Dowell M. E., Shortridge, V. D. (2003). Emergence of macrolide resistance during treatment of pneumococcal pneumonia. *New England Journal of Medicine, 346,* 630-631.

Neralla, S. & Meyer, K. C. (2004). Drug treatment of pneumococcal pneumonia in the elderly. *Drugs & Aging, 21,* 851-864.

Niederman, M. S. (2004). Review of treatment guidelines for community-acquired pneumonia. *American Journal of Medicine, 117*(suppl 3A), 51S-57S.

Niederman, M. S., Mandell, L. A., & Anzueto A. (2001). Guidelines for the management of adults with community-acquired pneumonia. *American Journal of Respiratory and Critical Care Medicine,* 163, 1730-1754.

Okamoto, T., Akuta, T., Tamura, F., van, D. V. & Akaike, T. (2004). Molecular mechanism for activation and regulation of matrix metalloproteinases during bacterial infections and respiratory inflammation. *Biological Chemistry,* 385, 997-1006.

Osmon, S. B. & Kollef, M. H. (2005). Prevention of pneumonia in the hospital setting. *Clinics in Chest Medicine,* 26, 135-142.

Ploutte, J. F. Jr. & Martin, D. R. (2004). Re-evaluation of the therapy of severe pneumonia caused by *Streptococcus pneumoniae. Infectious Disease Clinics of North America,* 18, 963-974.

Rello, J., Diaz, E., & Rodriguez, A. (2005). Etiology of ventilator-associated pneumonia. *Clinics in Chest Medicine,* 26, 87-95.

Restrepo, M. I. & Anzueto, A. (2005). Antimicrobial treatment of community-acquired pneumonia. *Clinics in Chest Medicine,* 26, 65-73.

Schwartz, D. B. (2004). Hospital-acquired pneumonia-evolving knowledge. *Current Opinion in Pulmonary Medicine,* 10(suppl 1), S9-S13.

Shorr, A. F. (2005). Preventing pneumonia: the role for pneumococcal and influenza vaccines. *Clinics in Chest Medicine,* 26, 123-134.

Shulman, L. & Ost, D. (2000). Managing infection in the critical care unit: how can infection control make the ICU safe? *Critical Care Clinics,* 21, 111-128.

Stalam, M. & Kaye, D. (2004). Antibiotic agents in the elderly. *Infectious Disease Clinics of North America,* 18, 533-549.

Steele, C., Shellito, J. E., & Kolls, J. K. (2005). Immunity against the opportunistic fungal pathogen Pneumocystis. *Medical Mycology,* 43, 1-19.

Stevens, D. L., Dotter, B., & Madaras-Kelly, K. (2004). A review of linezolid: the first oxazolidinone antibiotic. *Expert Review of Antiinfective Therapy,* 2, 51-59.

Szabo, D., Silveira, F., Fujitani, S., & Paterson, D. L. (2005). Mechanisms of resistance of bacteria causing ventilator-associated pneumonia. *Clinics in Chest Medicine,* 26, 75-79.

Thomas, C. F. Jr., & Limper, A. H. (2004). *Pneumocystis* pneumonia. *New England Journal of Medicine,* 350, 2487-2498.

Waterer, G. W. (2005). Monotherapy versus combination antimicrobial therapy for pneumococcal pneumonia. *Current Opinion in Infectious Diseases,* 18, 157-163.

Waterer, G. W. & Wunderink, R. G. (2005). Genetic susceptibility to pneumonia. *Clinics in Chest Medicine,* 26, 29-38.

Wazir, J. F., & Ansari, N. A. (2004). *Pneumocystis carinii* infection. Update and review. *Archives of Pathology & Laboratory Medicine,* 128, 1023-1027.

Wellington, K. & Noble, S. (2004). Telithromycin. *Drugs,* 64, 1683-1694.

Weyers, C. M. & Leeper, K. V. (2005). Nonresolving pneumonia. *Clinics in Chest Medicine,* 26, 143-158.

Whitney, C. G. & Harper, S. A. (2004). Lower respiratory tract infections: prevention using vaccines. *Infectious Disease Clinics of North America,* 18, 899-917.

Woodhead, M. (2004). Community-acquired pneumonia: severity of illness evaluation. *Infectious Disease Clinics of North America,* 18, 791-807.

Wunderink, R. G. & Waterer, G. W. (2004). Community-acquired pneumonia: pathophysiology and host factors with focus on possible new approaches to management of lower respiratory tract infections. *Infectious Disease Clinics of North America,* 18, 743-759.

Pneumonia

INITIAL HISTORY

- 63-year-old female bank manager presents to the clinic in November.
- 1-week history of upper respiratory symptoms; 2-day history of increasing fever, malaise, nausea.
- Cough productive "rusty"-colored sputum.
- Right-sided pleuritic chest pain.

Question 1. *What other questions would you like to ask?*

ADDITIONAL HISTORY

- No rashes, headache, or vomiting; no hemoptysis; some friends recently ill.
- Nonsmoker; denies HIV risk (husband died 10 years ago; has not been sexually active since his death).
- Negative past medical history.
- No known allergies.
- Usual childhood immunizations; had a flu shot this year.

Question 2. *What is your differential diagnosis based on the history?*

PHYSICAL EXAMINATION

- Alert, flushed, coughing, and using accessory muscles; in moderate respiratory distress.
- T = 39.2° C orally; P = 128 and regular; RR = 32; BP = 110/80, no orthostatic changes.
- Skin warm, moist, and flushed without rashes.

HEENT, Neck

- PERRLA, fundi without lesions; nares slightly flared, purulent drainage visible; ears with slight serous fluid seen behind both tympanic membranes.
- Pharynx erythematous with purulent postnasal drainage, no tonsillar exudate, mucous membranes moist; neck with mild anterior cervical adenopathy.

Lungs

- Normal chest configuration; mild use of accessory muscles; decreased expansion (splinting) over right chest; dullness to percussion and increased fremitus at the right anterior axillary line.
- Inspiratory crackles (rales), egophony, and whispered pectoriloquy at right anterior axillary line; clear left lung, right upper and right lower lobes.

Cardiac, Abdomen, Extremities, Neurologic

- Regular rate and rhythm, tachycardic with I/VI SEM left lower sternal border.
- Abdomen soft, nontender; no organomegaly; bowel sounds present.
- Extremities warm and flushed without cyanosis or edema, no clubbing.
- Alert and oriented; strength, sensation, and deep tendon reflexes 2+ and symmetric.

Question 3. *What are the significant findings on physical exam and what might they mean?*

Question 4. *What laboratories should now be obtained?*

LABORATORY RESULTS

- ABG: pH = 7.56, $PaCO_2$ = 26, PaO_2 = 90 on room air; HCT 42%; WBC 15,000; 5% bands, 83% PMNs, 10% lymphocytes, 3% monocytes, 1% eosinophils; LFTs normal.

Question 5.   *What is the A-a gradient?*

Question 6.   *What do the rest of the laboratory test results indicate?*

CHEST RADIOGRAPH

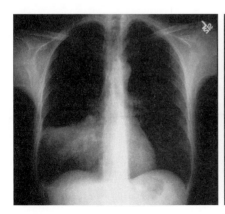 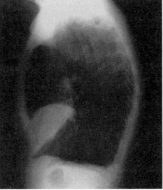

Question 7.   *What are the major findings on the chest radiograph?*

Question 8.   *What are the possible diagnoses now?*

Question 9.   *How should this patient be managed?*

Lung Cancer

DEFINITION

- Malignant neoplasms arising from the bronchial epithelium.
- The World Health Organization pathologic classification scheme for lung tumors includes more than 100 subcategories, but generally, lung cancer can be classified as non–small cell lung carcinoma (NSCLC, 85% of all lung cancers) and small cell lung carcinoma (SCLC, 15% of all lung cancers).
- NSCLC can be further divided into three subtypes:
    - Adenocarcinoma (including bronchoalveolar carcinoma).
    - Squamous cell carcinoma.
    - Large cell undifferentiated carcinoma.

EPIDEMIOLOGY

- Number one cancer killer of men and women in the United States (>172,000 cases estimated for 2005 with >163,000 deaths) and in the world.
- Lung cancer death rates in U.S. men have declined significantly since 1990; however, rates for women have only just begun to level off (increased 600% between 1930 and 1997). Although improvements in short-term survival for advanced-stage cancers have been achieved, overall survival for lung cancer remains at 15% to 17%.
- First-degree relatives who smoke have a 2.5-fold increase in risk over those who smoke who have no family history.
- 80% to 90% of lung cancer is caused by cigarette smoking. In the United States, smoking rates declined during recent decades, but have leveled off at about 25% of the overall population; 30% of high school students and 10% of middle school students continue to smoke. There is a dose-response relationship between the number of cigarettes smoked over time and cancer risk. The number of years smoked has the greatest effect (e.g., tripling the duration of smoking results in a 100-fold increase in cancer risk), thus people who begin smoking at an early age have a much higher risk for lung cancer. Low-tar, low-nicotine cigarettes are associated with changes in smoking patterns (e.g., increased puff rate and depth) such that the intake of these substances is not substantially different than from regular cigarettes.
- The risk of environmental tobacco smoke (passive smoking) has been estimated to be between 1.4 and 3 times the unexposed risk, especially if exposed as children. Nonsmoking spouses of smokers have a greater than 30% increase in lung cancer risk and may account for up to 3000 deaths in the United States per year.
- Other risks include outdoor and indoor air pollution, radiation, radon, and industrial exposure (e.g., asbestos, arsenic, sulfur dioxide, formaldehyde, silica, nickel, chloroethyl ethers, polycyclic aromatic hydrocarbons).
- Airflow obstruction as in chronic obstructive pulmonary disease (COPD) is an important indicator of increased risk for lung cancer. Fibrotic lung disease (e.g., pneumoconiosis) is also associated with an increased risk.

PATHOPHYSIOLOGY

Genetics

- Heritable vulnerability to lung cancer has been attributed to gene polymorphisms that make it more difficult for an affected individual to detoxify smoke carcinogens. Among those genes that have shown strong associations with lung cancer risk are polymorphisms of glutathione S-transferase M1, *CYP1A1, CYP2A6,* and *CYP2D6* genes. Inherited mutations in DNA repair genes such as *p53* and *XRCC1* have also been implicated.
- Chromosomal "instability" is common to many lung tumors, resulting in deletions from several chromosomes including 3p, 4q, 8p, and 17p. Translocations also are common.
- A lung tumor results from many exposures to carcinogens rather than one initiating event ("multi-hit"); it is estimated that it takes between 10 and 20 genetic mutations to create a tumor. Some of the more common acquired mutations that have been identified include:
    - Deletion of the short arm of chromosome 3.
    - Activation of oncogenes *(jun, fos, ras,* and *myc).*
    - Inactivation of tumor suppressor genes *(p53, p16, RB, DKN2).*
    - Activation of growth factor genes *ERBB* and *EGFR.*

Tumor Progression

- Cigarette smoke contains many potential carcinogens (nitrosamines [NNK], and polycyclic aromatic hydrocarbons [PAH]) that can cause deoxyribonucleic acid (DNA) mutations (Figure 8-1).
- These mutations lead to increasingly anaplastic-appearing cells that gradually develop the ability for uncontrolled cell division (including loss of telomerase), insensitivity to antigrowth signals, evasion of apoptosis, angiogenesis, tissue invasion, and metastasis.
- The bronchial epithelium goes through several stages, from hyperplasia to dysplasia to carcinoma in situ to invasive carcinoma.
- The type of lung cancer depends on the cell of origin.
    - NSCLC.
        1. Adenocarcinoma arises from glandular cells in bronchial epithelium and is often peripheral in location and metastasizes early.
            a. Most common type of lung cancer, especially in women. The pathologic appearance of this tumor can be difficult to distinguish from metastasis from another primary adenocarcinoma (e.g., colon, breast, prostate).

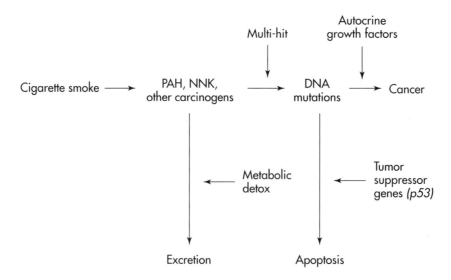

FIGURE **8-1 Pathogenesis of Lung Cancer.**

b. Includes bronchoalveolar carcinoma, which arises from the smallest bronchioles and alveolar septae. This tumor often appears as an infiltrate rather than a mass on radiograph. It is not associated with smoking.

2. Squamous cell carcinoma arises from squamous bronchial epithelium and is often central in location. It is a frequent cause of occult cancer found on chest radiograph and metastasizes late. It frequently metastasizes to bone and can often cause hypercalcemia.

3. Large cell carcinoma is composed of highly anaplastic cells and is an aggressive tumor with early metastasis.

- SCLC arises from neuroendocrine cells in bronchi; it is a very aggressive tumor and has usually metastasized by the time of diagnosis. It is frequently associated with paraneoplastic production of hormones such as antidiuretic hormone (syndrome of inappropriate antidiuretic hormone [SIADH]) and adrenocorticotropic hormone (Cushing syndrome).

PATIENT PRESENTATION

- A few patient presentation "pearls":
  - 90% of patients with lung cancer are symptomatic at presentation.
  - Hemoptysis in the absence of bronchitis, pneumonia, or sinus infection must be evaluated for possible bronchogenic cancer.
  - An enlarged supraclavicular node is suggestive of cancer in a smoker.
  - Patients may present with a pneumonia that does not clear with antibiotics. Smokers always need follow-up after treatment for pneumonia or bronchitis.
  - Patients may present with what appears to be an endocrine disorder (e.g., Cushing syndrome, SIADH). The underlying cancer is often found late.

History

History of smoking; family history; asbestos exposure; other industrial exposures; pulmonary radiation; history of COPD.

Symptoms

Result from tumor invasion of specific sites or systemic reaction: (1) *endobronchial:* cough, hemoptysis, dyspnea, atelectasis, postobstructive pneumonia; (2) *peripheral (pleura and chest wall):* chest discomfort, pleural effusions; (3) *regional spread:* dysphagia, stridor, chest pain, syncope, face and arm pain or swelling, hoarseness; (4) *metastasis:* pain in involved organs, edema, bone pain, seizures, headache; (5) *endocrine (paraneoplastic):* hyperpigmentation, centripetal obesity, syncope; and (6) *constitutional:* weight loss, anorexia, weakness, fever.

Examination

Cachexia, fever, stridor, vocal cord paralysis, dullness to percussion; localized wheeze, crackles that do not clear with antibiotics, adenopathy (supraclavicular, axillary); decreased strength or sensation in arm, digital clubbing, and focal neurologic findings.

DIFFERENTIAL DIAGNOSIS

- Benign lung tumors (hematomas, granulomas).
- Other primary tumor metastatic to the lung (breast, prostate, colon, testicular, etc.).
- COPD.
- Pneumonia.
- Tuberculosis.
- Inhaled foreign body.
- Endocrine disorder.

KEYS TO ASSESSMENT

- The goals of assessment are to (1) establish the presence of a primary lung cancer, (2) determine its cell type, and (3) stage the tumor.
- Many cancers remain occult until late stage.
- Although it is clear that diagnosing and treating lung cancer early in its development are crucial for long-term survival, screening for the presence of asymptomatic tumors in high-risk individuals remains controversial.
    - The U.S. Preventive Services Task Force in 2004 concluded that the evidence remains insufficient to recommend for or against screening asymptomatic individuals with sputum cytology, chest radiograph, or low-dose helical (spiral) computed tomography (LDCT). The National Lung Screening Trial is now underway to further evaluate whether screening should be recommended.
    - LDCT is more sensitive than radiograph or sputum cytology and did detect potentially curable lesions in several studies (tumors caught early have a much-improved prognosis in response to treatment).
    - There is evidence that high-risk patients (i.e., >40 years old, >30 pack/years smoking, airway obstruction, symptoms) benefit from screening; however, effects on mortality and cost effectiveness remain unclear.
- Lung cancer is often first suspected in someone due to the finding of a mass lesion on chest radiograph.
    - Unfortunately, chest radiograph has a relatively low sensitivity and can miss a significant number of small tumors.
    - A solitary pulmonary nodule is common, but some nodules have features suggestive of invasive carcinoma (high-risk lesions are not densely calcified and have spiculations).
    - The radiograph should be evaluated for evidence of hilar or mediastinal adenopathy, pleural disease (e.g., effusions for which thoracentesis might be diagnostic), and bone lesions.
- Sputum cytology sensitivity has been estimated to be only 20% to 30% overall. Sensitivity is improved when this test is used in individuals who have a proximally located tumor on radiograph or who have hemoptysis. In addition, the use of monoclonal antibody and specialized staining techniques can help in diagnosis.
- Bronchoscopy can often visualize endobronchial and relatively proximal tumors and may allow for biopsy. Transbronchial needle aspiration (TBNA) also can be used. Other techniques include fluorescence bronchoscopy (identify very early endobronchial lesions) and endoscopic ultrasound (define the size and depth of the lesion).
- Computed tomography (CT) with transthoracic needle aspiration (TTNA) of the tumor is used for small and peripheral lesions that are not likely to be seen via bronchoscopy.
- Serum laboratory results may include pancytopenia from marrow involvement, electrolyte imbalances due to endocrine disorders (e.g., hypercalcemia, hyponatremia), and elevation of liver enzymes (from hepatic metastases).
- Once the diagnosis of lung cancer has been made, a careful staging work-up is crucial for appropriate choice of management.
    - Mediastinoscopy or positron emission tomography (PET) to evaluate for mediastinal involvement (PET can also be used to evaluate the primary tumor).
    - CT or magnetic resonance imagery (MRI) to evaluate for metastases to abdomen and bone (also consider bone scan). Combined whole-body CT and PET scanning has a high sensitivity for staging of lung cancer.
    - Bone marrow biopsy is indicated for SCLC (likelihood of bone marrow metastases).
    - Head CT or MRI to evaluate for brain metastases in SCLC (present in 10% at time of diagnosis).
- Staging.
    - Staging is crucial for determining best treatment and predicting outcomes.
    - NSCLC: The tumor, node, and metastasis (TNM) system for the evaluation of tumor size, nodal involvement, or metastases determines resectability and prognosis.

- • SCLC: Thorough metastatic work-up to find the few (<15%) that have "limited disease" versus "extensive stage disease" (metastasis at the time of diagnosis).
- Performance status testing (e.g., Karnofsky scale) is used to assess for operability and prognosis; ventilation/perfusion ($\dot{V}/\dot{Q}$) lung scanning can help to assess viability of tumor-involved lobe.
- Specific protein and hormone markers are becoming increasingly useful for following the cancer once the diagnosis is made, and are being evaluated for screening (e.g., tumor-liberated protein [TLP]), cytokeratin 19, CYFRA 21-1, neuron-specific enolase (NSE), and tissue polypeptide antigen (TPA).

KEYS TO MANAGEMENT

- Prevention.
    - Smoking cessation is the only truly effective preventive measure, although risk may take more than 40 years to return to normal (half of all new lung cancer diagnoses are in former smokers).
    - A diet high in fruits and vegetables has been associated with a reduction in cancer risk, but results have not been consistent among studies.
    - Antioxidants have had mixed results. Some studies have shown that retinoids and vitamin E levels can reduce risk; however, other studies have shown a significant increase in risk of cancer in smokers taking β-carotene.
    - Other experimental chemoprevention methods include cyclooxygenase (COX)-2 inhibitors, epidermal growth factor inhibitors, and angiogenesis inhibitors.
- General management.
    - A tissue diagnosis is important: NSCLC and SCLC are treated differently.
    - Once the diagnosis is established, a well-informed patient can best choose if and what kind of therapy is appropriate.
    - Treating the symptoms of the cancer can be as important as treating the cancer itself, especially in advanced disease. Maximizing nutrition and watching for depression and anxiety help prepare the patient for treatment. Cancer cachexia is a major contributor to morbidity; drugs that may be helpful include metoclopramide, tetrahydrocannabinol, megestrol, and steroids.
- Surgery.
    - In all types, lung cancer is treated surgically if at all possible. Complete resection of the tumor offers the best hope for cure.
    - The aggressiveness of the planned surgery depends on the patient's operability as well as the tumor's resectability. Optimizing the patient's strength and stamina preoperatively is important.
    - In NSCLC, relatively healthy patients may be surgical candidates even if they are stage III; in SCLC, very few tumors are found to be resectable.
    - Surgical procedures range from thoracoscopic wedge resection to lobectomy to lung resection with mediastinal dissection.
- Chemotherapy.
    - Platinum-based chemotherapy, especially if used as adjuvant therapy for advanced stage tumors, can improve survival in NSCLC.
    - The most commonly used drug regimens include cisplatin in combination with etoposide or gemcitabine. Other regimens use vinorelbine, paclitaxel, docetaxel, adriamycin, cyclophosphamide, vincristine, carboplatin, irinotecan, topotecan, edatrexate, ifosfamide, or pemetrexed.
    - SCLC responds dramatically to platinum-based chemotherapy (with or without etoposide) with a tumor response rate of 75% to 80% and a marked increase in survival time (e.g., increases median survival from less than 3 months to 7 to 10 months in cases of extensive disease); however, relapse is inevitable in most patients.

- Radiation.
    - Radiation can be effective as an adjuvant to surgery and/or chemotherapy for NSCLC. It can also be used for palliative care.
    - SCLC responds well to radiation, but the extension of survival time is not as great as with chemotherapy. Prophylactic cranial irradiation can reduce relapse in the brain, but is associated with considerable toxicity and little survival benefit.
- Other therapies.
    - Endobronchial laser therapy, brachytherapy, photodynamic therapy, electrocoagulation, and bronchoplasty with stent placement can be considered in appropriate patients.
    - Biologic response modifiers such as growth factor inhibitors (e.g., gefitinib, an inhibitor of epidermal growth factor receptor [EGFR]), angiogenesis inhibitors (e.g., squalamine, protease inhibitors, interferon, carboxyamidotriazole [CAI]), and anti–vascular endothelial growth factor [VEGF]) have all been well tolerated. Biologic response modifiers have resulted in improvements in disease-related symptoms and have induced radiographic tumor regressions in patients with NSCLC unresponsive to standard chemotherapy.
    - A new class of antineoplastic agents that bind to retinoid receptors called rexinoids (e.g., bexarotene) is being studied.
    - Bisphosphonates (e.g., zoledronic acid) may be used to prevent and treat bone metastases.
    - Low-molecular-weight heparin (e.g., dalteparin) or warfarin should be used to treat those patients who develop venous thromboembolism in association with their cancer and/or cancer treatment.
    - Gene therapy and genomic surgery have shown promise; studies are ongoing.
        1. Prodrug therapy (e.g., herpes simplex virus thymidine kinase vector delivery and activation with ganciclovir).
        2. Gene transfer via vectorology (e.g., transfecting tumor cells with *p53*).
        3. Antisense therapy.
        4. Tumor vaccines.
        5. Genomic surgery.

PATHOPHYSIOLOGY ⟶	CLINICAL LINK
What is going on in the disease process that influences how the patient presents and how he or she should be managed?	*What should you do now that you understand the underlying pathophysiology?*
Most lung cancer arises from bronchial epithelial cells that have been exposed to cigarette smoke. ⟶	Smoking cessation is the most important step toward prevention; the risk increases with pack-years of smoking and takes many years to return to normal (if ever).
Multiple genetic mutations have been found in cancerous lung cells including oncogenes, loss of tumor-suppressor genes, chromosomal deletions, and other tumor growth and drug resistance–inducing gene abnormalities. ⟶	The ability to detect early genetic changes may lead to early detection of susceptible high-risk individuals, and may lead to gene therapies. Current work is around transplanting "wild" *p53* genes and monoclonal antibodies to growth factor receptors.
Lung tumors cause symptoms by endobronchial obstructions, pleural disease, metastases, endocrine abnormalities, and constitutional abnormalities, but may be asymptomatic until late stage. ⟶	Screening remains controversial, but studies using low-dose helical computed tomography (CT scanning) are increasingly positive.
Lung tumors produce a large number of tumor markers such as TLP, CYFRA 21-1, NSE, and TPA. ⟶	Although current methods of identifying tumor markers are not adequate for general screening, they are useful for following response to treatment, relapse, and prognosis.
Lung tumors depend upon numerous substances such as growth factors, angiogenesis factors, antiapoptosis factors, and proteases in order to grow, survive, and invade tissues. ⟶	Biologic response–modifying therapies and gene therapies are being investigated that interfere with the many features of malignancy in lung cancer.
NSCLC cells are relatively resistant to chemotherapy; complete tumor removal is the only hope for cure; SCLC is rarely adequately localized for surgery but responds dramatically to chemotherapy prolonging life even though it rarely cures. ⟶	Patients with NSCLC should be nutritionally, physically, educationally, and emotionally optimized to increase operability—a decision to add chemotherapy should take into account the likelihood of gain versus toxicity; those with SCLC should receive the same supportive care to minimize toxicity to chemotherapeutic agents.

SUGGESTED READINGS

Alberg, A. J. & Samet, J. M. (2003). Epidemiology of lung cancer. *Chest*, 123(suppl 1), 21S-49S.

American Society of Clinical Oncology. (2003). American Society of Clinical Oncology policy statement update: tobacco control—reducing cancer incidence and saving lives. *Journal of Clinical Oncology*, 21(14), 2777-2786.

Baselga, J. & Arteaga, C. L. (2005). Critical update and emerging trends in epidermal growth factor receptor targeting in cancer. *Journal of Clinical Oncology*, 23, 2445-2459.

Beckles, M. A., Spiro, S. G., Colice, G. L., & Rudd, R. M. (2003). Initial evaluation of the patient with lung cancer: symptoms, signs, laboratory tests, and paraneoplastic syndromes. *Chest*, 23(suppl 1), 97S-104S.

Bedor, M., Alexander, C., & Edelman, M. J. (2005). Management of common symptoms of advanced lung cancer. *Current Treatment Options in Oncology*, 6, 61-68.

Belani, C. P. (2005). Adjuvant and neoadjuvant therapy in non-small cell lung cancer. *Seminars in Oncology*, 32, S9-S15.

Benhamou, S. & Sarasin, A. (2005). ERCC2/XPD gene polymorphisms and lung cancer: a HuGE review. *American Journal of Epidemiology*, 161, 1-14.

Berenson, J. R. (2005). Recommendations for zoledronic acid treatment of patients with bone metastases. *Oncologist*, 10, 52-62.

Birnbaum, A. & Ready, N. (2005). Gefitinib therapy for non-small cell lung cancer. *Current Treatment Options in Oncology*, 6, 75-81.

Blum, R. (2004). Adjuvant chemotherapy for lung cancer—a new standard of care. *New England Journal of Medicine*, 350(4), 404-405.

Budde, L. S. & Hanna, N. H. (2005). Antimetabolites in the management of non-small cell lung cancer. *Current Treatment Options in Oncology*, 6, 83-93.

Chan, A. L., Yoneda, K. Y., Allen, R. P., & Albertson, T. E. (2003). Advances in the management of endobronchial lung malignancies. *Current Opinion in Pulmonary Medicine*, 9(4), 301-308.

Cullen, M. (2003). Lung cancer. 4: chemotherapy for non-small cell lung cancer: the end of the beginning. *Thorax*, 58(4), 352-356.

Dragnev, K., Stover, D., & Dmitrovsky, E. (2003). Lung cancer prevention: the guidelines. *Chest*, 123, 60S-71S.

Fong, K. M., Sekido, Y., Gazdar, A. F., & Minna, J. D. (2003). Lung cancer. 9: molecular biology of lung cancer: clinical implications. *Thorax*, 58(10), 892-900.

Franklin, W. A. (2001). Pathology of lung cancer. *Journal of Thoracic Imaging*, 15(1), 3-12.

Gadgeel, S. & Kalemkerian, G. (2003). Racial differences in lung cancer. *Cancer Metastasis Reviews*, 22(1), 39-46.

Gotay, C. C. (2005). Behavior and cancer prevention. *Journal of Clinical Oncology*, 23, 301-310.

Granville, C. A. & Dennis, P. A. (2005). An overview of lung cancer genomics and proteomics. *American Journal of Respiratory Cell and Molecular Biology*, 32, 169-176.

Hege, K. & Carbone, D. (2003). Lung cancer vaccines and gene therapy. *Lung Cancer*, 41(suppl 1), S103-S113.

Henschke, C. I., Yankelevitz, D. F., McCauley, D. I., Libby, D. M., Pasmantier, M. W., & Smith, J. P. (2003). Guidelines for the use of spiral computed tomography in screening for lung cancer. *European Respiratory Journal—Supplement*, 39, 45s-51s.

Horiike, A. & Saijo, N. (1954). Small-cell lung cancer: current therapy and novel agents. *Oncology (Huntington)*, 19, 47-52.

Humphrey, L. L., Teutsch, S., & Johnson, M. (2004). U.S. Preventive Services Task Force. Lung cancer screening with sputum cytologic examination, chest radiography, and computed tomography: an update for the U.S. Preventive Services Task Force. *Annals of Internal Medicine*, 140(9), 740-753.

Kelley, M. & McCrory, D. (2003). Prevention of lung cancer. Summary of published evidence. *Chest*, 123, 50S-59S.

Maciag, A. & Anderson, L. M. (2005). Reactive oxygen species and lung tumorigenesis by mutant K-ras: a working hypothesis. *Experimental Lung Research*, 31, 83-104.

Malaiyandi, V., Sellers, E. M., & Tyndale, R. F. (2005). Implications of CYP2A6 genetic variation for smoking behaviors and nicotine dependence. *Clinical Pharmacology and Therapeutics*, 77, 145-158.

Mascaux, C., Iannino, N., Martin, B., Paesmans, M., Berghmans, T., Dusart, M., Haller, A., Lothaire, P., Meert, A. P., Noel, S., Lafitte, J. J., & Sculier, J. P. (2005). The role of RAS oncogene in survival of patients with lung cancer: a systematic review of the literature with meta-analysis. *British Journal of Cancer*, 92, 131-139.

Mavi, A., Lakhani, P., Zhuang, H., Gupta, N. C., & Alavi, A. (2000). Fluorodeoxyglucose-PET in characterizing solitary pulmonary nodules, assessing pleural diseases, and the initial staging, restaging, therapy planning, and monitoring response of lung cancer. *Radiologic Clinics of North America*, 43, 1-21.

Mountain, C. (1997). Revisions in the international system for staging lung cancer. *Chest*, 11(6), 1710.

Oyama, T., Osaki, T., Baba, T., Nagata, Y., Mizukami, M., So, T., Nakata, S., Ichiki, Y., Uramoto, H., Sugaya, M., Yoshimatsu, T., Morita, M., Hanagiri, T., Sugio, K., Kawamoto, T., & Yasumoto, K. (2005). Molecular genetic tumor markers in non-small cell lung cancer. *Anticancer Research*, 25, 1193-1196.

Pao, W. & Miller, V. A. (2005). Epidermal growth factor receptor mutations, small-molecule kinase inhibitors, and non-small-cell lung cancer: current knowledge and future direction. *Journal of Clinical Oncology*, 23, 2556-2568.

Patel, J., Bach, P., & Kris, M. (2004). Lung cancer in U.S. women: a contemporary epidemic. *Journal of the American Medical Association*, 291, 1763-1768.

Petty, T. L. (2003). Sputum cytology for the detection of early lung cancer. *Current Opinion in Pulmonary Medicine*, 9(4), 309-312.

Raez, L., Samuels, M., & Lilenbaum, R. (2005). Combined modality therapy for limited-disease small cell lung cancer. *Current Treatment Options in Oncology*, 6, 69-74.

Reck, M. & Gatzemeier, U. (2005). Gefitinib ("Iressa"): a new therapy for advanced non-small-cell lung cancer. *Respiratory Medicine*, 99, 298-307.

Rigas, J. R. & Dragnev, K. H. (2005). Emerging role of rexinoids in non-small cell lung cancer: focus on bexarotene. *Oncologist*, 10, 22-33.

Rivera, M. P., Detterbeck, F., & Mehta, A. C. (2003). Diagnosis of lung cancer. The guidelines. *Chest*, 123, 129S-136S.

Saba, N. & Khuri, F. (2005). The role of bisphosphonates in the management of advanced cancer with a focus on non-small-cell lung cancer. Part 1: Mechanisms of action, role of biomarkers and preclinical applications. *Oncology*, 68, 10-17.

Saba, N. & Khuri, F. (2005). The role of bisphosphonates in the management of advanced cancer with a focus on non-small-cell lung cancer. Part 2: Clinical studies and economic analyses. *Oncology*, 68, 18-22.

Saha, D., Pyo, H., & Choy, H. (2003). COX-2 inhibitor as a radiation enhancer: new strategies for the treatment of lung cancer. *American Journal of Clinical Oncology*, 26(4), S70-S74.

Sandler, A. B. (2003). Chemotherapy for small cell lung cancer. *Seminars in Oncology*, 30(1), 9-25.

Scagliotti, G. V. (2005). Pemetrexed plus carboplatin or oxaliplatin in advanced non-small cell lung cancer. *Seminars in Oncology*, 32, S5-S8.

Schrump, D. S. (2004). Genomic surgery for lung cancer. *Journal of Surgical Research*, 117(1), 107-113.

Sekido, Y., Fong, K. M., & Minna, J. D. (2003). Molecular genetics of lung cancer. *Annual Review of Medicine, 54*, 73-87.

Seve, P. & Dumontet, C. (2005). Chemoresistance in non-small cell lung cancer. *Current Medicinal Chemistry—Anti-Cancer Agents, 5*, 73-88.

Simon, G. R. & Wagner, H. (2003). American College of Chest Physicians. Small cell lung cancer. *Chest, 123*(suppl 1), 259S-271S.

Smith, W. & Khuri, F. (2004). The care of the lung cancer patient in the 21st century, a new age. *Seminars in Oncology, 31* (2 suppl 4), 11-15.

Socinski, M. A. (2005). Pemetrexed (Alimta) in small cell lung cancer. *Seminars in Oncology, 32*, S1-S4.

Socinski, M. A., Stinchcombe, T. E., & Hayes, D. N. (2005). The evolving role of pemetrexed (Alimta) in lung cancer. *Seminars in Oncology, 32*, S16-S22.

Spira, A. & Ettinger, D. S. (2004). Multidisciplinary management of lung cancer. *New England Journal of Medicine, 350*(4), 379-392.

Tarro, G., Perna, A., & Esposito, C. (2005). Early diagnosis of lung cancer by detection of tumor liberated protein. *Journal of Cellular Physiology, 203*, 1-5.

Tibes, R., Trent, J., & Kurzrock, R. (2005). Tyrosine kinase inhibitors and the dawn of molecular cancer therapeutics. *Annual Review of Pharmacology and Toxicology, 45*, 357-384.

Tomida, S., Yatabe, Y., Yanagisawa, K., Mitsudomi, T., & Takahashi, T. (2005). Throwing new light on lung cancer pathogenesis: updates on three recent topics. *Cancer Science, 96*, 63-68.

Travis, W. D., Colby, T. V., Corrin, B., Shimosato, Y., & Brambilla, E. (1999). Histological Typing of Tumours of Lung and Pleura. In Sobin, L. H. (editor). *World Health Organization International Classification of Tumours,* ed. 3, Berlin, Heidelberg, New York: Springer-Verlag.

van der Hoijdon, H. F. & Heijdra, Y. F. (2005). Extrapulmonary small cell carcinoma. *Southern Medical Journal, 98*, 345-349.

Vignot, S., Spano, J. P., Lantuejoul, S., Andre, F., Le Chevalier, T., & Soria, J. C. (2005). Chemoprevention of lung cancer. *Recent Results in Cancer Research, 166*, 145-165.

Wieder, R. (2005). Insurgent micrometastases: sleeper cells and harboring the enemy. *Journal of Surgical Oncology, 89*, 207-210.

Winterhalder, R. C., Hirsch, F. R., Kotantoulas, G. K., Franklin, W. A., & Bunn, P. A., Jr. (2004). Chemoprevention of lung cancer—from biology to clinical reality. *Annals of Oncology, 15*(2), 185-196.

Zacharski, L. R., Prandoni, P., & Monreal, M. (2005). Warfarin versus low-molecular-weight heparin therapy in cancer patients. *Oncologist, 10*, 72-79.

Lung Cancer

INITIAL HISTORY

- 52-year-old female smoker with a history of emphysema comes in for routine yearly checkup.
- Over the past year she has experienced a mild increase in her chronic dyspnea, with a dramatic worsening over the past 4 months.
- She has begun coughing more frequently.

Question 1.   *Based on this limited history, what is your differential diagnosis?*

Question 2.   *What questions about her symptoms would you like to ask this patient?*

ADDITIONAL HISTORY

- Patient is now dyspneic on walking to her bathroom and back.
- Denies change in her chronic production of scant white sputum.
- Denies fever.
- Denies hemoptysis.
- Has had increasing discomfort in her left chest with deep breathing and cough.
- Denies substernal chest pain, palpitations, or edema.
- Admits to a 10-pound weight loss over the past year.

Question 3. *What questions about her past medical history would you like to ask?*

MEDICAL HISTORY

- 60 pack/year smoker.
- Emphysema diagnosed 5 years ago; managed with inhaled β-agonist and ipratropium.
- Latest pulmonary function testing was at the time of emphysema diagnosis; patient does not know results.
- Had pneumonia 3 years ago; treated at home.
- Seen in the emergency department with bronchitic exacerbation of her emphysema last year.
- Denies ever having angina or congestive heart failure (CHF) symptoms.
- No known allergies.
- Takes no other medications.
- Had influenza vaccine last year and pneumococcal vaccine 2 years ago.

PHYSICAL EXAMINATION

- Alert, thin woman who looks older than stated age; in mild respiratory distress; became dyspneic moving from chair to examination table.
- T = 37° C orally; P = 90 and regular; RR = 22 and mildly labored; BP = 124/74.
- Pursed-lip breathing, no cyanosis.

HEENT, Skin, Neck
- PERRLA, pharynx clear, pursed-lip breathing.
- No rashes.
- No thyromegaly or bruits.

Lungs
- Increase in anteroposterior (AP) diameter of the thorax.
- Use of accessory muscles of respiration.
- Chest tympanitic without dullness.
- Diaphragms low with decreased excursion bilaterally.
- Scattered wheezes without crackles or rhonchi.
- No rubs.

Cardiac
- Apical pulse felt at fifth intercostal space at the midclavicular line.
- Regular rate and rhythm; no murmurs or gallops.

Abdomen, Extremities, Neurologic
- Bowel sounds present, no masses, tenderness, or organomegaly.
- No edema, pulses full, no bruits, no digital clubbing.
- Cognition intact; strength, sensation, and reflexes normal and symmetric; gait steady.

Question 4.   *What are the pertinent positives and negatives on the examination and what might they mean?*

Question 5.   *How has your differential diagnosis changed?*

Question 6.   *What diagnostic tests would be indicated now?*

INITIAL DIAGNOSTICS

- Arterial blood gases: pH = 7.42, $PaCO_2$ = 48, PaO_2 = 68 on room air.
- Electrocardiogram (ECG) reveals sinus tachycardia without evidence of ischemia.
- Pulmonary function testing shows forced expiratory volume in 1 second (FEV_1) = 55% of predicted.
- Electrolytes, liver function tests, and CBC reveal an elevated bicarbonate level, but are otherwise normal.

CHEST RADIOGRAPH AND READING

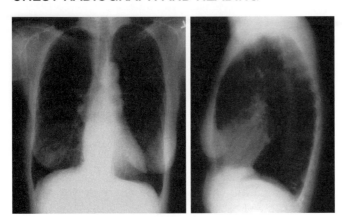

Small, peripheral, noncalcified, and spiculated lesion in the upper left lobe.
- No evidence of hilar adenopathy.
- No evidence of soft tissue or bone disease.
- Lungs otherwise show hyperexpansion, bullae, and scarring consistent with emphysema.

SPUTUM CYTOLOGY

- Atypical cells are suggestive of carcinoma but not diagnostic.

Question 7.   *What is your interpretation of these findings?*

Question 8.   *What other studies might be indicated?*

ADDITIONAL EVALUATION

- Patient is referred to a pulmonologist.
- CT scan reveals the lesion seen on radiograph, no mediastinal disease.
- Bronchoscopy cannot visualize the lesion; CT-guided fine-needle aspiration reveals adenocarcinoma.
- Stage is 1.
- V̇/Q̇ scanning and functional status testing indicates operability.
- There is no evidence of another primary tumor.

Question 9.   *The patient returns for advice prior to surgery, what should she be told?*

POSTOPERATIVE FOLLOW-UP

- Three weeks after left upper lobectomy, the patient returns feeling weak and still having pain at the incision site.
- Dyspnea is gradually improving after getting much worse immediately postop.
- Patient reports that she was told that the operation was a success; there were no complications.
- Patient is concerned about whether she will need chemotherapy and about her prognosis.

Question 10.   *What can you tell the patient now?*

Breast Cancer

DEFINITION

- Neoplastic proliferation of breast cells.
- Classification of breast tumors includes the following most common types.
    - Ductal.
        1. Carcinoma in situ (DCIS).
        2. Infiltrating ductal.
        3. Others include medullary, tubular, mucinous, papillary, adenocystic, carcinosarcoma.
    - Lobular.
        1. Carcinoma in situ (LCIS).
        2. Infiltrating lobular.

EPIDEMIOLOGY

- It is the most common cancer affecting women in the United States and is the cause of 32% of all cancers in women (estimated 211,240 cases in 2005) and 15% of all cancer deaths in women (estimated 40,410 deaths in 2005).
- One in every seven women in the United States develops breast cancer by the age of 85.
- Half of all cases of breast cancer occur in women older than 65 years of age, but breast cancer is the major cause of death for women ages 35 to 54.
- Risk factors.
    - Age.
    - Family history: having a first-degree relative with breast cancer confers a relative risk of 1.4 to 13.6 (risk increases if relative was young at the time of diagnosis).
    - Genetics.
        1. Hereditary (approximately 10% of cases).
            a. Mutation of *BRCA1* gene.
                i. Multiple types of mutations have been described in this tumor suppressor gene located on the long arm of chromosome 17.
                ii. Occurs in approximately 1 in 500 women in the United States and can be inherited from either parent.
                iii. Confers a 50% to 65% lifetime risk for breast cancer and a 40% lifetime risk for ovarian cancer.
                iv. Also increases the risk of a second breast cancer to 20% at 5 years and 15% at 15 years.
            b. Mutation of *BRCA2* gene.
                i. Located on chromosome 13.
                ii. Confers an 85% lifetime risk for female breast cancer and 10% to 20% risk of ovarian cancer.

        iii. Confers a 6% lifetime risk of male breast cancer (100-fold increase in risk over the general population).

        iv. Also associated with an increased risk for pancreatic cancer.

     c. Li Fraumeni syndrome.

        i. A germline deletion of *p53* (a tumor suppressor gene that normally induces apoptosis in mutated cells).

        ii. Risk for breast cancer is 49% by age 44 and 60% lifetime risk.

        iii. Also confers an increased risk for brain, lung, and adrenal tumors, as well as sarcomas and leukemias.

     d. Genetic screening is indicated if:

        i. Known mutation in family.

        ii. Personal or family history of breast cancer before age 35.

        iii. Personal or family history of ovarian cancer.

        iv. Multiple family history of pancreatic cancer.

        v. Patient without known breast cancer but strong family history of breast cancer and no available relatives for testing.

  2. Sporadic (approximately 90% of cases).

     a. Multiple mutations have been identified including oncogenes HER2/*neu* (*ERBB2*), *MYC, CPY17,* and *CCND1* and tumor suppressor genes *p53, RB1,* and *CDKN2.*

     b. Acquired mutations in *BRCA1* and *BRCA2* are rare in sporadic tumors, but there may be some depression in these tumor suppressor gene products.

     c. Hypermethylation of tumor suppressor genes and hypomethylation of proto-oncogenes have also been implicated in the genetics of breast cancer.

- Reproductive and hormonal.
  1. Increased risk due to increased estrogen exposure to breast tissue.
     a. Early menarche (younger than age 12) or late menopause (older than age 55).
     b. High levels of serum estradiol especially in postmenopausal women.
     c. Hormone replacement therapy with conjugated equine estrogen and medroxyprogesterone acetate.
  2. Increased risk due to prolonged time of Lob 1 tissue vulnerability (see below).
     a. Nulliparity or late first pregnancy (older than age 30).
     b. No breast-feeding.
  3. No effect on risk.
     a. Termination of pregnancy.
     b. Oral contraceptive use (even in *BRCA1*-positive individuals).
  4. Decreased risk.
     a. Pregnancy.
     b. Breast-feeding.
- **Environmental:** Incidence of breast cancer cannot be fully explained by genetic and reproductive and hormonal risks, but direct links to environmental toxins have been difficult to prove.
  1. Dietary fats: Still controversial; recent data continue to suggest obesity is a risk factor.
  2. Smoking: Data are suggestive that nicotine and *N*-nitrosamines (carcinogens in cigarette smoke) concentrate in breast tissue, and that postmenopausal women smokers with a polymorphism of the gene responsible for detoxifying these carcinogens (slow acetylators) have an increased risk for breast cancer.
  3. Alcohol: Risk increases at a level of two drinks per day (folate may ameliorate this risk).
  4. Radiation: Chest radiation increases breast cancer risk three to eight times normal depending on the location and intensity of the treatment (30% risk at 20 years' postradiation).

5. Antibiotics: Cause and effect not yet established, but previous use of antibiotics is associated with a significantly increased risk for breast cancer.
        6. Other potential carcinogens are being evaluated.
   • Proliferative breast disease (including fibrocysts).
        1. Affects 1.2 million women in the United States.
        2. Atypical hyperplasia is a step along the continuum from normal breast tissue to carcinoma in situ and increases risk for breast cancer fourfold.
        3. Increased mammographic density is an independent risk factor.
   • **History of breast cancer:** Nearly half of women will develop carcinoma in situ in contralateral breast, with 1% per year developing invasive carcinoma.
   • **Gail model** can be used to estimate overall breast cancer risk; see http://bcra.nci.nih.gov/brc. Other models include Cuzick and Claus.

PATHOPHYSIOLOGY

• Gene mutation.
   • Acquired mutation of proto-oncogenes (formation of oncogenes) and tumor suppressor genes begins the process of uncontrolled cellular proliferation.
        1. The tumor suppressor gene *p53* is a transcription regulator, genomic stabilizer, participant in deoxyribonucleic acid (DNA) repair, inhibitor of cell cycle progression, and a facilitator of apoptosis of damaged cells.
        2. Homozygous *p53* mutation results in a loss of these critical barriers to tumor formation and is a commonly acquired mutation in breast cancer as well as many other tumors such as lung cancer.
   • Likelihood of homozygous mutations of tumor suppressor genes is enhanced if there is an inherited mutation of the gene (e.g., *BRCA1*).
        1. *BRCA1* gene product is a growth inhibitor that controls proliferation of breast cells; this gene product is lost if the gene is mutated at both alleles (homozygous mutation).
        2. The amount of abnormal cellular proliferation seen with mutation of *BRCA1* is influenced by the presence of other modifier genes, location of the mutation on the gene, and life-style factors.
        3. Breast tissue from individuals with mutated *BRCA1* gene contains high levels of actively dividing cells (Lob 1 [see below]) even after pregnancy.
   • Other mutations occur that contribute to tumor growth and invasion (multi-hit) including those that support:
        1. Autocrine growth factor stimulation.
        2. Increased growth factor receptors.
        3. Angiogenesis.
        4. Cellular invasion and metastasis.
        5. Evasion of the immune system.
• Progressive cellular and tissue changes.
   • Mammary cancer originates in areas of the breast called Lob 1, which are undifferentiated terminal structures of the mammary gland.
        1. Lob 1 contains many undifferentiated cells with high proliferation rates and is particularly sensitive to carcinogens. This type of breast tissue is present in greatest amounts between the onset of menarche and the first pregnancy, making that the most vulnerable time for mutagenesis.
        2. Pregnancy, especially with breast-feeding, reduces the amount of Lob 1 in the breast. Most of Lob 1 matures to what is called Lob 2 or Lob 3, which is more differentiated and less vulnerable to mutagenesis.
   • Progressive tissue changes include atypical hyperplasia followed by carcinoma in situ (CIS), followed by invasive carcinoma; characterized by increasing numbers of mutations leading to invasion and metastasis.

- Cell adhesion molecules.
    1. One of the most important adhesion molecules in breast tissue is E-cadherin, which is down-regulated in breast cancer.
    2. Tumor cells escape normal cell–basement membrane adhesion molecules, which allows them to invade surrounding tissues.
- Matrix metalloproteinases and cathepsins.
    1. Breast cancers are high in these extracellular proteinases that modulate cell–basement membrane interactions and degrade the basement membrane itself.
    2. This allows for invasion of surrounding tissues and blood vessels and facilitates metastasis.
- Parathyroid-related hormone is often produced by tumor cells and increases osteoclastic activity, thus facilitating bone metastasis.
- Tumor cells secrete growth factors that stimulate neovascularization of tumor (angiogenesis factors), allowing for increased primary tumor size and access to blood vessels for metastasis.
- Immune system evasion.
    1. Breast cancer is associated with a progressive cellular immune deficiency with decreased number and function of T lymphocytes, macrophages, and natural killer cells.
    2. Some oncogenic peptides (e.g., MUC-1) can induce T cell apoptosis and may inhibit tumor-infiltrating lymphocyte function.
    3. Many tumor cells mutate such that they lose their tumor-specific immunogenic antigens and are therefore undetectable to the immune system.
- Multidrug resistance genes code for glycoprotein "efflux pump" that decreases intracellular concentration of anticancer agents.
- Growth factors and their receptors.
    - Estrogen.
        1. Estrogen is a growth factor for breast cell proliferation, is required for normal breast cell function, and causes breast maturation and proliferation. Withdrawal of estrogen, such as with menopause, results in apoptosis of breast cells.
        2. Estrogen receptors (ERs) are cytosol proteins present in normal breast cells and on many cancer cells of primary breast tumors and their metastases.
        3. In cancer cells with ERs, estrogen stimulation of these receptors results in increased cell proliferation.
        4. 60% of primary tumors are considered ER positive (ER+), which means that the majority of cancer cells in the tumor have ERs present. These tumors have slower growth rates, better prognoses, and better responses to hormone manipulation therapy than tumors made up of cancer cells lacking ERs.
        5. The loss of the ERs results from methylation of the cellular DNA. These ER negative (ER–) tumors are capable of autocrine stimulation independent of estrogen and thus are resistant to endocrine therapy and tend to be more aggressive. Experimentally, blocking of DNA methylation can restore ERs, which may improve tumor responsiveness to hormone therapy.
        6. Progesterone receptors are also found on normal breast cells and 50% of ER+ tumors, and indicate tumors that are most responsive to endocrine therapy.
    - Insulin-like growth factors.
        1. Insulin-like growth factor-1 (IGF_1) is important for normal mammary development, but is also a mitogen for cancer cells and promotes anchorage-independent growth.
        2. Insulin-like growth factor-2 (IGF_2) regulates IGF_1 activity; receptors for these growth factors are found on ER+ tumors and are suggestive of increased responsiveness to endocrine therapy.
    - Epidermal growth factor (EGF).

1. EGF leads to increased mitosis and resistance to tamoxifen.
2. It binds via HER receptors and increases HER2/*neu* expression (present on 20% to 30% of breast tumors).

- Cyclooxygenase (COX)-2 is found in increased amounts in breast cancer tissue and can serve as a growth factor, decreases apoptosis, and enhances angiogenesis.

PATIENT PRESENTATION

History

Medical history of breast disease; reproductive history (age of onset of menses, number of pregnancies and age at first pregnancy, age of onset of menopause); history of hormone use; family history of breast cancer; alcohol consumption, smoking history, diet. Risk assessment (consider Gail or Claus model).

Symptoms

Breast and axillary symptoms (mass, pain, nipple discharge or retraction, skin changes, arm swelling); symptoms of metastasis (headache, seizure, bone pain, dyspnea); fatigue; weight loss.

Examination

Breast mass (size, location, consistency, fixation to skin); skin changes (erythema, dimpling, edema); nipple changes (retraction, thickening, discharge); nodal status (axillary—size, location fixation, supraclavicular nodes).

DIFFERENTIAL DIAGNOSIS

- Fibroadenoma.
- Mastitis.
- Metastasis from another primary tumor.

KEYS TO ASSESSMENT

- Screening for breast cancer in the general public:
  - Monthly self-examination plus yearly clinical examination and mammography.
  - All major health care groups recommend beginning screening at age 40. Overall, mammographic screening reduces breast cancer mortality by 20% to 35%, but 95% of women with an abnormal mammogram do not have breast cancer—risks of false negatives and false positives continue to be discussed. Digital mammography is more sensitive and specific, especially in women with large, dense breasts.
- Screening of women with an inherited predisposition (*BRCA1, BRCA2*, Li Fraumeni) for breast cancer.
  - Monthly self-examination beginning at age 18; semiannual clinical examination after age 25.
  - Annual magnetic resonance imaging (MRI) is more sensitive and specific than mammogram for *BRCA*-positive individuals.
  - Ovarian cancer surveillance with yearly transvaginal ultrasound and serum CA-125 (not very sensitive, new markers being tested).
- Assessment once a breast mass is discovered.
  - Careful history of risk factors and family history.
  - Further diagnostic tests.
    1. Mammography: Digital mammography is more sensitive (88% to 95%).
    2. Ultrasound: Differentiates cystic versus solid masses; helps to find palpable masses not seen on mammogram (especially in young women) and can be used to guide biopsy.
    3. MRI: Especially useful for finding other foci of cancer in patients with a known primary tumor as well as for guiding biopsy of small lesions and for staging.

    4. Mammoscintigraphy: Highly sensitive but does not differentiate malignant from benign and cannot be used to guide biopsy.

    5. Positron emission tomography: Still being tested but highly sensitive.

- Tissue diagnosis.
    1. Fine-needle aspiration (FNA): 98% accuracy if combined with examination and mammogram.
    2. Core biopsy, excisional biopsy (lumpectomy).
    3. Ductal lavage: Provides very early detection in high-risk patients.
    4. Micro-array analysis of tissue allows for genetic analysis and may influence treatment decisions.
- Assessing nodal status.
    1. Sentinel node biopsy: If the sentinel node is negative, then it is highly likely that the rest of the axillary nodes are negative, thus it may eliminate the need for more extensive axillary biopsies; cytokeratin immunohistochemical staining can pick up micrometastases, further increasing the sensitivity of this procedure.
    2. Axillary dissection: If sentinel node is positive, full axillary dissection to assess the extent of nodal involvement is indicated.
    3. If axilla is clinically positive, fine-needle aspiration of a suspicious node before surgery is indicated.
- Recent reports suggest that testing for circulating tumor cells may be useful in determining prognosis in advanced breast cancer.
- Chest radiograph and bone scan are indicated if symptomatic for metastases or if alkaline phosphatase level is elevated.
- Staging: Tumor, nodes, and metastasis (TNM) system; determines type of surgery and adjuvant therapies.

KEYS TO MANAGEMENT

- Prevention of breast cancer.
    - Smoking cessation, decrease alcohol intake.
    - Exercise and weight loss.
    - Diet.
        1. Increase intake of ω-3 fatty acids and monounsaturated fats.
        2. Results of vitamin and antioxidant studies mixed; increased folate intake helpful.
        3. Studies on fiber intake are mixed.
        4. Phytoestrogens/isoflavones: Epidemiologic studies have suggested that these may compete for estrogen receptors and be protective, but studies are mixed and some investigators are concerned about a potential proestrogenic effect of some of these compounds.
    - Selective estrogen receptor modulators (SERMs).
        1. Tamoxifen: Approved in 1998 for the primary prevention of breast cancer in high-risk patients; clearly reduces risk for breast cancer but increases the risk of endometrial cancer and thromboembolic disease.
        2. Latest data suggest raloxifene for 8 years can decrease the risk of invasive breast cancer by as much as 60% (Continuing Outcomes Relevant to Evista [CORE] trial).
        3. Fluvestrant is a new SERM with no agonist effects at the estrogen receptors; being evaluated for treatment but may be considered for prevention.
    - Aromatase inhibitors.
        1. Anastrozole (Arimidex), exemestane (Aromasin), and letrozole (Femara).
        2. The Arimidex, Tamoxifen, Alone or in Combination (ATAC) study compared anastrozole to tamoxifen in women with known breast cancer and found that anastrozole reduced the risk of the developing breast cancer in the contralateral breast more effectively than tamoxifen.

3. Aromatase inhibitors have no estrogen agonist properties and are not a risk for endometrial cancer, thromboembolic disease, or vaginal bleeding, whereas at the same time are associated with fewer hot flashes than tamoxifen but do have an increase in bone fracture risk over tamoxifen.

4. A primary prevention trial with exemestane (National Cancer Institute of Canada Clinical Trials Group MAP.3) is under way.

- COX-2 inhibitors: The Women's Health Initiative found that use of aspirin and nonsteroidal anti-inflammatory drugs (NSAIDs) was associated with a significant reduction in the risk for breast cancer.

    1. Two or more NSAIDs per week for 5 to 9 years reduced risk by 21%.
    2. Aspirin 325 mg/day reduced the risk by 22%, ibuprofen 200 mg/day reduced the risk by nearly 50%.
    3. Phase II trials with combination aromatase inhibitor and celecoxib are continuing (MAP.3).

- Prophylactic mastectomy reduces risk of breast cancer by more than 90% in high-risk women (but obviously does not protect against ovarian cancer in *BRCA1*- or *BRCA2*-positive individuals).

- Oophorectomy can be used to reduce the risk of breast cancer in high-risk individuals by as much as 50%.

- Surgical management.
    - Lumpectomy: Used when the tumor is small and there is no obvious axillary involvement; results clearly show survival similar to mastectomy, even if axillary nodes are positive.
    - Modified radical mastectomy: Preserves pectoralis muscles with improved cosmesis over radical mastectomy; it is used for stage II to stage III if there is no tumor fixation to muscle.
    - Total mastectomy (simple mastectomy): No axillary dissection; it is used for CIS, prophylactic removal of a contralateral breast, local recurrence after lumpectomy, and palliation of bulky tumor.
    - Radical mastectomy: The breast is removed en bloc, along with all axillary nodes and both pectoralis muscles. It is used if the tumor is fixed to the pectoralis muscle or if there is bulky axillary involvement.

- Radiation.
    - Local breast radiation after breast-conserving surgery reduces the risk of local recurrence. Newer accelerated hypofractionated radiotherapy equally effective but administered over a shorter time frame. Locoregional irradiation (includes regional lymph nodes) improves outcomes in large primary tumors after mastectomy.
    - Concern for increased risk of secondary breast cancers.

- Endocrine therapy (hormone manipulation).
    - It is used as adjuvant therapy after surgery for both pre- and postmenopausal women with ER+ tumors.
    - It increases survival and disease-free survival, and decreases the risk for disease in the contralateral breast.
    - Aromatase inhibitors block estrogen synthesis and have been found to be more effective and safer than tamoxifen in postmenopausal women in most studies.
    - Tamoxifen: Significant decrease in recurrence rate (47%) and death rate (26%) and reduces the risk of recurrence in the contralateral breast in pre- and postmenopausal individuals with ER+ tumors. Tamoxifen continues to be the endocrine treatment of choice for premenopausal women. It should not be used for more than 5 years because there is no additional benefit. It confers an increased risk of endometrial cancer and thromboembolic disease.
    - Raloxifene probably has equal antitumor effects when compared with tamoxifen and with less risk of endometrial cancer; studies ongoing.
    - Others: Luteinizing hormone–releasing hormone agonists and ovarian ablation can be considered in selected individuals.

- Chemotherapy.
    - Adjunctive chemotherapy substantially improves long-term, disease-free survival in both pre- and postmenopausal women up to age 70 with node-positive and node-negative disease.
    - Doxorubicin (Adriamycin), cyclophosphamide (Cytoxan), and docetaxel are widely used agents for most regimens. Many patients receive combination chemotherapy containing an anthracycline (e.g., doxorubicin) or a fluoropyrimidine (e.g., capecitabine). Vinlorelbine is also used. Dose-dense regimens are used to maximize effects while minimizing side effects.
    - High-dose chemotherapy plus supporting granulocyte colony–stimulating factor (G-CSF) and blood stem cells has been found to be an effective and safe outpatient regimen for selected patients.
    - Preoperative chemotherapy can shrink tumors and make lumpectomy a surgical option in some patients with a relatively large primary tumor.
    - High-dose chemotherapy and an autologous bone marrow transplant provide dramatic results in a few patients, but are associated with high morbidity and mortality and cannot be recommended for most patients.
- Trastuzumab (Herceptin): Monoclonal antibody to HER2/*neu* growth factor receptor can be used alone or with chemotherapy for tumors that have a mutation of this receptor. It improves response rates and survival time but is associated with significant myocardial toxicity when used with some chemotherapeutic agents. It recently has been approved for use as adjuvant therapy for node-positive breast cancer.
- Bisphosphonates reduce the risk of skeletal metastases; alendronate has been used, but clodronate, pamidronate, zoledronate, and ibandronate are more effective in preventing and treating bone metastases and for reducing serum hypercalcemic complications.
- Targeted therapy for specific types of tumors based on molecular genetics is increasingly possible.
- Tumor vaccines for tumor-associated antigens, matrix metalloproteinase and cathepsin blockers, and antiangiogenic drugs are under investigation.

PATHOPHYSIOLOGY $\longrightarrow$	CLINICAL LINK
What is going on in the disease process that influences how the patient presents and how he or she should be managed?	*What should you do now that you understand the underlying pathophysiology?*
Strong genetic component to risk including *BRCA1*, *BRCA2*, and Li Fraumeni. $\longrightarrow$	The family history is important, and genetic screening should be considered.
Between puberty and pregnancy, the breast contains high amounts of Lob 1. Breast cancer is most likely to arise in Lob 1 tissue. $\longrightarrow$	Nulliparous women are at greater risk; pregnancy, especially with lactation, reduces risk. The interval between puberty and the first pregnancy may be the most vulnerable time for exposure to carcinogens.
Numerous environmental toxins accumulate in breast tissue and are associated with carcinogenesis. $\longrightarrow$	Women should be counseled to exercise and avoid smoking and should consider dietary modification including reduced fat and alcohol intake. These measures may be most important between puberty and the first pregnancy.
Mutation of the *BRCA1* gene leads to loss of an important growth inhibitor and is associated with high amounts of Lob 1 even in multiparous women. $\longrightarrow$	Patients with *BRCA1* gene require careful screening beginning at age 25.
When estrogen receptors are stimulated, they cause the production of growth factors that induce cell division. $\longrightarrow$	Tamoxifen and raloxifene are selective estrogen receptor modulators (SERMs) that block estrogens effect on the breast and can be used in both prevention and treatment. Raloxifene may turn out to be better and safer. Aromatase inhibitors prevent the production of estrogen in postmenopausal women and are more effective than SERMs for many postmenopausal women.
Positive axillary nodes indicate spread of the primary tumor. $\longrightarrow$	Axillary sentinel node biopsy or full axillary dissection is crucial to proper staging for treatment.
When the tumor is small, there is less likelihood of tumor spread. $\longrightarrow$	Early stage tumors should be treated with lumpectomy; most patients will also be treated with adjuvant endocrine, radiation, and/or chemotherapy.

SUGGESTED READINGS

Arthur, D. W. & Vicini, F. A. (2005). Accelerated partial breast irradiation as a part of breast conservation therapy. *Journal of Clinical Oncology, 23,* 1726-1735.

Arun, B. & Goss, P. (2004). The role of COX-2 inhibition in breast cancer treatment and prevention. *Seminars in Oncology, 31,* 22-29.

Bartus, C. M., Schreiber, J. S., & Kurtzman, S. H. (2000). Palliative approaches to the patient with breast cancer. *Surgical Oncology Clinics of North America, 13,* 517-530.

Baum, M. (2004). The endocrine management of postmenopausal women with early breast cancer. *Breast Cancer, 11,* 15-19.

Benda, R. K., Mendenhall, N. P., Lind, D. S., Cendan, J. C., Shea, B. F., Richardson, L. C., & Copeland, E. M., III (2004). Breast-conserving therapy (BCT) for early-stage breast cancer. *Journal of Surgical Oncology, 85,* 14-27.

Beral, V., Bull, D., Doll, R., Peto, R., Reeves, G., & Collaborative Group on Hormonal Factors in Breast Cancer. (2004). Breast cancer and abortion: collaborative reanalysis of data from 53 epidemiological studies, including 83,000 women with breast cancer from 16 countries. *Lancet, 363,* 1007-1016.

Berenson, J. R. (2005). Recommendations for zoledronic acid treatment of patients with bone metastases. *Oncologist, 10,* 52-62.

Biganzoli, L., Minisini, A., Aapro, M., & Di Leo, A. (2004). Chemotherapy for metastatic breast cancer. *Current Opinion in Obstetrics & Gynecology, 16,* 37-41.

Biglia, N., Defabiani, E., Ponzone, R., Mariani, L., Marenco, D., & Sismondi, P. (2004). Management of risk of breast carcinoma in postmenopausal women. *Endocrine-Related Cancer, 11,* 69-83.

Bold, R. J. (2005). Standardization of sentinel lymph node biopsy in breast carcinoma. *Cancer, 103,* 444-446.

Burstein, H. J., Polyak, K., Wong, J. S., Lester, S. C., & Kaelin, C. M. (2004). Ductal carcinoma in situ of the breast. *New England Journal of Medicine, 350,* 1430-1441.

Campos, S. M. (2004). Aromatase inhibitors for breast cancer in postmenopausal women. *Oncologist, 9,* 126-136.

Carmichael, A. R. & Bates, T. (2004). Obesity and breast cancer: a review of the literature. *Breast, 13,* 85-92.

Carrick, S., Ghersi, D., Wilcken, N., & Simes, J. (2004). Platinum containing regimens for metastatic breast cancer. *Cochrane Database of Systematic Reviews* CD003374.

Chang, J. C., Hilsenbeck, S. G., & Fuqua, S. A. (2005). Genomic approaches in the management and treatment of breast cancer. *British Journal of Cancer, 92,* 618-624.

Cooper, C. R., Sikes, R. A., Nicholson, B. E., Sun, Y. X., Pienta, K. J., & Taichman, R. S. (2004). Cancer cells homing to bone: the significance of chemotaxis and cell adhesion. *Cancer Treatment & Research, 118,* 291-309.

Coradini, D. & Daidone, M. G. (2004). Biomolecular prognostic factors in breast cancer. *Current Opinion in Obstetrics & Gynecology, 16,* 49-55.

Coyle, Y. M. (2004). The effect of environment on breast cancer risk. *Breast Cancer Research and Treatment, 84,* 273-288.

Cuzick, J. (2005). Aromatase inhibitors for breast cancer prevention. *Journal of Clinical Oncology, 23,* 1636-1643.

Dellapasqua, S. & Castiglione-Gertsch, M. (2005). The choice of systemic adjuvant therapy in receptor-positive early breast cancer. *European Journal of Cancer, 41,* 357-364.

Dellapasqua, S. Colleoni, M., Gelber, R. D., & Goldhirsch, A. (2005). Adjuvant endocrine therapy for premenopausal women with early breast cancer. *Journal of Clinical Oncology, 23,* 1736-1750.

Duffy, M. J. (2005). Predictive markers in breast and other cancers: a review. *Clinical Chemistry, 51,* 494-503.

Duncan, A. M. (2004). The role of nutrition in the prevention of breast cancer. *AACN Clinical Issues, 15,* 119-135.

Dunn, B. K., Wickerham, D. L., & Ford, L. G. (2005). Prevention of hormone-related cancers: breast cancer. *Journal of Clinical Oncology, 23,* 357-367.

Edwards, A. G., Hailey, S., & Maxwell, M. (2004). Psychological interventions for women with metastatic breast cancer. *Cochrane Database of Systematic Reviews* CD004253.

Elmore, J. G., Armstrong, K., Lehman, C. D., & Fletcher, S. W. (2005). Screening for breast cancer. *Journal of the American Medical Association, 293,* 1245-1256.

Eng-Wong, J. & Zujewski, J. A. (2004). Raloxifene and its role in breast cancer prevention. *Expert Review of Anticancer Therapy, 4,* 523-532.

Esteva, F. J. (2004). Monoclonal antibodies, small molecules, and vaccines in the treatment of breast cancer. *Oncologist, 9*(suppl 3), 4-9.

Eubank, W. B. & Mankoff, D. A. (2004). Current and future uses of positron emission tomography in breast cancer imaging. *Seminars in Nuclear Medicine, 34,* 224-240.

Fabian, C. J. & Kimler, B. F. (2005). Selective estrogen-receptor modulators for primary prevention of breast cancer. *Journal of Clinical Oncology, 23,* 1644-1655.

Foulkes, W. D. (2004). *BRCA1* functions as a breast stem cell regulator. *Journal of Medical Genetics, 41,* 1-5.

Freedman, O. C., Verma, S., & Clemons, M. J. (2005). Using aromatase inhibitors in the neoadjuvant setting: evolution or revolution? *Cancer Treatment Reviews, 31,* 1-17.

Galvao, D. A. & Newton, R. U. (2005). Review of exercise intervention studies in cancer patients. *Journal of Clinical Oncology, 23,* 899-909.

Hamilton, A. & Hortobagyi, G. (2005). Chemotherapy: what progress in the last 5 years? *Journal of Clinical Oncology, 23,* 1760-1775.

Hodgson, S. V., Morrison, P. J., & Irving, M. (2004). Breast cancer genetics: unsolved questions and open perspectives in an expanding clinical practice. *American Journal of Medical Genetics, 129C,* 56-64.

Hylton, N. (2005). Magnetic resonance imaging of the breast: opportunities to improve breast cancer management. *Journal of Clinical Oncology, 23,* 1678-1684.

Jackson, V. P. (2000). Diagnostic mammography. *Radiologic Clinics of North America, 42,* 853-870.

Jerome, L., Shiry, L., & Leyland-Jones, B. (2004). Anti-insulin-like growth factor strategies in breast cancer. *Seminars in Oncology, 31,* 54-63.

Jordan, V. C. (2005). Chemoprevention in the 21st century: is a balance best or should women have no estrogen at all? *Journal of Clinical Oncology, 23,* 1598-1600.

Kaklamani, V. & O'Regan, R. M. (2004). New targeted therapies in breast cancer. *Seminars in Oncology, 31,* 20-25.

Kelley, M. C., Hansen, N., & McMasters, K. M. (2004). Lymphatic mapping and sentinel lymphadenectomy for breast cancer. *American Journal of Surgery, 188,* 49-61.

Koomen, M., Pisano, E. D., Kuzmiak, C., Pavic, D., & McLelland, R. (2005). Future directions in breast imaging. *Journal of Clinical Oncology, 23,* 1674-1677.

Kuerer, H. M. & Newman, L. A. (2005). Lymphatic mapping and sentinel lymph node biopsy for breast cancer: developments and resolving controversies. *Journal of Clinical Oncology, 23,* 1698-1705.

Kurebayashi, J., Okubo, S., Yamamoto, Y., & Sonoo, H. (2004). Inhibition of HER1 signaling pathway enhances antitumor effect of endocrine therapy in breast cancer. *Breast Cancer, 11,* 38-41.

Limer, J. L., & Speirs, V. (2004). Phyto-oestrogens and breast cancer chemoprevention. *Breast Cancer Research, 6,* 119-127.

Lin, N. U. & Winer, E. P. (2004). New targets for therapy in breast cancer: small molecule tyrosine kinase inhibitors. *Breast Cancer Research, 6,* 204-210.

Lucassen, A. & Watson, E. (2005). Family history of breast cancer. *British Medical Journal, 330,* 26.

Mamounas, E. P. (2005). Continuing evolution in breast cancer surgical management [comment]. *Journal of Clinical Oncology, 23,* 1603-1606.

Martino, S., Costantino, J., McNabb, M., Mershon, J., Bryant, K., Powles, T., & Secrest, R. J. (2004). The role of selective estrogen receptor modulators in the prevention of breast cancer: comparison of the clinical trials. *Oncologist, 9,* 116-125.

McKeage, K., Curran, M. P., & Plosker, G. L. (2004). Fulvestrant: a review of its use in hormone receptor-positive metastatic breast cancer in postmenopausal women with disease progression following antiestrogen therapy. *Drugs, 64,* 633-648.

Mincey, B. A. & Perez, E. A. (2004). Advances in screening, diagnosis, and treatment of breast cancer. *Mayo Clinic Proceedings, 79,* 810-816.

Moffat, F. L., Jr. (2005). Lymph node staging surgery and breast cancer: potholes in the fast lane from more to less. *Journal of Surgical Oncology, 89,* 53-60.

Mokbel, K., Escobar, P. F., & Matsunaga, T. (2005). Mammary ductoscopy: current status and future prospects. *European Journal of Surgical Oncology, 31,* 3-8.

Morabito, A., Sarmiento, R., Bonginelli, P., & Gasparini, G. (2004). Antiangiogenic strategies, compounds, and early clinical results in breast cancer. *Critical Reviews in Oncology-Hematology, 49,* 91-107.

Muti, P. (2005). The role of endogenous hormones in the etiology and prevention of breast cancer: the epidemiological evidence. *Recent Results in Cancer Research, 166,* 245-256.

Narod, S. A. & Offit, K. (2005). Prevention and management of hereditary breast cancer. *Journal of Clinical Oncology, 23,* 1656-1663.

Newman, L. A. & Kuerer, H. M. (2005). Advances in breast conservation therapy [see comment]. *Journal of Clinical Oncology, 23,* 1685-1697.

Noguchi, M. (2004). Current controversies concerning sentinel lymph node biopsy for breast cancer. *Breast Cancer Research & Treatment, 84,* 261-271.

Oluwole, S. F., Ali, A. O., Shafaee, Z., & DePaz, H. A. (2005). Breast cancer in women with HIV/AIDS: report of five cases with a review of the literature. *Journal of Surgical Oncology, 89,* 23-27.

Osborne, C. K. & Schiff, R. (2005). Estrogen-receptor biology: continuing progress and therapeutic implications. *Journal of Clinical Oncology, 23,* 1616-1622.

Peek, M. E. & Han, J. H. (2004). Disparities in screening mammography. Current status, interventions and implications. *Journal of General Internal Medicine, 19,* 184-194.

Pegram, M. D., Pietras, R., Bajamonde, A., Klein, P., & Fyfe, G. (2005). Targeted therapy: wave of the future. *Journal of Clinical Oncology, 23,* 1776-1781.

Quon, A. & Gambhir, S. S. (2005). FDG-PET and beyond: molecular breast cancer imaging [see comment]. *Journal of Clinical Oncology, 23,* 1664-1673.

Ring, A., Smith, I. E., & Dowsett, M. (2004). Circulating tumour cells in breast cancer. *Lancet Oncology, 5,* 79-88.

Robertson, J. F., Come, S. E., Jones, S. E., Beex, L., Kaufmann, M., Makris, A., Nortier, J. W., Possinger, K., & Rutqvist, L. E. (2005). Endocrine treatment options for advanced breast cancer—the role of fulvestrant. *European Journal of Cancer, 41,* 346-356.

Rosen, L. S. (2004). New generation of bisphosphonates: broad clinical utility in breast and prostate cancer. *Oncology (Huntington), 18,* 26-32.

Schneider, B. P., & Miller, K. D. (2005). Angiogenesis of breast cancer. *Journal of Clinical Oncology, 23,* 1782-1790.

Sengupta, S. & Wasylyk, B. (2004). Physiological and pathological consequences of the interactions of the p53 tumor suppressor with the glucocorticoid, androgen, and estrogen receptors. *Annals of the New York Academy of Sciences, 1024,* 54-71.

Shao, W. & Brown, M. (2004). Advances in estrogen receptor biology: prospects for improvements in targeted breast cancer therapy. *Breast Cancer Research, 6,* 39-52.

Simpson, D., Curran, M. P., & Perry, C. M. (2004). Letrozole: a review of its use in postmenopausal women with breast cancer. *Drugs, 64,* 1213-1230.

Simpson, P. T., Reis-Filho, J. S., Gale, T., & Lakhani, S. R. (2005). Molecular evolution of breast cancer. *Journal of Pathology, 205,* 248-254.

Stewart, A. F. (2005). Clinical practice. Hypercalcemia associated with cancer. *New England Journal of Medicine, 352,* 373-379.

Strasser-Weippl, K. & Goss, P. E. (2005). Advances in adjuvant hormonal therapy for postmenopausal women. *Journal of Clinical Oncology, 23,* 1751-1759.

Szyf, M., Pakneshan, P., & Rabbani, S. A. (2004). DNA methylation and breast cancer. *Biochemical Pharmacology, 68,* 1187-1197.

Toi, M., Takada, M., Bando, H., Toyama, K., Yamashiro, H., Horiguchi, S., & Saji, S. (2004). Current status of antibody therapy for breast cancer. *Breast Cancer, 11,* 10-14.

Vergote, I. & Robertson, J. F. (2004). Fulvestrant is an effective and well-tolerated endocrine therapy for postmenopausal women with advanced breast cancer: results from clinical trials. *British Journal of Cancer, 90*(suppl 1), S11-S14.

Wang, D. & Dubois, R. N. (2004). Cyclooxygenase-2: a potential target in breast cancer. *Seminars in Oncology, 31,* 64-73.

Whelan, T. J. (2005). Use of conventional radiation therapy as part of breast-conserving treatment. *Journal of Clinical Oncology, 23,* 1718-1725.

Wilkinson, K. (2004). Anastrozole (Arimidex). *Clinical Journal of Oncology Nursing, 8,* 87-88.

Winer, E. P., Hudis, C., Burstein, H. J., Wolff, A. C., Pritchard, K. I., Ingle, J. N., Chlebowski, R. T., Gelber, R., Edge, S. B., Gralow, J., Cobleigh, M. A., Mamounas, E. P., Goldstein, L. J., Whelan, T. J., Powles, T. J., Bryant, J., Perkins, C., Perotti, J., Braun, S., Langer, A. S., Browman, G. P., & Somerfield, M. R. (2005). American Society of Clinical Oncology technology assessment on the use of aromatase inhibitors as adjuvant therapy for postmenopausal women with hormone receptor-positive breast cancer: status report 2004. *Journal of Clinical Oncology, 23,* 619-629.

Yoneda, T. & Hiraga, T. (2005). Crosstalk between cancer cells and bone microenvironment in bone metastasis. *Biochemical and Biophysical Research Communications, 328,* 679-687.

Breast Cancer

INITIAL HISTORY

- 62-year-old white, postmenopausal woman.
- Presents for annual examination after "call-back" on mammogram
- States her breasts are cystic.
- History of 2- to 3-year use of hormone replacement therapy.
- Denies pain, nipple discharge, or skin changes of her breasts.

Question 1.   *What is your differential diagnosis based on the information you now have?*

Question 2.   *What other questions would you like to ask this patient?*

ADDITIONAL HISTORY

- The patient does practice breast self-examination, but not routinely.
- Latest mammogram 2 years ago.
- Has noticed no changes in her breasts.
- Maternal grandmother was diagnosed with breast cancer at age 78.
- No previous breast biopsies.
- One child, age 34; has never breast-fed.
- No significant health history, no medications, exercises three times a week.
- Menarche at age 12, gave birth to first child at age 28.

Question 3.   *What are the major risk factors for breast cancer?*

□ **Kathleen R. Haden, RN, MSN, ANP-C contributed this case study.**

Question 4.   *What are the controversial risk factors associated with breast cancer?*

PHYSICAL EXAMINATION

- Well-appearing, 62-year-old, white female in no acute distress.
- Afebrile, vital signs stable.
- Weight stable at 150 pounds.
- Height 5 feet, 4 inches.

HEENT
- Head examination normal.
- Neck supple, no JVD.
- No palpable cervical, supraclavicular, infraclavicular, or axillary adenopathy.
- Thyroid nonpalpable.

Breast Examination
- Symmetric breasts.
- No dimpling, puckering, or nipple discharge.
- Skin appears normal.
- Diffuse, small mobile cystic nodules palpable in the upper outer quadrants of both breasts.

Chest, Cardiac, Abdomen, Gynecologic
- Examination unremarkable.

Question 5.   *What do you think of her examination findings?*

Question 6.   *What would you do at this point?*

Question 7.   *What would you tell the patient about her examination and the scheduled testing?*

ADDITIONAL FINDINGS

- Because "call-back" mammogram showed a new calcification, a diagnostic mammogram is ordered. This mammogram reveals a 1.5-cm spiculated mass with irregular borders within the left upper outer quadrant of the left breast.
- During her examination, the radiologist informs you about the findings, and the patient agrees to undergo a core biopsy of the lesion.
- Results reveal an infiltrating ductal carcinoma.

Question 8.   *What do you do now?*

ADDITIONAL INFORMATION

- All laboratory test results and chest radiograph are normal.
- Breast surgeon educates patient about two surgical options including:
  - Lumpectomy with axillary dissection followed by local irradiation.
  - Mastectomy with axillary lymph node dissection with or without reconstruction surgery.

PATIENT AND RADIATION ONCOLOGIST DISCUSS POTENTIAL SIDE EFFECTS OF RADIATION THERAPY

- Acute changes such as skin changes (erythema and desquamation), lymphedema of the breast, and fatigue.
- Chronic problems such as rib fracture, breast retraction, scarring of lumpectomy incision, and the potential of pneumonitis.

Question 9.   *On what basis is breast conservation therapy (lumpectomy) based?*

MORE INFORMATION

- The patient elects breast conservation therapy (lumpectomy) and axillary dissection with RT.
- The pathology results reveal a 1.1-cm infiltrating ductal carcinoma.
- Graded II/III
  - None of the 12 lymph nodes is positive.
  - All surgical margins are clear.
  - ERs and PRs are positive.
  - HER2/*neu is* negative.
- Stage IA.

Question 10.   *The patient is seen and evaluated by a medical oncologist. What therapy would be recommended?*

Question 11.   *What side effects would be discussed with the patient?*

ADDITIONAL INFORMATION

- Patient elects treatment with the aromatase inhibitor anastrozole (Arimidex) only, followed by 6 weeks of radiation treatment because she had breast-conserving therapy.
- Following therapy, the patient will be followed every 3 to 4 months for the first 2 years, then every 6 months until 5 years, and then annually.
- Only routine yearly chest radiograph, routine chemistries, and mammography are ordered for follow-up, unless clinical suspicion for recurrence.

Question 12.   *Where are the most common sites of breast cancer recurrence that would be important to ask about during routine review of system history taken during follow-up visits?*

Cutaneous Malignant Melanoma

DEFINITION

- Intraepidermal proliferation of malignant melanocytes with or without extension into the subcutaneous layers.
- Melanoma types include the following:
    - Superficial spreading melanoma.
    - Acral lentiginous melanoma.
    - Lentigo maligna.
    - Nodular melanoma.

EPIDEMIOLOGY

- It is the seventh most common cancer in the United States. It accounts for only 4% of all skin cancers, but most of the skin cancer deaths. In 2005 there were an estimated 59,580 cases of melanoma, with 7770 deaths. Early localized disease has a >85% 10-year survival rate, but disseminated disease has only a 6% 10-year survival.
- Incidence increased 125% between 1973 and 1994 but has leveled off to a rate of increase of approximately 3% per year. The greatest increase in incidence is in older men.
- Risk factors.
    - Sun exposure: Intermittent intense sun exposures (especially repeated sunburns as children) have the highest risk (blistering sunburns between the ages of 15 and 20 increase risk 2.2-fold); occupational exposure and tanning beds have also been implicated.
    - Pigment traits: Blue eyes, fair complexion, red hair, freckling, sunburns easily.
    - Nevi: The total number of benign melanocytic nevi has been related to up to a 10-fold increased melanoma risk; dysplastic nevi are the precursor lesion to melanoma; the dysplastic nevus syndrome is an inherited entity associated with 25 to 75 such nevi per individual and a high risk for melanoma.
    - Family history: One relative = 2 times the risk; two relatives = 14 times the risk. Heritable risk includes germline mutations of *CDKN2A* (90% lifetime risk) and *CDK4* (see following).
    - Immunosuppression: Risk is increased by four- to eightfold.

PATHOPHYSIOLOGY

Genetics

- Inherited: Accounts for about 10% of all cases. Two gene mutations have been clearly identified in heritable melanoma, *CDKN2A* and *CDK4*. *CDKN2A* codes for two proteins, p16 and p14; p16 regulates *CDK4* activity, which in turn regulates the tumor suppressor gene *RB,* and p14 enhances the tumor suppressor activity of *p53.* Thus mutations of these two genes contribute to unregulated tumor growth though inactivation of tumor suppressor activity. Another germline mutation that has been identified in melanoma is the gene *MC1R* (melanocortin-1 receptor gene).

- Acquired: Commonly acquired mutations seen in melanoma include B-*raf,* N-*ras, p53, APAF1,* melanoma differentiation associated-7 (MDA-7), and mitogen-activated protein (MAP) kinase genes.

Tumor Activation and Progression

- 30% of melanoma arises from dysplastic nevi that occur in about 10% of the white population.
- Melanin functions to absorb ultraviolet protons; skin that is low in melanin is more vulnerable to ultraviolet damage; in most individuals, melanomas occur in areas that are not usually tanned but have been severely burned intermittently (e.g., trunk on men, legs on women).
- Ultraviolet radiation acts as an initiator, a promoter, a cocarcinogen, and an immunosuppressive agent. Ultraviolet A (UVA) and ultraviolet B (UVB) radiation is absorbed by deoxyribonucleic acid (DNA), resulting in DNA mutations.
- Mutation of the B-*raf* gene leads to activation of the mitogen-activated protein kinase pathway, which is a primary step in activating melanocyte proliferation. Mutated melanocytes also produce high levels of basic fibrinogen growth factor (bFGF), which stimulates autonomous melanocyte proliferation asic fibrinogen growth factor (bFGF), which stimulates autonomous melanocyte proliferation.
- Melanocytes have high levels of the antiapoptotic protein Bcl-2, thus mutations do not result in apoptosis, and damaged melanocytes can continue to divide with little or no DNA repair.
- Numerous other autocrine and paracrine growth factors further stimulate melanoma cell proliferation including insulin-like growth factor-1 (IGF$_1$); interleukin (IL)-1, IL-8, and IL-10; platelet-derived growth factor; epidermal growth factors; vascular endothelial growth factors; and angiogenesis factors.
- Disordered cellular "cross-talk" by cadherins, connexins, and adhesion receptors results in abnormalities in cell growth and differentiation, apoptosis, and migration.
- Melanoma cells frequently express specific tumor antigens such as the melanoma antigen encoding gene (MAGE) antigens.
- Intraepidermal proliferation of malignant melanocytes (radial growth phase) is followed by malignant cell nests and single cells spreading outward and down through the dermis and into the subcutaneous fat. There is often stepwise progression from a symmetric, uniformly pigmented macule to an increasingly asymmetric, variegated, elevated lesion with atypia and patchy lymphocyte invasion.
- The intraepidermal phase is not associated with metastasis; once growth is vertical (nodular with penetration through the dermis), then metastasis is likely.
- There are three primary pathways of melanoma metastasis: (1) to regional lymph nodes (50%), (2) in-transit satellite lesions (20%), and (3) immediately distant metastases (30%). Neovascularization (angiogenesis) of the primary tumor is followed by adhesion to vessels and invasion into the bloodstream or lymphatics. Tumor cell embolization in tissues may result in preferred tumor cell binding to cytokine receptor ligands (e.g., CCR1D, CXCR4, CXCR7) that promote local proliferation of tumor in selected organs (tropism).
- Primary tumors on the trunk, upper arm, neck, or scalp (TANS) are most likely to metastasize to distant sites, especially skin, lymph nodes, subcutaneous tissues, lung, liver, brain, and bone.

PATIENT PRESENTATION

History

Fair skinned with a history of frequent sunburns as a child; multiple nevi; outdoor occupation; residence in sunny location; family history; immunosuppression.

Symptoms

Enlarging pigmented lesion commonly on the trunk in men and on the legs in women; also occurs on the neck, head or arms, genitalia, mucous membranes; occasionally on palms, soles, or nail plate; may present with dyspnea, diarrhea, or neurologic symptoms from pulmonary, gastrointestinal, or central nervous system involvement.

Examination (Palpate for Satellite Nodules and Lymph Nodes)

- *Superficial spreading:* Lesions occur on the back or the legs with irregular, asymmetric borders and color variegation; size is generally 6 to 8 mm.
- *Acral lentiginous:* Occurs on soles, palms, and beneath the nail plate with irregular pigmentation and large size (≥3 cm); pigmentation of the proximal or lateral nail folds (Hutchinson sign) is diagnostic of subungual melanoma.
- *Lentigo maligna:* Often occurs in the older adult with lesions on head, neck, and arms occurring in a previously benign lesion (often present for numerous years); tan or brown patch with hypopigmented areas and nodular areas.
- *Nodular melanoma:* Located on the back and the trunk with rapid growth and the presence of a raised dark nodule with frequent bleeding and ulceration.

DIFFERENTIAL DIAGNOSIS

- Seborrheic keratoses.
- Common acquired melanocytic nevi.
- Traumatized benign nevi (bleeding mole).
- Blue nevus.
- Spitz nevus.
- Congenital melanocytic nevi.
- Dysplastic nevi.

KEYS TO ASSESSMENT

- Visually recognize suspicious nevi.
    - Recent change and/or location in unusual areas (palms, soles, under breasts).
    - ABCD criteria = *A*symmetry, *B*order irregularity, *C*olor variegation, and *D*iameter >6 mm.
    - Recently suggested that E be added for *E*volving (i.e., change in size).
- Dermoscopy, computer-aided techniques, scanning laser microscopy, and ultrasound can all help to characterize a suspicious lesion.
- Full-thickness punch biopsy for large lesions; excisional biopsy with 1- to 2-mm margin for small or medium lesions.
- Determination of prognostic indicators include the following:
    - Anatomic level of invasion (Clark): Five levels of invasion based on anatomic landmarks (e.g., I is intraepidermal only, V is infiltration of the subcutaneous fat).
    - Linear depth of invasion (Breslow): Millimeters from the top to the deepest tumor cell.
    - Histiogenic type (superficial spreading, acral lentiginous).
    - Evidence of regression or ulceration.
- Sentinel node biopsy.
    - Lymphoscintigraphy is used to identify lymphatic basins draining the primary melanoma followed by sentinel node biopsy.
    - Indications include presence of a tumor greater than 1 mm and less than 4 mm in thickness without clinical evidence of metastasis.
    - Sensitivity is high (especially with special stains of the node specimen) and if positive, regional elective lymph node dissection (ELND) is indicated in most patients.
- Polymerase chain reaction (PCR) detection of melanoma markers detect nodal micrometastases (can also use PCR to detect circulating melanoma cells in the blood).

- Staging is according to the 2002 American Joint Committee on Cancer TNM Staging System for Malignant Melanoma of the Skin: tumor thickness, Clark levels (vertical penetration), and the presence of ulceration determine stage.
- Chest radiograph; liver function tests, complete blood count.
- Chest, head, or abdominal computed tomography (CT) or magnetic resonance imaging (MRI) is used to evaluate symptoms that may be related to metastases.
- Positron emission tomography can be used to detect metastases and for recurrent melanoma; its use in primary diagnosis is not yet determined.

KEYS TO MANAGEMENT

Prevention
- Avoidance of excessive sunlight exposure, especially before age 20 is the most effective prevention.
- Sunscreens may be helpful, but studies are not conclusive. Hats and clothing are more effective.
- Thorough skin self-examination (TSSE) is recommended, and in one study reduced melanoma mortality by 63%.
- Regular primary care or dermatologic screening results in lesions being diagnosed at thinner (earlier) stages.

Surgical Management
- Wide excision of primary lesion (1- to 4-cm margins, depending on the thickness of the lesion).
- Sentinel node biopsy after lymphatic mapping: if negative, the procedure is terminated; if positive, regional ELND is performed. Complications include postoperative lymphedema.
- Local recurrences are widely excised.
- Resection of distant metastases is indicated if there are few lesions (<4) and a disease-free interval after primary resection of 1 to 2 years: subcutaneous, pulmonary, and gastrointestinal.
- Stereotactic radiosurgery may be used for palliation of brain metastases.

Adjuvant Therapy
- Used for moderate- to high-risk tumors.
- Interferon-α (INF)-2b is used as adjuvant therapy in patients at high risk for recurrence. It increases 5-year survival in patients with positive nodes, but has a high toxicity. Use in patients with negative nodes is controversial and has not been definitively shown to change outcomes. Interferons are also used for metastatic disease, alone or in combination with other chemotherapy agents. This drug is highly toxic.
- IL-2 results in only a 15% to 22% response rate, but can achieve long-term remission and even cure in 85% of those patients who achieve a complete response. Toxicities are severe with this drug, however, and correct dosing and expert care are vital.
- Chemotherapy for metastatic disease consists of single agent or combinations of dacarbazine, cisplatin, nitrosoureas, or taxanes and IL-2 or INF. Toxicity is high and response rates are variable. Temozolomide is commonly used for central nervous system metastases.
- Radiation is used as primary therapy for inoperable tumors, as adjuvant therapy for mucosal and uveal melanomas, and as palliation for unresectable locoregional disease and brain metastases.
- Isolated limb perfusion or infusion with melphalan with or without tumor necrosis factor or interferon for limb recurrence improves survival and decreases the need for major amputation.
- Immunotherapy.
  - The detection of tumor-specific melanoma-associated antigens (MAA) such as MAGE-1, melanoma antigen recognized by T cells (MART), and gp100 has led to the development of several immunotherapy strategies.

1. Tumor vaccination with peptide and heat shock vaccines administered with interleukins or granulocyte-macrophage colony-stimulating factor (GM-CSF) can generate a vigorous immune response. Although clinical responses are limited at this time, this area of treatment continues to be studied extensively in melanoma patients.
2. Other types of vaccines being studied include virus vectors (e.g., vaccinia), dendritic cells, and autologous and allogenic whole cell vaccines.
3. Monoclonal antibodies can bring in targeted cytotoxic factors and block growth factor receptors.

- Nonspecific immunotherapy with bacille Calmette-Guérin (BCG) via intralesional injection controls local disease and continues to play a role as an adjuvant to vaccine therapy.

- Future agents.
  - B-*raf* blockers.
  - Gene therapy (e.g., antisense blockade of *Bcl-2* with oblimersen).
  - Cytokine blockers (e.g., CCR7 and CXCR4 blockers).

PATHOPHYSIOLOGY $\longrightarrow$	CLINICAL LINK
What is going on in the disease process that influences how the patient presents and how he or she should be managed?	*What should you do now that you understand the underlying pathophysiology?*
UVA and UVB radiation, especially when associated with recurrent childhood sunburns, causes changes in melanocyte DNA and increases melanoma risk. $\longrightarrow$	Protection from excessive sun exposure, especially in children, is essential for the prevention of melanoma.
Melanin functions to absorb ultraviolet (UV) radiation and is protective of the skin. $\longrightarrow$	Malignant melanomas tend to arise in areas that are not normally tanned but that have been burned intermittently.
Many melanomas arise from dysplastic nevi, especially in inherited dysplastic nevus syndrome. $\longrightarrow$	Patients with multiple nevi require frequent examinations to screen for malignancy.
Melanocytes possess high levels of antiapoptotic proteins and lack the ability for effective DNA repair. $\longrightarrow$	Damaged melanocytes can be long lived and proliferate even when there is significant DNA mutation, with the possibility of tumor progression years after initial exposure to ultraviolet radiation.
Both inherited and acquired mutations of specific genes (e.g., *CDKN2A, CDK4,* B-*raf*) have been identified. $\longrightarrow$	New treatments such as antisense therapy and protein kinase blockade are in development.
Malignant lesions initially spread within the epidermis and have little risk of metastasis. Once intradermal invasion occurs with formation of a nodular lesion, there is significant risk for distant spread. $\longrightarrow$	Careful biopsy to evaluate for Clark level and depth of invasion (Breslow) is essential to staging and prognostic evaluation.
Melanoma usually spreads first through the lymphatics, and outcomes can be improved with lymph node removal if positive nodes are found on biopsy. $\longrightarrow$	Lymphoscintigraphy and sentinel node biopsy are used to determine the appropriate extent of surgical removal.
Melanoma cells are relatively responsive to immunologic intervention. $\longrightarrow$	Interferons, interleukins, monoclonal antibodies, tumor vaccines, and passive immunotherapy are all being used as adjunctive treatment for malignant melanoma.

SUGGESTED READINGS

Abbasi, N. R., Shaw, H. M., Rigel, D. S., Friedman, R. J., McCarthy, W. H., Osman, I., Kopf, A. W., & Polsky, D. (2004). Early diagnosis of cutaneous melanoma: revisiting the ABCD criteria. *Journal of the American Medical Association, 292,* 2771-2776.

Bafaloukos, D., & Gogas, H. (2004). The treatment of brain metastases in melanoma patients. *Cancer Treatment Reviews, 30,* 515-520.

Balch, C. M., Soong, S. J., Atkins, M. B., Buzaid, A. C., Cascinelli, N., Coit, D. G., Fleming, I. D., Gershenwald, J. E., Houghton, A., Jr., Kirkwood, J. M., McMasters, K. M., Mihm, M. F., Morton, D. L., Reintgen, D. S., Ross, M. I., Sober, A., Thompson, J. A., & Thompson, J. F. (2004). An evidence-based staging system for cutaneous melanoma. *Ca: A Cancer Journal for Clinicians, 54,* 131-149.

Ballo, M. T., & Ang, K. K. (2004). Radiotherapy for cutaneous malignant melanoma: rationale and indications. *Oncology (Huntington), 18,* 99-107.

Bastiaannet, E., Beukema, J. C., & Hoekstra, H. J. (2005). Radiation therapy following lymph node dissection in melanoma patients: treatment, outcome and complications. *Cancer Treatment Reviews, 31,* 18-26.

Bastian, B. C. (2004). Molecular genetics of melanocytic neoplasia: practical applications for diagnosis. *Pathology, 36,* 458-461.

Bauer, J., Blum, A., Strohhacker, U., & Garbe, C. (2005). Surveillance of patients at high risk for cutaneous malignant melanoma using digital dermoscopy. *British Journal of Dermatology, 152,* 87-92.

Berwick, M. (2005). Toward reduction of misclassification in the biology of melanoma. *Journal of Investigative Dermatology, 124,* xiv.

Bradbury, P. A., & Middleton, M. R. (2004). DNA repair pathways in drug resistance in melanoma. *Anti-Cancer Drugs, 15,* 421-426.

Buzaid, A. C. (2004). Management of metastatic cutaneous melanoma. *Oncology (Huntington), 18,* 1443-1450.

Bystryn, J. C., & Reynolds, S. R. (111). Melanoma vaccines: what we know so far. *Oncology (Huntington), 19,* 97-108.

Chung, E. S., Sabel, M. S., & Sondak, V. K. (2004). Current state of treatment for primary cutaneous melanoma. *Clinical and Experimental Medicine, 4,* 65-77.

Day, T. A., Hornig, J. D., Sharma, A. K., Brescia, F., Gillespie, M. B., & Lathers, D. (2005). Melanoma of the head and neck. *Current Treatment Options in Oncology, 6,* 19-30.

Denkins, Y., Reiland, J., Roy, M., Sinnappah-Kang, N. D., Galjour, J., Murry, B. P., Blust, J., Aucoin, R., & Marchetti, D. (2004). Brain metastases in melanoma: roles of neurotrophins. *Neuro-Oncology, 6,* 154-165.

Elliott, B., & Dalgleish, A. (2004). Melanoma vaccines. *Hospital Medicine (London), 65,* 668-673.

Flaherty, K. T. (2004). New molecular targets in melanoma. *Current Opinion in Oncology, 16,* 150-154.

Friedman, K. P., & Wahl, R. L. (2004). Clinical use of positron emission tomography in the management of cutaneous melanoma. *Seminars in Nuclear Medicine, 34,* 242-253.

Gandini, S., Sera, F., Cattaruzza, M. S., Pasquini, P., Picconi, O., Boyle, P., & Melchi, C. F. (2005). Meta-analysis of risk factors for cutaneous melanoma: II. Sun exposure. *European Journal of Cancer, 41,* 45-60.

Gershenwald, J. E., & Bar-Eli, M. (2004). Gene expression profiling of human cutaneous melanoma: are we there yet? *Cancer Biology & Therapy, 3,* 121-123.

Gogas, H., Bafaloukos, D., & Bedikian, A. Y. (2004). The role of taxanes in the treatment of metastatic melanoma. *Melanoma Research, 14,* 415-420.

Grossman, D. (2004). Imatinib mesylate for melanoma: will a new target be revealed? *Journal of Investigative Dermatology, 123,* xi-xiii.

Haass, N. K., Smalley, K. S., & Herlyn, M. (2004). The role of altered cell-cell communication in melanoma progression. *Journal of Molecular Histology, 35,* 309-318.

Healy, E. (2004). Melanocortin 1 receptor variants, pigmentation, and skin cancer susceptibility. *Photodermatology, Photoimmunology & Photomedicine, 20,* 283-288.

Heenan, P. J. (2004). Local recurrence of melanoma. *Pathology, 36,* 491-495.

Heymann, W. R. (2004). The genetics of melanoma. *Journal of the American Academy of Dermatology, 51,* 801-802.

Hussein, M. R. (2004). Genetic pathways to melanoma tumorigenesis. *Journal of Clinical Pathology, 57,* 797-801.

Ingram, S. B., & O'Rourke, M. G. (2004). DC therapy for metastatic melanoma. *Cytotherapy, 6,* 148-153.

Johnson, T. M., Bradford, C. R., Gruber, S. B., Sondak, V. K., & Schwartz, J. L. (2004). Staging workup, sentinel node biopsy, and follow-up tests for melanoma: update of current concepts. *Archives of Dermatology, 140,* 107-113.

Komenaka, I., Hoerig, H., & Kaufman, H. L. (2004). Immunotherapy for melanoma. *Clinics in Dermatology, 22,* 251-265.

Kumar, R., Mavi, A., Bural, G., & Alavi, A. (2005). Fluorodeoxyglucose-PET in the management of malignant melanoma. *Radiologic Clinics of North America, 43,* 23-33.

Lahn, M. M., & Sundell, K. L. (2004). The role of protein kinase C-alpha (PKC-alpha) in melanoma. *Melanoma Research, 14,* 85-89.

Lawson, D. H. (2004). Update on the systemic treatment of malignant melanoma. *Seminars in Oncology, 31,* 33-37.

Lee, K. K., Vetto, J. T., Mehrany, K., & Swanson, N. A. (2004). Sentinel lymph node biopsy. *Clinics in Dermatology, 22,* 234-239.

Leiter, U., Meier, F., Schittek, B., & Garbe, C. (2004). The natural course of cutaneous melanoma. *Journal of Surgical Oncology, 86,* 172-178.

Lewis, J. J. (2004). Therapeutic cancer vaccines: using unique antigens. *Proceedings of the National Academy of Sciences of the United States of America, 101*(suppl 2), 14653-14656.

Linette, G. P., Carlson, J. A., Slominski, A., Mihm, M. C., & Ross, J. S. (2005). Biomarkers in melanoma: stage III and IV disease. *Expert Review of Molecular Diagnostics, 5,* 65-74.

Macapinlac, H. A. (2004). FDG PET and PET/CT imaging in lymphoma and melanoma. *Cancer Journal, 10,* 262-270.

Macapinlac, H. A. (2004). The utility of 2-deoxy-2-[18F]fluoro-D-glucose-positron emission tomography and combined positron emission tomography and computed tomography in lymphoma and melanoma. *Molecular Imaging & Biology, 6,* 200-207.

Mosca, P. J., Tyler, D. S., & Seigler, H. F. (2004). Surgical management of cutaneous melanoma: current practice and impact on prognosis. *Advances in Surgery, 38,* 85-119.

Murakami, T., Cardones, A. R., & Hwang, S. T. (2004). Chemokine receptors and melanoma metastasis. *Journal of Dermatological Science, 36,* 71-78.

Nguyen, T. H. (2004). Mechanisms of metastasis. *Clinics in Dermatology, 22,* 209-216.

Penmatcha, S., Rovinsky, S. A., Cockerell, C. J., & Hsu, M. Y. (2004). Advances in prognostication of cutaneous malignant melanoma. *Advances in Dermatology, 20,* 323-343.

Perlis, C. & Herlyn, M. (2004). Recent advances in melanoma biology. *Oncologist, 9,* 182-187.

Petro, A., Schwartz, J., & Johnson, T. (2004). Current melanoma staging. *Clinics in Dermatology, 22,* 223-227.

Pfeifer, G. P., You, Y. H., & Besaratinia, A. (2005). Mutations induced by ultraviolet light. *Mutation Research, 571,* 19-31.

Poochareon, V. N., Federman, D. G., & Kirsner, R. S. (2004). Primary prevention efforts for melanoma. *Journal of Drugs in Dermatology: JDD, 3,* 506-519.

Queirolo, P., Taveggia, P., Gipponi, M., & Sertoli, M. R. (2004). Sentinel lymph node biopsy in melanoma patients: the medical oncologist's perspective. *Journal of Surgical Oncology, 85,* 162-165.

Reintgen, D., Pendas, S., Jakub, J., Swor, G., Giuliano, R., Bauer, J., Cassall, R., Duhaime, L., Alsarrai, M., & Shivers, S. (2004). National trials involving lymphatic mapping for melanoma: the Multicenter Selective Lymphadenectomy Trial, the Sunbelt Melanoma Trial, and the Florida Melanoma Trial. *Seminars in Oncology, 31,* 363-373.

Roberts, A. A., & Cochran, A. J. (2004). Pathologic analysis of sentinel lymph nodes in melanoma patients: current and future trends. *Journal of Surgical Oncology, 85,* 152-161.

Rodolfo, M., Daniotti, M., & Vallacchi, V. (2004). Genetic progression of metastatic melanoma. *Cancer Letters, 214,* 133-147.

Schaffer, J. V., Rigel, D. S., Kopf, A. W., & Bolognia, J. L. (2004). Cutaneous melanoma—past, present, and future. *Journal of the American Academy of Dermatology, 51,* S65-S69.

Schmollinger, J. C., & Dranoff, G. (2004). Targeting melanoma inhibitor of apoptosis protein with cancer immunotherapy. *Apoptosis, 9,* 309-313.

Schoder, H., Larson, S. M., & Yeung, H. W. (2004). PET/CT in oncology: integration into clinical management of lymphoma, melanoma, and gastrointestinal malignancies. *Journal of Nuclear Medicine, 45*(suppl 1), 72S-81S.

Scolyer, R. A., Thompson, J. F., Stretch, J. R., Sharma, R., & McCarthy, S. W. (2004). Pathology of melanocytic lesions: new, controversial, and clinically important issues. *Journal of Surgical Oncology, 86,* 200-211.

Strungs, I. (2004). Common and uncommon variants of melanocytic naevi. *Pathology, 36,* 396-403.

Swetter, S. M., Geller, A. C., & Kirkwood, J. M. (2004). Melanoma in the older person. *Oncology (Huntington), 18,* 1187-1196.

Tarhini, A. A., & Agarwala, S. S. (2004). Management of brain metastases in patients with melanoma. *Current Opinion in Oncology, 16,* 161-166.

Testori, A., Stanganelli, I., Della, G. L., & Mahadavan, L. (2004). Diagnosis of melanoma in the elderly and surgical implications. *Surgical Oncology, 13,* 211-221.

Thomas, J. M., & Clark, M. A. (2004). Selective lymphadenectomy in sentinel node-positive patients may increase the risk of local/in-transit recurrence in malignant melanoma [see comment]. *European Journal of Surgical Oncology, 30,* 686-691.

Thompson, J. F., & Kam, P. C. (2004). Isolated limb infusion for melanoma: a simple but effective alternative to isolated limb perfusion. *Journal of Surgical Oncology, 88,* 1-3.

Thompson, J. F., Scolyer, R. A., & Kefford, R. F. (2005). Cutaneous melanoma. *Lancet, 365,* 687-701.

Tsao, H., Atkins, M. B., & Sober, A. J. (2004). Management of cutaneous melanoma. *New England Journal of Medicine, 351,* 998-1012.

Tsao, H. & Niendorf, K. (2004). Genetic testing in hereditary melanoma. *Journal of the American Academy of Dermatology, 51,* 803-808.

Wang, S. Q., Rabinovitz, H., Kopf, A. W., & Oliviero, M. (2004). Current technologies for the in vivo diagnosis of cutaneous melanomas. *Clinics in Dermatology, 22,* 217-222.

Melanoma

INITIAL HISTORY

- 39-year-old white, red-haired, green-eyed male with light, freckled skin.
- History of numerous nevi since childhood.
- Presents with a large, dark, irregular-shaped skin lesion on his midback.
- Physical education teacher.
- Positive family history of dysplastic nevus syndrome.

Question 1.   *What of this patient's history are considered risk factors for melanoma, and what are other warning signs?*

Question 2.   *Is there a relationship between dysplastic nevus syndrome and melanoma?*

Question 3.   *What is the relationship between sunlight and melanoma for this patient?*

□ **Patrice Y. Neese, RN, MSN, CS, ANP contributed this case study.**

PHYSICAL EXAMINATION

HEENT, Neck, Lungs, Cardiac, Abdomen, Neurologic
- Conjunctival and funduscopic examination without lesions.
- No supraclavicular or cervical adenopathy.
- Clear to auscultation and percussion, no axillary adenopathy.
- Regular rate and rhythm (RRR) without murmurs.
- Soft, nontender, no liver enlargement.
- Strength and reflex +2 and equal bilaterally.

Integument
- Numerous nevi and freckles.
- 5-mm, irregularly shaped, darker lesion, midback.
- Moderate sun damage to face, neck, chest, and back.

Question 4.   *What are the pertinent positive and negative findings of this patient's physical examination?*

Question 5.   *Does melanoma always appear on the skin?*

Question 6.   *What are the most common sites of metastases?*

Question 7.   *What type of biopsy should be done for this patient?*

BIOPSY RESULTS

- Clark level IV.
- Breslow 2.2 mm.
- Superficial spreading melanoma.

Question 8.   *What does this tell you about his prognosis?*

Question 9.   *What is the significance of this histologic subgroup of melanoma?*

Question 10.   *What tests should be ordered for staging?*

SURGICAL MANAGEMENT

• Wide local excision and sentinel lymph node biopsy.

Question 11.   *What is the role of sentinel lymph node mapping and biopsy in melanoma for this patient?*

RESULTS OF SURGERY

• Lymphoscintigraphy results: One hotspot identified in right axilla.
• Lymph node biopsy: Negative.
• Scar and inflammatory changes in remainder of wide local excision.

Question 12.   *Should adjuvant therapy be offered to this patient?*

Question 13.   *What is the pertinent patient education the practitioner should convey?*

Question 14.   *What is the appropriate follow-up for this patient?*

Type 2 (Non–Insulin-Dependent) Diabetes Mellitus

DEFINITION

- In 1997, the Expert Committee on the Diagnosis and Classification of Diabetes Mellitus in the United States recommended replacing the term *non–insulin-dependent diabetes mellitus* (NIDDM) with *type 2 diabetes,* although both are still used throughout the world literature.
- As defined by the National Diabetes Data Group and the World Health Organization, type 2 diabetes is carbohydrate intolerance characterized by insulin resistance, relative (rather than absolute) insulin deficiency, excessive hepatic glucose production, and hyperglycemia. Because complete insulin deficiency seldom occurs, ketoacidosis is unusual in this form of diabetes.

EPIDEMIOLOGY

- Type 2 diabetes mellitus is the most common endocrine disease and the most common form of diabetes.
- Its overall prevalence in the United States is approximately 7%, and is present in 10% to 12% of people older than 65 years of age. Approximately 18 million people in the United States have been diagnosed with diabetes, of whom 90% have type 2 diabetes. It is estimated that the number of individuals with diabetes will increase by 165% between 2000 and 2050.
- There is an emerging epidemic of type 2 diabetes in youth that parallels the rise of obesity and sedentary life-style in this age-group.
- The epidemic of type 2 diabetes is also becoming an international problem, particularly in countries that adopt Western life-styles and dietary patterns.
- Because of the lengthy latent onset, the estimated average time from onset of type 2 diabetes to diagnosis is 7 to 12 years; many patients already have long-term complications at diagnosis.
- Type 2 diabetes mellitus is the seventh leading cause of death in the United States, causing 17% of all deaths in people older than 25 years of age; it is responsible for 300,000 deaths annually.
- It is the leading cause of blindness, end-stage renal disease, and lower extremity amputations.
- It increases the risk of coronary disease and stroke two to five times.

□ Eugene C. Corbett, Jr., MD, FACP contributed this chapter.

PATHOPHYSIOLOGY

- *Genetics:* Carbohydrate tolerance is controlled by myriad genetic and dietary influences. Type 2 diabetes, therefore, is a polygenic disorder with multiple metabolic factors that interact with exogenous influences to produce the phenotype. Genetic concordance for type 2 diabetes in identical twins approaches 90%.
- Insulin resistance.
    - Resistance to the metabolic effect of one's own insulin exists throughout the body, particularly within the major glucose processing organs, the skeletal muscle, and the liver.
    - The major mechanisms of insulin resistance in skeletal muscle include impairments in glycogen synthase activation, metabolic regulatory dysfunction, receptor down-regulation, and glucose transport abnormalities.
    - These mechanisms of insulin resistance result in reduced insulin-mediated cellular glucose uptake and hyperglycemia.
    - The liver also becomes resistant to insulin. The liver would normally respond to hyperglycemia with a decrease in its endogenous glucose production. In type 2 diabetes, hepatic glucose production continues despite hyperglycemia, leading to inappropriately raised basal hepatic glucose output, which contributes further to hyperglycemia.
    - Obesity, particularly abdominal obesity, is directly correlated with increasing degrees of insulin resistance. This is a major underlying reason for the relationship between increased body fat and an increased incidence of glucose intolerance and type 2 diabetes.
- β-cell dysfunction.
    - β-cell dysfunction refers to the inability of the pancreatic islet cells to respond appropriately to a rise in blood sugar. This is partly due to the greater degree of insulin output required in the insulin-resistant individual. It is also caused by an increasing limitation in the absolute amount of insulin that can be produced by the islet cells, particularly in the postingestion (postprandial) period, as the natural history of the disease progresses.
    - Persistent hyperglycemia may also render β-cells increasingly unresponsive to an elevated glucose level in the blood. This is termed "glucose toxicity."
    - Insulin secretion normally occurs in two phases following carbohydrate ingestion. The first phase occurs within minutes of glucose intake and represents release of preformed insulin stored in the β-cells. In the second phase newly synthesized insulin continues to be released over a period of hours postingestion. In type 2 diabetes the first phase of insulin release is predominantly and progressively impaired.
- β-cell dysfunction (including early-phase insulin secretion) and insulin resistance are reversible biochemical processes and are improved with weight loss and increased physical activity.

PATIENT PRESENTATION

Symptoms

- Type 2 diabetes is generally asymptomatic for many years before the symptoms of an elevated blood sugar become evident. This includes the lengthy period of insulin resistance and early postprandial hyperglycemia.
- Because of the very gradual way in which hyperglycemia develops over time, many patients can sustain extended periods of significant hyperglycemia without experiencing a loss of a sense of well-being or recognizing the significance of early symptoms of the disease.
- Classic symptoms of hyperglycemia include inappropriate levels of fatigue, polyuria, polydipsia, new or increasing nocturia, subtle losses of visual acuity, delayed wound healing, and numbness or tingling sensations and decreased sensory perception of the feet (neuropathy). Weight gain or loss can occur. Yeast infections of the skin and vagina are common.

Difficulty with bladder emptying or with perceiving the presence of a full bladder can indicate motor or sensory autonomic neuropathy. Early presentation can occasionally include symptoms of diabetic complications such as visual blurring or loss (retinopathy) or acute localized motor weakness (peripheral motor neuropathy).

Personal and Family History

- Progressive and long-standing overweight condition.
    - Physical activity levels are frequently reported to be chronically low, resulting in a low level of caloric expenditure.
    - Nutritional patterns generally include chronic excessive consumption of caloric nutrients, including sweets, processed carbohydrates, alcohol, and fat.
- Look for a history of gestational diabetes in women, and for associated cardiovascular risk factors (hypertension, dyslipidemia, smoking).
- A positive family history of type 2 diabetes is found in the large majority of cases.

Examination

- The patient may have the general appearance of being unwell. Obesity with increased waist-to-hip ratio, weight gain or loss; signs of dehydration in the acute setting; sensory or vibration sense impairment (neuropathy) of the feet; localized motor weakness; yeast skin rashes, particularly in skin-to-skin areas (axilla, beneath the breast); skin ulcers, particularly on the soles of the feet; multiple hyperpigmented lesions, especially of the lower extremities; decrease in visual acuity or abnormalities of the retinal examination; hypertension; loss of peripheral pulses.

DIFFERENTIAL DIAGNOSIS

- Type 1 diabetes (insulin-dependent diabetes mellitus).
- Latent autoimmune diabetes in adults (very rare).
- Gestational diabetes mellitus.
- Secondary diabetes mellitus: pancreatic disorder (hemochromatosis, chronic pancreatitis, pancreatectomy), hormonal disorder (Cushing syndrome, acromegaly), medication-induced (steroids, thiazides).
- There are several other rare clinical and genetic syndromes associated with diabetes such as chromium deficiency.

KEYS TO ASSESSMENT

- Screening for diabetes.
    - All patients, particularly those who:
        1. Are obese (>120% ideal body weight) or who have gained a significant amount of weight.
        2. Have relatives with type 2 diabetes.
        3. Are members of a high-risk ethnic population (black, Hispanic, Native American, Pacific Islander).
        4. Have a history of gestational diabetes.
        5. Are hypertensive and/or have dyslipidemia (high-density lipoprotein [HDL] <35, triglyceride >250).
        6. Have any kind of symptoms of diabetes, including unexplained fatigue.
        7. Have recurrent infections, especially of the skin, urinary tract, and vagina.
- Establishing the diagnosis.
    - The diagnosis of diabetes can be established by any one of five criteria:
        1. Fasting plasma glucose (FPG) level ≥7 mmol/L (126 mg/dL).
        2. Any casual plasma glucose concentration ≥11.1 mmol/L (200 mg/dL).
        3. A 2-hour plasma glucose level of ≥11.1 mmol/L during an oral glucose tolerance test (OGTT).

   4. A glycosylated hemoglobin (HgbA$_{1c}$) level >6%.
   5. Identification of characteristic diabetic retinopathy.
- The HgbA$_{1c}$ measures the percentage of hemoglobin molecules in the blood that have a glucose molecule bonded onto their structure, a process that takes place in the circulation. This percentage is a direct reflection of the average level of blood sugar in an individual over the preceding 2 to 3 months. This period corresponds to the average lifetime of the red blood cell. Generally, a glycosylated (glycated) hemoglobin level greater than 6% is considered an abnormal blood sugar average, and is consistent with the diagnosis of diabetes.
- The **C-peptide** is the inactive fragment which is cleaved from proinsulin, resulting in the production of the active insulin molecule. Measurement of C-peptide helps to establish the insulin-making capacity of β-cells, thus offering a test that helps to distinguish type 1 from type 2 diabetes. Individuals with type 2 diabetes generally have normal or elevated levels of C-peptide, whereas individuals with type 1 make very little, if any.
- Looking for associated complications.
  - Look for proteinuria or albuminuria (>30 mg/24 hr) as well as glycosuria in the urine analysis. A 24-hour urine collection for creatinine clearance and total protein and albumin evaluates for the degree of intact renal function and the presence of diabetic nephropathy. The albumin/creatinine ratio (normally less than 30 mg/g), which can be measured in a single specimen of urine, is an alternative and more convenient method for identifying the presence of diabetic renal disease.
  - For blood studies, evaluate renal function (blood urea nitrogen [BUN], creatinine) and lipids (total cholesterol, low-density lipoprotein [LDL], HDL, triglyceride levels).
  - Look for signs of retinal abnormalities, preferably with a careful, dilated ophthalmologic examination.

KEYS TO MANAGEMENT

- Prevention.
  - Prevention of type 2 diabetes mellitus is based on the control of factors known to directly influence the development and reversal of insulin resistance and β-cell dysfunction.
    1. Maintenance of body weight within 120% of ideal body weight, particularly when family history is positive for the disease.
    2. Maintain an exercise program throughout one's lifetime.
    3. Limit the excessive intake of simple carbohydrates such as sweets, alcohol, and snacks.
  - The second-most important preventive strategy pertains to the early detection and therefore prevention of the complications of type 2 diabetes. Strict glycemic control has been demonstrated to prevent all of the following:
    1. Retinopathy and lens cataract (annual ophthalmologic examination).
    2. Nephropathy (annual assessment for degree of albuminuria and renal function, and the administration of renal protective drugs such as angiotensin-converting enzyme inhibitors and angiotensin receptor blockers).
    3. Nephropathy: meticulous prevention and control of hypertension.
    4. Neuropathy (monitoring for evidence of early sensory impairment, particularly of the feet).
  - In addition, careful management of comorbid cardiovascular risk factors is essential.
    1. Avoidance of cigarette smoke.
    2. Optimal management of cholesterol and triglyceride levels.
    3. Observation of peripheral pulses for signs of peripheral vascular impairment.
    4. Observation for silent ischemic cardiac and cerebrovascular disease (e.g., electrocardiogram, carotid artery Doppler examination).

- *Therapeutic goals* include optimizing blood glucose control, reducing body weight, increasing physical activity, normalizing lipid disturbances, and reducing hypertension. Identifying organ-system complications as early as possible so that they may be treated is also fundamental. Improving the patient's sense of well-being, self-care attitude, and life-style habits are critical for ensuring the healthiest long-term outcomes.
- *Goals for glycemic control* include fasting and preprandial serum glucose level of <126 mg/dL, postprandial glucose level <160, and a glycosylated hemoglobin level of <6%.
- *Self-monitoring of blood glucose* is most desirable in patients with type 2 diabetes to obtain optimal glycemic control.
- *Exercise:* Within the limits guided by one's potential cardiovascular ability, the patient should begin an individualized exercise regimen emphasizing aerobic exercise for 30 minutes at least 3 days per week. The regimen should be begun gradually and built up as exercise capacity increases. Exercise significantly enhances improved caloric balance and reduces insulin resistance.
- *The diabetic diet* aims to normalize blood glucose and lipid levels, as well as obtain and maintain optimal body weight and balance caloric intake with caloric expenditure.
    - Current dietary recommendations advocate:
        1. Carbohydrates should be complex and rich in fiber and should make up 55% to 60% of the total energy intake.
        2. Total fat should be reduced to 30% to 35% of total energy intake; animal fats should be replaced with monounsaturated or polyunsaturated fats.
        3. Protein should equate to 10% of total caloric intake.
        4. Cholesterol intake should be limited to 300 mg/day.
        5. Alcohol consumption should be limited to the equivalent of 4 ounces of wine per day.
    - Recent studies have reported a more favorable lipid, glucose, and insulin profile following the ingestion of a diet that predominates in monounsaturated fats.
- Oral hypoglycemics.
    - When glycemic control is not sufficiently achieved with dietary and exercise interventions, oral hypoglycemic agents are warranted. In this setting, glucose self-monitoring is essential when striving for glycemic control and the avoidance of hypoglycemia.
    - There are five categories of oral hypoglycemic drugs.
        1. *Sulfonylureas* (tolbutamide, acetohexamide, chlorpropamide, glyburide, glipizide).
            a. Sulfonylureas primarily stimulate insulin release from β-cells during the pharmacologic life of the drug (4 to 24 hours).
            b. They are often successful when used alone.
            c. Side effects include weight gain and hypoglycemia.
            d. Drug interactions: Sulfonamides, salicylates, probenecid, and β-blockers may enhance hypoglycemia.
            e. They are contraindicated in insulin deficiency (type 1 diabetes), pregnancy, and lactation. The perioperative patient is also best managed with insulin.
        2. *Biguanides* (metformin).
            a. Biguanides lower blood glucose by enhancing insulin sensitivity and peripheral glucose uptake, and inhibiting hepatic glucose production.
            b. They do not cause hypoglycemia.
            c. Other benefits include decreased levels of total cholesterol, triglyceride, and LDL.
            d. Because of the occasional side effects of reduced appetite and weight loss, this drug is preferred in the treatment of the obese patient.
            e. Side effects include minor gastrointestinal effects that can be controlled by decreasing the dosage. A rare serious consequence is lactic acidosis; this usually occurs when a contraindication such as renal insufficiency has been overlooked.
            f. Biguanides are contraindicated in renal impairment, pregnancy, and insulin deficiency, and should be used with caution in patients who have liver, heart, or lung disease; cimetidine increases serum levels of metformin.

 3. *Secretagogues* (nateglinide, repaglinide).
   a. Secretagogues are structurally distinct from sulfonylureas but similar in their insulin secretion stimulation mechanism.
   b. They are short acting and designed to increase mealtime insulin secretion and should be taken at mealtime.
 4. α-glucosidase inhibitors (acarbose, miglitol).
   a. α-glucosidase inhibitors interfere with enzymes in the intestine that break down complex sugars. As a result, they limit the absorption of simple sugar (glucose) from the gastrointestinal tract. They have been shown to improve postprandial blood glucose levels and lower levels of glycosylated hemoglobin.
   b. They do not cause hypoglycemia.
   c. Side effects are similar to those of lactose intolerance because of the effect of undigested sugars upon colonic bacteria (diarrhea, abdominal distention and pain, flatus).
 5. *Thiazolidinediones* (rosiglitazone, pioglitazone).
   a. Thiazolidinediones enhance hepatic insulin sensitivity and reduce insulin resistance.
   b. Side effects include fluid retention and occasional, reversible increases in liver function enzymes. Because of concerns for hepatic impairment, the latter is an indication for discontinuation of the drug.

- Insulin.
  - Because the typical patient with type 2 diabetes is insulin resistant and usually has an elevated basal insulin level, the administration of additional exogenous insulin is a last choice for achieving blood sugar control. It is often used when there is an urgent need for immediate blood sugar control, during a perioperative period, and as a last resort in longer-term glycemic control.
  - Exogenous insulin substitutes for the β-cell defect by reducing glucose levels, suppressing hepatic glucose production, and increasing glucose uptake into cells.
  - Insulin treatment is initiated after insufficient metabolic control is obtained with maximal doses of oral hypoglycemic agents; small doses are begun (10 to 20 units) and gradually increased until the fasting blood sugar becomes normal (or $HgbA_{1c} <6\%$); large doses (200 to 300 units daily) may sometimes be required to overcome insulin resistance.
  - Side effects of insulin administration include weight gain and hypoglycemia. Chronic hyperinsulinemia is a known risk factor for cardiovascular disease.
  - Insulin may be useful during acute medical or surgical events when more careful management of blood glucose is needed.

- *For general management,* treatment is initiated with one of the oral hypoglycemic agents (metformin, sulfonylurea, secretagogue). If ineffective, two- or three-drug therapy using multiple classes of oral agents is indicated. Because of cost factors, thiazolidinediones are more selectively used although they can be effective as monotherapy.
- *Combinations* of oral agents and selected insulin regimens (NPH, Glargine) have been shown to have benefit in type 2 diabetes.
- *Monitoring and management of diabetic complications.*
  - Microvascular disease, including retinopathy, nephropathy, and neuropathy, may all be delayed or prevented by tight glycemic control (HbA_{1c} averaging 6% or less) and aggressive treatment of hypertension when present.
    1. Retinopathy includes microaneurysms, vitreous and retinal hemorrhage, and proliferative retinopathy. Yearly eye examinations are recommended. Laser photocoagulation may be beneficial in the early stages of disease.
    2. Nephropathy results in early urinary albumin excretion in excess of 30 mg in 24 hours due to glomerular injury. The use of angiotensin-converting enzyme inhibitors and angiotensin receptor blockers has been shown to delay the progress of diabetic renal disease in both normotensive and hypertensive patients, reverse albuminuria, and delay the decline in glomerular filtration rate.

3. Neuropathy, both sensory and motor, is best avoided and treated with tight glycemic control. It is the primary factor in the pathogenesis of diabetic foot ulcers. Practicing consistent foot observation and care, and avoiding physical injury decrease the risk of foot ulcers, potential infection, and the likelihood of amputation.

4. Neurogenic bladder, usually in the form of a flaccid dilating bladder, frequently gives rise to recurrent urinary tract infection because of the existence of a post-void residual volume of urine. Silent urinary infections are frequent because of the presence of an autonomic sensory lesion, resulting in a diminished or absent perception of bladder symptoms.

5. Poor glucose control results in increased bacterial and fungal infections, itching, and eventually more severe variations in diabetic skin disease.

6. Diabetic foot infections account for nearly half of all nontraumatic lower-extremity amputations in the United States. Patients should examine their feet daily and wear appropriate footwear. Foot examination with particular attention to vascular and neurologic function and nail integrity should be done regularly.

7. Atherosclerosis is accelerated in the individual with diabetes. Careful attention to other cardiovascular risk factors including smoking, hypertension, lipid abnormalities, and sedentary life-style is mandatory. Observation for evidence of developing cardiac, cerebral, and peripheral vascular disease is important for the purpose of early detection and treatment. The silent nature of vascular disease in its early stages is complicated in the patient with diabetes because of the occurrence of autonomic sensory neuropathy, which diminishes the ability of the patient to perceive the symptoms of organ dysfunction.

PATHOPHYSIOLOGY →	CLINICAL LINK
What is going on in the disease process that influences how the patient presents and how he or she should be managed?	*What should you do now that you understand the underlying pathophysiology?*
There is clear evidence of the genetic profile that predisposes an individual to the development of type 2 diabetes.	Type 2 diabetes is a familial disorder; patients with a family history (especially a first-degree relative) should be counseled and screened regularly.
Insulin resistance results from a variety of mechanisms including genetic predisposition, excessive caloric storage volume, metabolic dysfunction, receptor down-regulation, and glucose transport abnormalities.	Diabetes is heterogeneous in its pathogenesis, and management techniques must be multifaceted in nature; reversal of insulin resistance is essential; newer oral hypoglycemic drugs target several of these mechanisms.
Obesity, particularly abdominal obesity, is directly correlated with insulin resistance.	Weight loss is the most effective management strategy for reversing diabetes type 2 metabolic abnormalities such as insulin resistance.
Caloric restriction decreases body weight, insulin demand, and hepatic glucose production.	Caloric dietary management is essential to the reversibility of diabetic processes.
End-organ effects from diabetes occur frequently in patients before their diagnosis and may begin early in the course of the disease.	At-risk patients should be screened regularly for eye disease, albuminuria, and peripheral neuropathy. Criteria for diagnosis are designed to identify patients with early diabetic evidence.
Diabetes affects many organ systems including skin, eyes, kidneys, nerves, and blood vessels.	Patients with diabetes require careful screening for skin infections, foot ulcers, retinopathy, microalbuminuria, neuropathy, and atherosclerosis (ischemic heart disease, cerebrovascular disease, and peripheral vascular disease).

SUGGESTED READINGS

Centers for Disease Control and Prevention. (2004). Primary prevention of type 2 diabetes mellitus by lifestyle intervention: implications for health policy. *Annals of Internal Medicine, 140,* 951-957.

Cooper, M. E. & Johnston, C. I. (2000). Optimizing treatment of hypertension in patients with diabetes. *Journal of the American Medical Association, 283*(24), 3177-3179.

DeFronzo, R. A. (1999). Pharmacologic therapy for type 2 diabetes mellitus. *Annals of Internal Medicine, 131*(4), 281-303.

Donnelly, R., Emslie-Smith, A. M., Gardner, I. D., & Morris, A. D. (2000). ABC of arterial and venous disease: vascular complications of diabetes. *British Medical Journal, 320*(7241), 1062-1066.

Edelman, D., Olsen, M. K., Dudley, T. K., Harris, A. C., & Oddone, E. Z. (2004). Utility of hemoglobin A1c in predicting diabetes risk. *Journal of General Internal Medicine, 19,* 1175-1180.

Ferris, F. L., III, Davis, M. D., & Aiello, L. M. (1999). Treatment of diabetic retinopathy. *New England Journal of Medicine, 341*(9), 667-678.

Folsom, A. R., Kushi, L. H., Anderson, K. E., Mink, P. J., Olson, J. E., Hong, C. P., Sellers, T. A., Lazovich, D., & Prineas, R. J. (2000). Associations of general and abdominal obesity with multiple health outcomes in older women: the Iowa Women's Health Study. *Archives of Internal Medicine, 160*(14), 2117-2128.

Gaster, B. & Hirsch, I. B. (1998). The effects of improved glycemic control on complications in type 2 diabetes. *Archives of Internal Medicine, 158*(2), 134-140.

Gibbons, G. R. & Newton, W. (2000). Noninvasive glucose monitoring. *Journal of Family Practice, 49*(2), 110-111.

Goldberg, R. B. (2000). Cardiovascular disease in diabetic patients. *Medical Clinics of North America, 84*(1), 81-93.

Griffin, S. & Kinmonth, A. L. (2000). Diabetes care: the effectiveness of systems for routine surveillance for people with diabetes. *Cochrane Database of Systematic Reviews* (2), CD000541.

Herman, W. H., Hoerger, T. J., Brandlem, M., Hicks, K., Sorensen, S., Zhang, P., Hamman, R. F., Ackermann, R. T., Engelgau, M. M., Ratner, R. E., & Diabetes Prevention Program Research Group. (2005). The cost effectiveness of lifestyle modification or metformin in preventing type 2 diabetes in adults with impaired glucose tolerance. *Annals of Internal Medicine, 142,* 323-332.

Klonoff, D. C. (2005). Pharmacologic treatment of type 2 diabetes mellitus. *American Journal of Medicine,* 118s.

Kopelman, P. G. & Hitman, G. A. (1998). Diabetes. Exploding type II. *Lancet, 352*(suppl 4), SIV5.

Lovell, H. G. (2000). Angiotensin converting enzyme inhibitors in normotensive diabetic patients with microalbuminuria. *Cochrane Database of Systematic Reviews,* (2), CD002183.

Mak, K. H. & Topol, E. J. (2000). Emerging concepts in the management of acute myocardial infarction in patients with diabetes mellitus. *Journal of the American College of Cardiology, 35*(3), 563-568.

Mangan, D., Selwitz, R. H., & Genco, R. (2000). Infections associated with diabetes mellitus. *New England Journal of Medicine, 342*(12), 896.

Narayan, K. M., Boyle, J. P., Thompson, T. J., Sorensen, S. W., & Williamson, D. F. (2003). Lifetime risk for diabetes mellitus in the United States. *Journal of the American Medical Association, 290,* 14, 1884-1890.

Rosenbloom, A. L., Joe, J. R., Young, R. S., & Winter, W. E. (1999). Emerging epidemic of type 2 diabetes in youth. *Diabetes Care, 22*(2), 345-354.

Seidell, J. C. (2000). Obesity, insulin resistance and diabetes—a worldwide epidemic. *British Journal of Nutrition, 83* (suppl 1), S5-S8.

Sumpio, B. E. (2000). Foot ulcers. *New England Journal of Medicine, 343*(11), 787-793.

White, W. B., Prisant, L. M., & Wright, J. T., Jr. (2000). Management of patients with hypertension and diabetes mellitus: advances in the evidence for intensive treatment. *American Journal of Medicine, 108*(3), 238-245.

Type 2 Diabetes Mellitus

INITIAL HISTORY

- 52-year-old black female.
- Diagnosed with type 2 diabetes 6 years ago but did not follow up with recommendations for care.
- Now complaining of weakness in her right foot and an itching rash in her groin area.

Question 1.   *What questions would you like to ask her about her symptoms?*

ADDITIONAL HISTORY

- Patient says her foot has been weak for about a month and is difficult to dorsiflex; it also feels numb.
- Denies any other weakness, numbness, difficulty speaking or walking, syncope, or seizures. She finds that watching television particularly in the evening, is becoming a problem because her eyes "are tired" more.
- Has had some increased thirst and gets up more often at night to urinate, sometimes excessively.
- Says she has had the rash on and off for many years. It is worse when the weather is warm. It also occurs in her armpits. She gets some relief from salt baths. She occasionally gets a boil in these areas.
- Denies any chest pain, shortness of breath, edema, change in bowel habits, or skin ulcers.

Question 2.   *What other personal and family-related questions would you like to ask her about her diabetes?*

DIABETES HISTORY

- Patient remembers being told her blood sugar was "around 200" when she was first diagnosed. She had gone for a work physical and felt fine at the time and saw no need for expensive drugs.
- Her mother and sister have diabetes. Both of them were diagnosed in their 40s and are on pills and injections.
- Has been completely asymptomatic, except for the rash, until the foot weakness.
- Has gained 18 pounds over the past year and eats a diet high in fats and refined sugars.
- Employed as a banking executive and gets little exercise.

Question 3. *What would you like to ask about her medical history?*

PHYSICAL EXAMINATION

- Obese female in no acute distress.
- T = 37° C orally; P = 80 and regular; RR = 15 and unlabored; BP = 162/98 right arm (sitting); weight 84 kg.

Skin

- Erythematous moist rash in both inguinal areas, beneath both breasts, and in the axillae.
- No petechiae or ecchymoses.
- Many dime-sized hyperpigmented spots located on the anterior shins.

HEENT, Neck

- Pupils equal and round, fundi with mild arteriolar narrowing.
- Nares and tympanic membranes clear.
- Pharynx clear.
- Neck without bruits or thyromegaly.

Lungs, Cardiac

- Lungs clear to auscultation and percussion.
- Cardiac examination with distant heart tones, a regular rate and rhythm without murmurs or gallops.

Abdomen, Extremities

- Abdomen moderately obese with bowel sounds heard in all four quadrants; no abdominal bruits, tenderness, masses, or organomegaly.
- Extremities without edema; arterial pulses are diminished in volume but palpable in both feet.

Neurologic

- Alert and oriented.
- Cranial nerves II through XII intact (including normal visual acuity with glasses).
- Limb strength 5/5 throughout except 2/5 on dorsiflexion of the right foot.
- Sensory perception to light touch diminished on the soles of both feet along the metatarsal bar.
- Deep tendon reflexes 1+ and symmetric throughout.
- Gait normal except for accommodation to a right footdrop; negative Romberg test.

Question 4.   *What are the pertinent positives and negatives on the physical examination?*

Question 5.   *What laboratory tests would you order now?*

INITIAL LABORATORY RESULTS

- Serum electrolytes, including BUN and creatinine, calcium, and magnesium all within normal limits.
- Random glucose = 253 mg/dL (taken at 11 AM).
- HgbA$_{1c}$ = 9.1%.
- Urine dipstick positive for glucose, negative for protein; microscopic without significant cellular or infectious findings.
- Wet prep of smear from skin rash consistent with fungal spores and mycelia.
- Electrocardiogram with evidence of early left ventricular hypertrophy (LVH) by voltage.

PATIENT'S RETURN VISIT (THE FOLLOWING WEEK)

- BP = 150/100 both arms (sitting).
- Fasting glucose = 168 mg/dL.
- Fasting total cholesterol = 246 mg/dL with HDL = 28 mg/dL and triglycerides = 658 mg/dL.
- 24-hour urine for albumin = 160 mg/24 hr.
- Electromyography consistent with peripheral neuropathy of right foot (peroneal nerve palsy).

Question 6. *How would you interpret these laboratory findings?*

Question 7. *What would you recommend at this time?*

Anemia

DEFINITION

- A decrease in red blood cells (RBCs), often reported as a decrease in hematocrit (Hct) or a decrease in hemoglobin concentration (Hgb). The World Health Organization defines anemia as an Hgb concentration of less than 13 g/dL in men, less than 12 g/dL in women and in children ages 6 to 14 years, and less than 11 g/dL in children 6 months to 6 years old.
- Results in decreased oxygen carrying capacity of the blood.
- Selected causes of anemia.
    - Insufficient production.
        1. Microcytic anemia (iron deficiency, anemia of chronic disease [ACD], thalassemia).
        2. Macrocytic anemia (alcoholism, vitamin B_{12} or folate deficiency, pernicious anemia).
        3. Marrow disease (leukemia, aplastic anemia, other myelodysplastic diseases).
        4. Renal disease with decreased erythropoietin.
    - Increased destruction.
        1. Immune hemolytic anemia.
        2. Inherited hemolytic anemia.
            a. Hereditary spherocytosis.
            b. Sickle cell disease.

EPIDEMIOLOGY

- Iron deficiency is the most common form of anemia and occurs in an estimated 30% of the world's population. In the United States, 7% of toddlers ages 1 to 2 years, and up to 19% of adolescent girls and women of childbearing age are iron deficient; less than 1% of older male children and men are iron deficient.
- Anemia of chronic disease is associated with many inflammatory, infectious, and neoplastic conditions and is second in incidence to iron deficiency anemia.
- Thalassemia affects 3% to 10% of people from Asia, Africa, and the Mediterranean region.
- Vitamin B_{12} deficiency affects 10% to 15% of the U.S. population older than 60 years of age. Pernicious anemia occurs in an estimated 3% of the white U.S. population older than 60 years.
- Immune hemolytic anemias are common in hospitalized patients and result from many medications and conditions.
- Hereditary spherocytosis is the most common inherited anemia in people of northern European descent.
- Sickle cell trait occurs in about 8% of blacks, with sickle cell anemia present in 0.15%.

PATHOPHYSIOLOGY

Insufficient Production (Decreased Reticulocytes)

- Microcytic anemia.
  - Iron deficiency anemia.
    1. Normally, approximately 1 mg of iron is absorbed and lost per day; an imbalance between intake, requirements, and loss of iron leads to iron deficiency.
    2. Dietary iron deficiency is common in states of increased iron requirements such as infancy and pregnancy; inadequate iron absorption can occur after partial gastrectomy, atrophic gastritis (as with *Helicobacter pylori*) and in diseases of the intestine (celiac disease).
    3. Increased iron loss occurs in menstruation (up to 20 mg with each period) and with chronic blood loss (e.g., peptic ulcer disease, colon cancer, repetitive phlebotomy).
    4. Iron deficiency leads to decreased ferritin (in response to iron-regulatory protein 1 gene) and decreased bone marrow iron stores with resultant abnormal RBC production.
    5. RBCs are small (microcytic—decreased mean corpuscular volume [MCV]) and pale (hypochromic—decreased mean corpuscular hemoglobin concentration [MCHC]).
  - Anemia of chronic disease (ACD) is the most common anemia in hospitalized patients.
    1. Anemia is associated with underlying inflammatory and neoplastic conditions.
    2. Mechanisms of the anemia are not well understood but include impaired erythropoiesis, relative erythropoietin deficiency, decreased utilization of iron, abnormal hemoglobin synthesis, and decreased RBC survival.
    3. Because ferritin is an acute phase protein, it is frequently normal or elevated in ACD.
  - Thalassemia.
    1. Hereditary defects in hemoglobin synthesis.
    2. α-thalassemia occurs most commonly in Asia and results from a mutation in the α_1- and α_2-globin genes, resulting in decreased production of α-globin.
    3. β-thalassemia occurs most commonly in Mediterranean countries and can result from any one of 200 possible mutations in the β-globin gene, which results in abnormal β-globin synthesis.
    4. Ineffective erythropoiesis and premature death of erythroblasts lead to microcytic anemia; accumulation and precipitation of abnormal hemoglobin tetramers result in RBC apoptosis and splenic RBC destruction.
    5. Several forms of each thalassemia (including carrier, trait, and disease states) result in varying degrees of anemia with hemolysis.
    6. Extramedullary erythropoietic tissues may be stimulated to expand and lead to characteristic deformities of the skull and face and to osteopenia with fractures.
    7. Iron absorption is increased, resulting in significant iron overload with multiorgan damage, especially to the liver, heart, and endocrine glands. Cardiac toxicity can be severe with heart failure and death possible.
    8. Many individuals with thalassemia are infected with hepatitis C.
- Macrocytic anemia.
  - Alcoholism is the most common cause of macrocytic anemia. Alcohol interferes with RBC maturation and is associated with vitamin B_{12} and folate deficiency (poor diet and gastric dysfunction) thus is a common cause of macrocytic anemia (high MCV).
  - B_{12} and/or folate deficiency cause abnormal deoxyribonucleic acid (DNA) synthesis in RBC precursor marrow stem cells (megaloblastic) with inadequate and abnormal RBC production. RBCs are macrocytic and normochromic.
  - Pernicious anemia is a condition that results from autoimmune destruction of intrinsic factor and or the parietal cells of gastric mucosa that produce it. Intrinsic factor is

necessary for normal B_{12} absorption in the ileum. Patients with atrophic gastritis (as with *H. pylori*) or who are postgastrectomy may also present with pernicious anemia.

- Some medications (e.g., methotrexate), hepatic disease, and thyroid disorders can also cause macrocytic changes in RBCs.
- Marrow disease.
  - Abnormalities of the marrow lead to decreased RBC production and include:
    1. Displacement of erythropoietic stem cells by leukemic or metastatic tumor cells.
    2. Abnormal differentiation of the hematopoietic stem cells seen in myelodysplastic syndromes.
    3. Aplasia of the marrow (aplastic anemia).
  - The marrow becomes depleted of stem cells such that the anemia is accompanied by leukopenia and thrombocytopenia (pancytopenia).
  - Aplastic anemia refers to a condition that arises from failure of the bone marrow stem cells. Although there are rare congenital cases (e.g., Fanconi anemia), aplastic anemia is most often an acquired disorder resulting from infiltrative, autoimmune, infectious, or toxic insults to the marrow. Among the most commonly implicated toxins are drugs (chemotherapeutic agents, some antibiotics) and industrial chemicals. Intensive radiation also destroys marrow stem cells.
- Renal disease.
  - Patients with chronic renal disease synthesize inadequate amounts of erythropoietin with resultant diminished RBC production.
  - Treatment with recombinant erythropoietin is highly effective but can result in a state of relative iron deficiency requiring iron supplementation (may require parenteral iron).

Increased Destruction (Increased Reticulocytes)

- Immune hemolytic anemia.
  - 50% of cases are idiopathic; secondary causes include: (1) Neoplasia (chronic leukemia, lymphoma); (2) collagen vascular disorders (systemic lupus erythematosus, rheumatoid arthritis); (3) drugs (α-methyldopa, penicillin); (4) infections (mycoplasma, infectious mononucleosis).
  - Caused by binding of autoimmune antibodies and/or complement to RBC.
  - May be mediated by immunoglobulin G (IgG) antibody that reacts with RBC at body temperature (warm antibody) or by IgM that reacts with RBC at colder temperatures (cold antibody).
  - RBCs are lysed or are removed from the circulation by the spleen. On blood smear, see polychromasia (due to increased reticulocytes) and fragmented cells (schistocytes).
- Inherited hemolytic anemia.
  - Hereditary spherocytosis.
    1. Autosomal dominant inheritance; common in northern Europeans.
    2. Defect in the proteins of the red cell cytoskeleton results in spherocytes that have reduced membrane surface area compared with cell volume.
    3. Spherical RBCs are fragile and are removed by the spleen.
  - Sickle cell anemia.
    1. Inherited genetic defect that is the result of a single base mutation in the β-globin gene (Hgb S). Inheritance of one defective gene is called sickle cell trait, inheritance of two defective genes is called sickle cell anemia.
    2. Substitution of a single amino acid (valine for glutamic acid) results in intracellular polymerization of the hemoglobin molecule in response to deoxygenation, low temperature, and acidosis. In sickle trait, 40% of the total hemoglobin is Hgb S and anemia is mild. In sickle cell anemia, the majority of hemoglobin is defective.
    3. Another type of hemoglobin defect results in production of Hgb C, which often presents with Hgb S (Hgb SC). Hgb C also results in sickling.
    4. Sickled cells adhere to the endothelium and cause microvascular obstruction (vasoocclusive disease) with organ infarcts.

5. Vasoocclusive exacerbations can affect any organ (spleen, brain, heart, lung). Stroke is common in children. The acute chest syndrome results from vasoocclusion of pulmonary vessels causing pulmonary infiltrates, infarcts, effusions, and hypoxemia. Chronic leg ulcers are common, as is priapism.

6. Sickled cells are removed by the spleen, which can result in aplastic crisis with severe pain and profound anemia. Aplastic crises can occur when erythropoiesis cannot compensate for cellular destruction. It is interesting to note that transient aplastic crises, especially in children, have been linked to parvovirus B19 infection, which is cytopathic to red cell precursors.

7. Hepatomegaly with abnormal liver function occurs in 90% of individuals with sickle cell anemia; hepatitis, cholecystis, and acute hepatic crises are common.

8. Other complications include susceptibility to infection and sepsis (especially to *Streptococcus pneumoniae* due to splenic dysfunction), delayed growth and development, kidney dysfunction, bone necrosis, retinal hemorrhage, and narcotic addiction.

PATIENT PRESENTATION

History

Pregnancy; menorrhagia; unusual diet (e.g., strict vegetarian); Mediterranean or Asian descent; alcohol abuse; chronic underlying illness; gastric surgery; drugs; family history; history of pain crises or sepsis.

Symptoms

- Mild cases are often asymptomatic or may be associated with fatigue; dyspnea on exertion; weakness; palpitations; edema; or symptoms of underlying disease. More severe cases may present with congestive heart failure, transient ischemic attacks, syncope, or angina.
    - Iron deficiency may be associated with menometrorrhagia or other blood loss (melena, hematochezia, hematemesis, hematuria) and occasionally will present with pica for starch, ice, or clay.
    - Bone marrow disorders such as aplastic anemia with resultant pancytopenia are characterized by recurrent infections and bleeding.
    - Sickle cell disease is characterized by pain crises, skin ulcers, and organ infarcts that may be manifested by acute pain, neurologic deficits, or symptoms of other specific organ dysfunction. The acute chest syndrome is characterized by fever, pleuritic chest pain, and cough.

Examination

- Pallor and/or jaundice (from hemolysis); tachycardia; systolic murmurs; edema; splenomegaly; severe anemia may be manifested with evidence of congestive heart failure; signs of alcohol abuse; signs of specific underlying illnesses.
    - Iron deficiency is associated with glossitis, angular cheilitis, and brittle nails.
    - Bone marrow disorders such as aplastic anemia are associated with petechiae and evidence of infection (fever, tachycardia, cough, dysuria).
    - Sickle cell disease is associated with evidence of organ infarction including focal neurologic deficits, skin ulcers, evidence of infection or kidney disease, and pulmonary congestion with infiltrates and hypoxemia (acute chest syndrome).

KEYS TO ASSESSMENT

- Mild anemia may be asymptomatic and should be suspected in infants, women of menstrual age, and pregnant women.
- Alcohol abuse can be associated with direct marrow toxicity, vitamin deficiency, and upper gastrointestinal blood loss and is a common cause of a mixed microcytic and macrocytic anemia.

- A family history of anemia is common, especially in certain racial and ethnic groups.
- A logical progression of investigative studies should be undertaken (Figure 12-1).
- Specific tests.
  - Iron deficiency: Serum iron, iron-binding capacity, and marrow iron stores; serum ferritin, transferrin receptor assay, and reticulocyte hemoglobin concentration (differentiate iron deficiency anemia from anemia of chronic disease).
  - Aplastic anemia and other marrow disorders: Bone marrow biopsy.
  - Macrocytic anemia: Serum and RBC folate, serum B_{12}, and Schilling test (B_{12} absorption), bone marrow biopsy for megaloblasts; liver function and thyroid function tests if not megaloblastic or vitamin deficient.
  - Immune hemolysis: Measurement of specific warm and cold antibodies; Coombs test.
  - Hereditary anemias: Hemoglobin electrophoresis and genetic profiles.

KEYS TO MANAGEMENT

- Treatment of any underlying systemic disease is vital. Discontinuation of alcohol intake should be recommended for most patients.
- Transfusion should be limited to those patients with severe anemia and symptoms such as chest pain, dyspnea at rest, congestive heart failure, or neurologic complaints.
- Unexplained iron deficiency in adult males and postmenopausal women must be evaluated thoroughly, including a complete gastrointestinal work-up. Recent articles suggest that up to 12% of premenopausal women with iron deficiency have gastrointestinal lesions (not all of

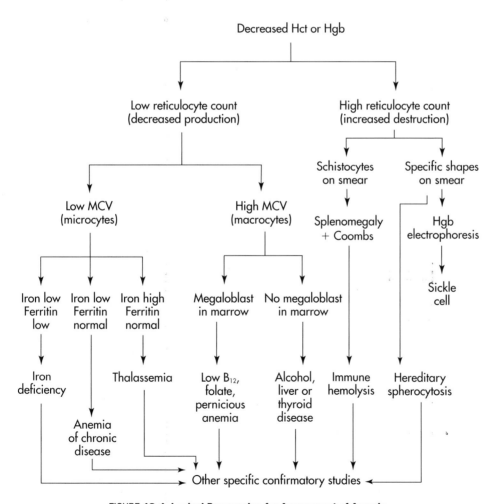

FIGURE **12-1 Logical Progression for Assessment of Anemia.**

their iron loss is via menstruation). Upper and lower endoscopy in premenopausal patients is indicated if there are any gastrointestinal complaints or guaiac-positive stools.

- Specific therapies.
  - Iron deficiency.
    1. Oral iron (60 mg three times a day): Gastrointestinal side effects such as dyspepsia and constipation are common. Normalization of Hct usually occurs in 6 to 8 weeks.
    2. For those intolerant or unresponsive to oral iron therapy or for those receiving recombinant erythropoietin therapy (e.g., renal disease), parenteral iron replacement is indicated. Choices include iron dextran, ferric gluconate, and iron sucrose. Iron dextran is associated with a significant risk for toxicity including fatal anaphylaxis, and patients should receive a test dose with epinephrine available at the bedside. Ferric gluconate and iron sucrose are generally safer with less toxicity.
    3. In patients with *H. pylori*–associated atrophic gastritis, treatment with appropriate antibiotic combinations may reverse the iron deficiency (see Chapter 15).
  - Anemia of chronic disease (ACD).
    1. Successful treatment of the underlying disease will often result in normalization of the Hct.
    2. Erythropoietin therapy has been used in rheumatoid arthritis and is being tested in other causes of ACD.
  - B_{12} and folate deficiency.
    1. Oral replacement is indicated in dietary insufficiency without malabsorption. Public health service guidelines recommend that all women of childbearing age consume a minimum of 400 mcg/day of folate.
    2. In patients with B_{12} malabsorption (pernicious anemia, postgastrectomy), B_{12} should be given monthly via intramuscular injection or via sublingual formulations.
  - Bone marrow disease (aplastic anemia).
    1. Treatment of the underlying disease may improve anemia; however, many of the indicated treatments (e.g., chemotherapy, bone marrow transplant) may result in a transient worsening of the RBC count and may necessitate transfusion.
    2. Myelodysplastic syndromes may respond to androgens, differentiating agents (retinoic acid), or growth factors (erythropoietin).
    3. Aplastic anemia is treated with bone marrow transplantation.
  - Thalassemia.
    1. Many patients require no treatment.
    2. Plasmapheresis with transfusions followed by iron chelation therapy (deferoxamine, deferiprone, desferrithiocin) is indicated in severe anemia.
    3. Bone marrow transplant has been successful in selected extreme cases.
    4. If thalassemia is diagnosed in utero, successful cord blood transplantation has been reported.
    5. Gene therapy is being explored.
  - Chronic renal disease.
    1. Recombinant erythropoietin with iron supplementation when indicated.
    2. Parenteral iron administration is often necessary (iron dextran, ferric gluconate, or iron sucrose).
  - Immune hemolysis.
    1. Removal of causative drugs and treatment of underlying disease.
    2. Splenectomy may be necessary in some chronic diseases.
    3. Plasmapheresis has been used in cold antibody immune hemolysis.
    4. Steroids and cytotoxic agents (e.g., cyclosporin) may be indicated in severe cases.
    5. Monoclonal antibodies against CD20 antigen (rituximab) and CD53 antigen (alemtuzumab) have been shown in early clinical trials to be safe and effective in reducing autoimmune RBC destruction.

- Hereditary spherocytosis.
    1. Splenectomy; vaccination to reduce the risk of infection after splenectomy.
    2. A new procedure called "near-total splenectomy" (NTS) preserves some splenic parenchyma that partially regenerates and allows for normal immune function without recurrence of significant anemia.
- Sickle cell disease.
    1. Pain crises: Oxygen, hydration, pain control (patient-controlled analgesia has been effective in emergency department and clinic settings).
    2. Severe anemia (aplastic crisis) is treated with oxygen and transfusion.
    3. Vasoocclusive episodes are treated with hydration, oxygen, and may soon include consideration for a new drug (phase III trials) called purified poloxamer 188, which lowers blood viscosity, decreases RBC aggregation, and decreases friction between RBCs and vessel walls to increase microvascular blood flow.
    4. Chronic therapy with hydroxyurea, 5-azacitidine, or decitibine (increase Hgb F) decreases symptoms and extends time between transfusions.
    5. Clotrimazole and magnesium help retain RBC water content by reducing potassium and water efflux; early trials have documented decreased sickling when these are used.
    6. Nitric oxide inhalation may be beneficial for acute chest syndrome.
    7. Phytomedicines (e.g., Niprisan) have been documented to reduce pain crises.
    8. Bone marrow transplant has been successful in children and can be increasingly considered for adults with severe disease.
    9. Monitor and treat the many potential complications; patient education is crucial; daily penicillin for patients ages 3 months to 5 years; pneumococcal vaccine.
    10. Neonatal screening is available; regular transfusions in children may decrease the risk of stroke but remains controversial.
    11. Gene therapy is being investigated.

PATHOPHYSIOLOGY $\longrightarrow$	CLINICAL LINK
What is going on in the disease process that influences how the patient presents and how he or she should be managed?	*What should you do now that you understand the underlying pathophysiology?*
Iron deficiency can result from increased requirement for iron, decreased intake of iron, or increased loss of iron.	Patients at risk for iron deficiency anemia include infants, women of menstrual age, pregnant women, those with atrophic gastritis, postgastrectomy patients, and patients with chronic blood loss.
Normally, iron is recycled in the body after RBC destruction and is reused to make new RBCs such that only 1 g of iron is lost and needs to be replaced per day.	Men and postmenstrual women who become iron deficient should be evaluated for sites of blood loss, especially from the gastrointestinal tract (ulcers, cancers). Iron deficient premenopausal women with gastrointestinal complaints should also be evaluated.
Macrocytosis can result from direct toxicity from alcohol, or from abnormal RBC maturation due to B_{12} and/or folate deficiency, which are common in alcoholism. Vitamin deficiency results in megaloblastic changes in the marrow.	A patient with macrocytic anemia should be questioned about alcohol use and have B_{12} and folate levels measured in the blood.
Intrinsic factor is produced in the stomach and is necessary for adequate B_{12} absorption in the ileum. Some patients have autoimmune antibodies to parietal cells or intrinsic factor (pernicious anemia); other patients have atrophic gastritis or are postgastrectomy and have low levels of intrinsic factor.	Patients with autoimmune pernicious anemia can be diagnosed by measuring intrinsic factor antibodies. Patients who cannot absorb B_{12} will have an abnormal Schilling test. Treatment for these patients requires intramuscular injection or sublingual administration of B_{12}.
Immune hemolytic anemias are associated with a variety of underlying conditions and the intake of certain drugs; patients will demonstrate autoimmune antibodies to their own RBCs.	Patients with lymphoma, chronic leukemia, rheumatoid arthritis, systemic lupus erythematosus, mycoplasma, or Epstein-Barr virus infections, or who are on penicillin or α-methyldopa who develop anemia should be evaluated with a Coombs test for autoantibodies.
Sickle cell disease and thalassemia result from specific mutations in hemoglobin genes.	Future therapy for these common and sometimes devastating disorders will most likely rest on gene therapy.

SUGGESTED READINGS

Bagby, G. C., Lipton, J. M., Sloand, E. M., & Schiffer, C. A. (2004). Marrow failure. *Hematology*, 318-336.

Bar-Or, D. & Kepros, J. P. (2004). Anemia associated with critical illness: is the erythropoietin receptor a culprit? *Critical Care Medicine*, 32, 1234-1235.

Bashiri, A., Burstein, E., Sheiner, E., & Mazor, M. (2003). Anemia during pregnancy and treatment with intravenous iron: review of the literature. *European Journal of Obstetrics, Gynecology, & Reproductive Biology*, 110, 2-7.

Bergman, M. P., Vandenbroucke-Grauls, C. M., Appelmelk, B. J., D'Elios, M. M., Amedei, A., Azzurri, A., Benagiano, M., & Del Prete, G. (2005). The story so far: *Helicobacter pylori* and gastric autoimmunity. *International Reviews of Immunology*, 24, 63-91.

Beutler, E., Hoffbrand, A. V., & Cook, J. D. (2003). Iron deficiency and overload. *Hematology*, 40-61.

Bolton-Maggs, P. H. (2004). Hereditary spherocytosis; new guidelines. *Archives of Disease in Childhood*, 89, 809-812.

Bolton-Maggs, P. H., Stevens, R. F., Dodd, N. J., Lamont, G., Tittensor, P., King, M. J., & General Haematology Task Force of the British Committee for Standards in Haematology. (2004). Guidelines for the diagnosis and management of hereditary spherocytosis. *British Journal of Haematology*, 126, 455-474.

Brodsky, R. A. & Jones, R. J. (2005). Aplastic anaemia. *Lancet*, 365, 1647-1656.

Brugnara, C. (2003). Iron deficiency and erythropoiesis: new diagnostic approaches. *Clinical Chemistry*, 49, 1573-1578.

Buchanan, G. R., DeBaun, M. R., Quinn, C. T., & Steinberg, M. H. (2004). Sickle cell disease. *Hematology*, 35-47.

Chinegwundoh, F. & Anie, K. A. (2004). Treatments for priapism in boys and men with sickle cell disease. *Cochrane Database of Systematic Reviews*, CD004198.

Clark, B. E. & Thein, S. L. (2004). Molecular diagnosis of haemoglobin disorders. *Clinical & Laboratory Haematology*, 26, 159-176.

Cohen, A. R., Galanello, R., Pennell, D. J., Cunningham, M. J., & Vichinsky, E. (2004). Thalassemia. *Hematology*, 14-34.

Cordeiro, N. J. & Oniyangi, O. (2004). Phytomedicines (medicines derived from plants) for sickle cell disease. *Cochrane Database of Systematic Reviews*, CD004448.

Davies, E. G., Riddington, C., Lottenberg, R., & Dower, N. (2004). Pneumococcal vaccines for sickle cell disease. *Cochrane Database of Systematic Reviews*, CD003885.

Dodd, J., Dare, M. R., & Middleton, P. (2004). Treatment for women with postpartum iron deficiency anaemia. *Cochrane Database of Systematic Reviews*, CD004222.

DuBois, S. & Kearney, D. J. (2005). Iron-deficiency anemia and *Helicobacter pylori* infection: a review of the evidence. *American Journal of Gastroenterology*, 100, 453-459.

Eber, S. & Lux, S. E. (2004). Hereditary spherocytosis—defects in proteins that connect the membrane skeleton to the lipid bilayer. *Seminars in Hematology*, 41, 118-141.

Elion, J. E., Brun, M., Odievre, M. H., Lapoumeroulie, C. L., & Krishnamoorthy, R. (2004). Vaso-occlusion in sickle cell anemia: role of interactions between blood cells and endothelium. *Hematology Journal*, 5(suppl 3), S195-S198.

Ferrone, F. A. & Rotter, M. A. (2004). Crowding and the polymerization of sickle hemoglobin. *Journal of Molecular Recognition*, 17, 497-504.

Fleming, R. E. (2005). Advances in understanding the molecular basis for the regulation of dietary iron absorption. *Current Opinion in Gastroenterology*, 21, 201-206.

Gallagher, P. G. (2004). Update on the clinical spectrum and genetics of red blood cell membrane disorders. *Current Hematology Reports*, 3, 85-91.

Garratty, G. (2004). Review: drug-induced immune hemolytic anemia—the last decade. *Immunohematology*, 20, 138-146.

Gibbs, W. J. & Hagemann, T. M. (2004). Purified poloxamer 188 for sickle cell vaso-occlusive crisis. *Annals of Pharmacotherapy*, 38, 320-324.

Goodman, S. R. (2004). The irreversibly sickled cell: a perspective. *Cellular & Molecular Biology*, 50, 53-58.

Grossi, A. (2004). Management of cancer anemia. *Journal of Chemotherapy*, 16(suppl 4), 112-116.

Hill, J., Walsh, R. M., McHam, S., Brody, F., & Kalaycio, M. (2004). Laparoscopic splenectomy for autoimmune hemolytic anemia in patients with chronic lymphocytic leukemia: a case series and review of the literature. *American Journal of Hematology*, 75, 134-138.

Hoppe, C. (2005). Defining stroke risk in children with sickle cell anaemia. *British Journal of Haematology*, 128, 751-766.

Keohane, E. M. (2004). Acquired aplastic anemia. *Clinical Laboratory Science*, 17, 165-171.

Keung, Y. K. & Owen, J. (2004). Iron deficiency and thrombosis: literature review. *Clinical & Applied Thrombosis/Hemostasis*, 10, 387-391.

Kwiatkowski, J. L. & Cohen, A. R. (2000). Iron chelation therapy in sickle-cell disease and other transfusion-dependent anemias. *Hematology-Oncology Clinics of North America*, 18, 1355-1377.

Lew, V. L. & Bookchin, R. M. (2005). Ion transport pathology in the mechanism of sickle cell dehydration. *Physiological Reviews*, 85, 179-200.

Marti-Carvajal, A., Dunlop, R., & Agreda-Perez, L. (2004). Treatment for avascular necrosis of bone in people with sickle cell disease. *Cochrane Database of Systematic Reviews* CD004344.

Panagiotou, J. P. & Douros, K. (2004). Clinicolaboratory findings and treatment of iron-deficiency anemia in childhood. *Pediatric Hematology & Oncology*, 21, 521-534.

Park, K. W. (2004). Sickle cell disease and other hemoglobinopathies. *International Anesthesiology Clinics*, 42, 77-93.

Perifanis, V., Sfikas, G., Tziomalos, K., Vakalopoulou, S., & Garipidou, V. (2005). Hereditary spherocytosis uncovered in adulthood due to concomitant lead poisoning. *Annals of Hematology*, 84, 131-132.

Petz, L. D. (2004). Review: evaluation of patients with immune hemolysis. *Immunohematology*, 20, 167-176.

Polychronopoulou, S. & Koutroumba, P. (2004). Telomere length variation and telomerase activity expression in patients with congenital and acquired aplastic anemia. *Acta Haematologica*, 111, 125-131.

Puthenveetil, G. & Malik, P. (2004). Gene therapy for hemoglobinopathies: are we there yet? *Current Hematology Reports*, 3, 298-305.

Ramanathan, S., Koutts, J., & Hertzberg, M. S. (2005). Two cases of refractory warm autoimmune hemolytic anemia treated with rituximab. *American Journal of Hematology*, 78, 123-126.

Rappaport, V. J., Velazquez, M., & Williams, K. (2000). Hemoglobinopathies in pregnancy. *Obstetrics & Gynecology Clinics of North America*, 31, 287-317.

Robak, T. (2004). Monoclonal antibodies in the treatment of autoimmune cytopenias. *European Journal of Haematology*, 72, 79-88.

Rocha, S., Rebelo, I., Costa, E., Catarino, C., Belo, L., Castro, E. M., Cabeda, J. M., Barbot, J., Quintanilha, A., & Santos-Silva, A. (2005). Protein deficiency balance as a predictor of clinical outcome in hereditary spherocytosis. *European Journal of Haematology*, 74, 374-380.

Rosse, W. F., Hillmen, P., & Schreiber, A. D. (2004). Immune-mediated hemolytic anemia. *Hematology,* 48-62.

Sadelain, M. (2004). Globin gene transfer as a potential treatment for the beta-thalassaemias and sickle cell disease. *Vox Sanguinis,* 87(suppl 2), 235-242.

Sadelain, M., Rivella, S., Lisowski, L., Samakoglu, S., & Riviere, I. (2004). Globin gene transfer for treatment of the beta-thalassemias and sickle cell disease. *Bailliere's Best Practice in Clinical Haematology,* 17, 517-534.

Sandoval, C., Jayabose, S., & Eden, A. N. (2000). Trends in diagnosis and management of iron deficiency during infancy and early childhood. *Hematology-Oncology Clinics of North America,* 18, 1423-1438.

Saunthararajah, Y. & DeSimone, J. (2004). Clinical studies with fetal hemoglobin-enhancing agents in sickle cell disease. *Seminars in Hematology,* 41, 11-16.

Shah, A. (2004). Thalassemia syndromes. *Indian Journal of Medical Sciences,* 58, 445-449.

Shah, S. & Vega, R. (2004). Hereditary spherocytosis. *Pediatrics in Review,* 25, 168-172.

Silverstein, S. B. & Rodgers, G. M. (2004). Parenteral iron therapy options. *American Journal of Hematology,* 76, 74-78.

Stabler, S. P. & Allen, R. H. (2004). Vitamin B_{12} deficiency as a worldwide problem. *Annual Review of Nutrition,* 24, 299-326.

Stevens, P. E. & Flossmann, O. (2003). Clinical management of anaemia pre-endstage renal failure. *Clinical Medicine,* 3, 503-508.

Stoehr, G. A., Stauffer, U. G., & Eber, S. W. (2005). Near-total splenectomy: a new technique for the management of hereditary spherocytosis. *Annals of Surgery,* 241, 40-47.

Stuart, M. J. & Nagel, R. L. (2004). Sickle-cell disease. *Lancet,* 364, 1343-1360.

Thein, S. L. (2004). Genetic insights into the clinical diversity of beta thalassaemia. *British Journal of Haematology,* 124, 264-274.

Toh, B. H. & Alderuccio, F. (2004). Pernicious anaemia. *Autoimmunity,* 37, 357-361.

Trent, J. T. & Kirsner, R. S. (2004). Leg ulcers in sickle cell disease. *Advances in Skin & Wound Care,* 17, 410-416.

Umbreit, J. (2005). Iron deficiency: a concise review. *American Journal of Hematology,* 78, 225-231.

Vicari, P., Achkar, R., Oliveira, K. R., Miszpupten, M. L., Fernandes, A. R., Figueiredo, M. S., & Bordin, J. O. (2004). Myonecrosis in sickle cell anemia. case report and review of the literature. *Southern Medical Journal,* 97, 894-896.

Voskaridou, E. & Terpos, E. (2004). New insights into the pathophysiology and management of osteoporosis in patients with beta thalassaemia. *British Journal of Haematology,* 127, 127-139.

Wada, H., Yata, K., Mikami, M., Suemori, S., Nakanishi, H., Kondo, T., Tsujioka, T., Suetsugu, Y., Otsuki, T., Sadahira, Y., Yawata, Y., & Sugihara, T. (2004). Multiple myeloma complicated by autoimmune hemolytic anemia. *Internal Medicine,* 43, 595-598.

Walters, M. C. (2004). Sickle cell anemia and hematopoietic cell transplantation: When is a pound of cure worth more than an ounce of prevention? *Pediatric Transplantation,* 8(suppl 5), 33-38.

Young, N. S. & Brown, K. E. (2004). Parvovirus B19. *New England Journal of Medicine,* 350, 586-597.

Zlotkin, S. (2003). Clinical nutrition: 8. The role of nutrition in the prevention of iron deficiency anemia in infants, children and adolescents. *CMAJ: Canadian Medical Association Journal,* 168, 59-63.

Anemia

INITIAL HISTORY

- 47-year-old male presents with the gradual onset of dyspnea on exertion and fatigue.
- Also complains of frequent dyspepsia with nausea and occasional epigastric pain.
- Has a history of alcohol abuse.

Question 1.   *What questions would you like to ask this patient about his symptoms?*

ADDITIONAL HISTORY

- Patient says he has not had his usual energy levels for several months; the dyspnea has become much worse in the past few weeks.
- Denies chest pain, orthopnea, edema, cough, wheezing, or recent infections.
- States he has had occasional episodes of hematemesis after drinking heavily, and subsequently had several days of dark stools.
- Consumes up to two six-packs of beer a day for the past 8 years since losing his job.
- Nothing seems to make his breathing any better, but antacids help his epigastric discomfort and dyspepsia.

Question 2.   *What questions would you like to ask about his past medical history?*

MEDICAL HISTORY

- Denies any history of cardiac or pulmonary disease.
- Diagnosed with a duodenal ulcer in the past and was on "three drugs at once" for a while 2 years ago, but stopped taking them due to expense.
- Only surgery was a childhood tonsillectomy.
- Nonsmoker.
- On no medications except over-the-counter antacids.
- Has no known allergies.

PHYSICAL EXAMINATION

- Thin, pale, white male in no acute distress; appears older than stated age.
- T = 37° C orally; P = 95 and regular; RR = 16 and unlabored; BP = 128/72 right arm (sitting).

Skin, HEENT, Neck

- Skin pale without rash; no spider angiomata.
- Sclera pale; no icterus.
- PERRLA, fundi without lesions.
- Pharynx clear without postnasal drainage.
- No thyromegaly or adenopathy.
- No bruits.

Lungs, Cardiac

- Good lung expansion; lungs clear to auscultation and percussion.
- PMI at the fifth ICS at the midclavicular line.
- RRR with a II/VI systolic ejection murmur at the left sternal border.
- No gallops, heaves, or thrills.

Abdomen, Rectal

- Abdomen nondistended; bowel sounds present.
- Liver 8 cm at the midclavicular line.
- Moderate epigastric tenderness without rebound or guarding.
- Prostate not enlarged and nontender.
- Stool guaiac positive.

Extremities, Neurologic

- No joint deformity or muscle tenderness.
- No edema.
- Alert and oriented ×3.
- Strength 5/5 throughout and sensation intact.
- Gait normal.
- DTR 2+ and symmetric throughout.

Question 3.   *What are the pertinent positives and negatives on examination?*

Question 4.   *What is your differential diagnosis at this time?*

Question 5.   *What laboratory studies should be obtained at this time?*

LABORATORY RESULTS

- WBC = normal with a normal differential; platelets normal.
- Hct = 29%; MCV = normal; MCHC = slightly decreased; RDW = markedly increased; reticulocyte count <2%.
- Smear with mixed microcytic/hypochromic and macrocytic/normochromic red blood cells; WBC and platelets appear normal.
- PT/PTT, liver function tests, electrolytes, and amylase normal.
- Upper endoscopy reveals 2-cm duodenal ulcer with evidence of recent but no acute hemorrhage.

Question 6.   *What might the hematologic findings indicate and what should be done to further evaluate them?*

ADDITIONAL LABORATORY RESULTS

- Serum iron, total iron-binding capacity, saturation, and ferritin all reduced.
- Bone marrow biopsy with megaloblastic changes and low iron stores.
- Serum folate and red cell folate low; B_{12} normal.

Question 7.   *Based on these findings, what are the diagnoses for this patient?*

Question 8.   *How should this patient be managed?*

Bleeding Disorders

DEFINITION

- Bleeding disorders can be divided into platelet disorders or coagulation disorders.
- They include many possible etiologies; a few common selected ones include the following:

Platelet Disorders
Thrombocytopenia
Platelet dysfunction
Liver dysfunction
Disseminated intravascular coagulation (DIC)

Coagulation Disorders
Hemophilia
von Willebrand syndrome

PATHOPHYSIOLOGY (Figures 13-1 through 13-3)

- Figure 13-1 provides an overview of the clotting cascade with the components that are frequently involved in bleeding disorders indicated by bold type (see Boxes 13-1 and 13-2).
- Bleeding disorders result from a defect in one or more of the steps in clot formation.
- Defects can be due to inadequate quantities of platelets and/or clotting factors, or to the abnormal function of these elements.
- Defects in clotting can be inherited or acquired.

PATIENT PRESENTATION

- In general, platelet disorders present with petechiae. Bleeding usually stops easily with local pressure and does not recur once the pressure is removed unless the platelet count is very low.
- In general, coagulation factor disorders present with ecchymoses and deep tissue hemorrhages (hematomas, hemarthroses). Bleeding is slow to stop with local pressure and tends to recur when pressure is removed.

History

History of easy bruising; history of bleeding after surgery or dental work; family history of bleeding disorder; history of alcohol abuse; history of medication use; history of one of the many diseases listed in Boxes 13-1 and 13-2.

Symptoms

"Rashes" (petechiae); bruises (purpura and ecchymoses); mucosal membrane bleeding; gum bleeding with toothbrushing; epistaxis; deep soft tissue hematomas; bleeding into joints; sustained bleeding after injury or surgery; menorrhagia; hematuria; symptoms of liver disease or other underlying systemic illness as in Boxes 13-1 and 13-2.

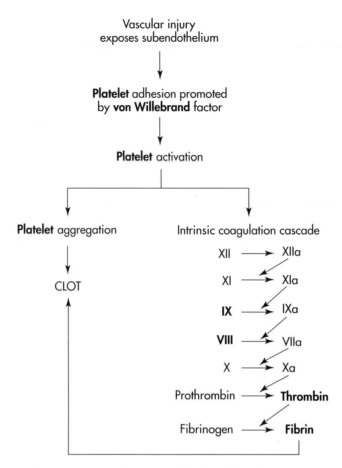

Vascular injury
exposes subendothelium

↓

Platelet adhesion promoted
by **von Willebrand** factor

↓

Platelet activation

Platelet aggregation   Intrinsic coagulation cascade

↓   XII ⟶ XIIa

CLOT   XI ⟶ XIa

                                    IX ⟶ IXa

                                    VIII ⟶ VIIa

                                    X ⟶ Xa

                                    Prothrombin ⟶ **Thrombin**

                                    Fibrinogen ⟶ **Fibrin**

FIGURE **13-1** The Clotting Cascade. Components frequently involved in bleeding disorders are indicated by bold type (see Boxes 13-1 and 13-2).

Examination

Petechiae; purpura and ecchymoses; hematomas; heme-positive stools; hemarthroses; evidence of liver disease or other underlying systemic illness as in Boxes 13-1 and 13-2.

DIFFERENTIAL DIAGNOSIS

• See Boxes 13-1 and 13-2.

KEYS TO ASSESSMENT

• The approach to the patient with bleeding disorders should be systematic and include a logical selection of laboratory evaluations (see Figure 13-4).
• Alcohol can cause thrombocytopenia, platelet dysfunction, and coagulation disorders and should be suspected in any bleeding patient.
• After a careful history, family history, and physical examination, basic laboratory evaluation for the majority of patients should include the following:
  • CBC
    1. Platelet count
    2. Hematocrit (Hct) and hemoglobin (Hgb) with RBC indices (mean corpuscular volume [MCV], mean corpuscular hemoglobin concentration [MCHC])
    3. Careful examination of the peripheral blood smear

BOX **13-1** Selected Platelet Problems

THROMBOCYTOPENIA

A. It first must be differentiated from pseudothrom-bocytopenia (spuriously low platelet count obtained from an automated complete blood count [CBC] counter) and dilutional thrombo-cytopenia caused by a transfusion greater than 10 to 12 units of red blood cells (RBCs)

B. "True" thrombocytopenia can be divided into three major causes
  1. Diminished production
     a. Congenital (Fechtner, Epstein, Wiskott-Aldrich, gray platelet syndrome, amegakaryocyitic, etc.)
     b. Viral infections (cytomegalovirus [CMV], human immunodeficiency virus [HIV], rubella, Epstein-Barr virus [EBV])
     c. Vitamin B_{12}, folate, or iron deficiency
     d. Aplastic anemia
     e. Malignant marrow replacement (e.g., leukemia, metastases)
     f. Drugs (chemotherapeutic agents, estrogens, thiazide diuretics)
     g. Toxins (ethanol, cocaine)
  2. Altered distribution
     a. Hypersplenism (cirrhosis, heart failure, portal hypertension)
  3. Increased destruction
     a. Primary autoimmune (immune thrombo-cytopenic purpura [ITP], HIV related) results from autoimmune antibodies that complex with platelet surface antigen resulting in splenic destruction of platelets.
     b. Secondary autoimmune (systemic lupus erythematosus, malignancy, drug induced [heparin, gold, quinidine, furosemide, anticonvulsants, penicillin, sulfonylurea, cimetidine], and infection induced).

For example, heparin-induced thrombo-cytopenia (HIT) is due to IgG binding to platelet factor 4, which becomes immunogenic when it binds to heparin. Paradoxically, these autoimmune-bound platelets can also activate the clotting cascade causing venous and arterial thromboembolic events.
     c. DIC (see following)
     d. Thrombotic thrombocytopenic purpura
     e. Extracorporeal circulation

PLATELET DYSFUNCTION

A. It can be divided into three main categories
  1. Hereditary
     a. Defects in platelet adhesion (Bernard-Soulier syndrome)
     b. Defects in platelet aggregation (Glanzmann thrombasthenia)
  2. Acquired
     a. Uremia
     b. Myeloproliferative syndromes (leukemia, multiple myeloma)
     c. Autoimmune diseases (collagen vascular disease, platelet antibodies)
     d. DIC
     e. Liver disease
  3. Drug induced
     a. Nonsteroidal anti-inflammatory drugs (NSAIDs)
     b. Aspirin
     c. Antibiotics
     d. Psychiatric drugs
     e. Cardiovascular drugs
     f. Anesthetics
     g. Antihistamines

- Chemistries including blood urea nitrogen (BUN) and creatinine (Cr); liver function tests (LFTs).
- Prothrombin time (PT) and activated partial thromboplastin time (aPTT).
- If thrombocytopenia is found:
  - A blood smear should be obtained.
    1. If the smear is normal and PT and aPTT are normal, suspect autoimmune or drug-induced thrombocytopenia (e.g., HIT—check for antibodies).
    2. If the smear is normal and the PT and aPTT are abnormal, suspect liver dysfunction and evaluate for acute or chronic hepatic disease and alcohol abuse (LFTs).
    3. If the smear is abnormal and hemolysis is present, suspect DIC (measure D-dimer, fibrin degradation products (FDPs), or antithrombin III levels) or autoimmune destruction (e.g., ITP—measure serum antibodies).
    4. If the smear is abnormal and the white blood cell (WBC) and RBC number or appearance is abnormal, suspect bone marrow disease and obtain bone marrow biopsy for diseases such as aplastic anemia, metastases, or leukemia.
- If platelet disorder is suspected, but platelet count is normal, suspect platelet dysfunction.
  - Template bleeding time or platelet function analyzer. Review medication history carefully; check BUN and Cr.

BOX **13-2** Selected Coagulation Disorders

HEMOPHILIA

A. Inherited coagulation factor deficiency; sex-linked recessive, primarily affecting males
B. 30% of cases are due to new mutations with no family history
   1. Hemophilia A: Factor VIII deficiency
   2. Hemophilia B: Factor IX deficiency
   3. Several more, rare hereditary factor deficiencies

von WILLEBRAND SYNDROME

A. von Willebrand factor (vWF) is necessary for proper adhesion between platelets and vascular subendothelial structures and between adjacent platelets
B. vWF is a protective carrier for factor VIII; without vWF, factor VIII has a very short half-life
   1. Inherited
      a. It is the most common inherited bleeding disorder in humans, affecting up to 2% of the population
      b. In women, frequently presents with menorrhagia and can cause mucosal bleeding and hemarthroses
      c. It is autosomal dominant with variable penetrance
      d. There are three types
         Type I (moderate decrease in vWF and factor VIII)
         Type II (functional abnormality in vWF)
         Type III (severe decrease in vWF and factor VIII)
   2. Acquired
      a. Antibodies to, and increase in proteolysis of, vWF
      b. It is associated with many disease states and some drugs: lymphoproliferative disease (leukemia, lymphoma); autoimmune disease (collagen vascular); solid tumors (Wilms tumor); hypothyroidism; valvular heart disease; viral infection; ciprofloxacin; and valproate

LIVER DYSFUNCTION

A. The liver synthesizes most of the factors of the clotting system except for vWF
B. It is also responsible for the clearance of activated clotting or fibrinolytic factors
C. Vitamin K is important in hepatic synthesis of functioning clotting factors
D. Liver disease causes coagulopathy
   1. Impaired factor synthesis
   2. Abnormally functioning clotting factors
   3. Increased consumption of coagulation factors
   4. Disturbed clearance of circulating components of the coagulation system
E. When accompanied by portal hypertension, hypersplenism and thrombocytopenia are common

DISSEMINATED INTRAVASCULAR COAGULATION

A. DIC is defined as an acquired syndrome characterized by the intravascular activation of coagulation with loss of localization arising from different causes
B. It is associated with infection, trauma, shock, anoxia, burns, transfusion reactions, and obstetric emergencies
C. Intense inflammation causes the systemic inflammatory response syndrome (SIRS), which is associated with the release of numerous cytokines and damage to the vascular endothelium
D. Diffuse activation of thrombin, fibrin deposition, and inhibition of the fibrinolytic system (inactivation of antithrombin III and protein C) leads to widespread coagulation
E. This results in depletion of clotting factors, increased clot lysis and production of fibrin degradation products (anticoagulants), thrombocytopenia, and subsequent bleeding

---

- Other specific tests of platelet function include aggregation to adenosine, epinephrine, collagen arachidonate, and thrombin; and the prothrombin consumption test.
- Platelets are normal in number and function but PT or aPTT is abnormal.
  - If both PT and aPTT are abnormal, suspect liver disease or DIC.
  - If only the PT is abnormal, suspect warfarin use or liver disease.
  - If only aPTT is abnormal, suspect inherited disease or heparin treatment; look again for a family history and measure von Willebrand antigen (or ristocetin cofactor activity) and factors VIII and IX levels.

KEYS TO MANAGEMENT

- The control of hemorrhage and the stabilization of the patient are of primary importance in acute bleeding.
- All patients should discontinue alcohol intake and nonessential medications (e.g., NSAIDs).

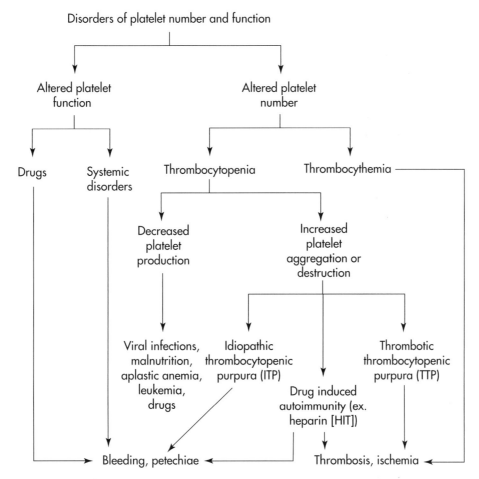

FIGURE **13-2 Summary of Disorders of Platelet Number and Function.**

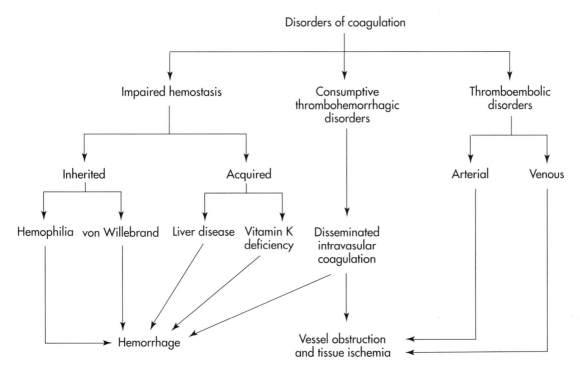

FIGURE **13-3 Summary of Disorders of Coagulation.**

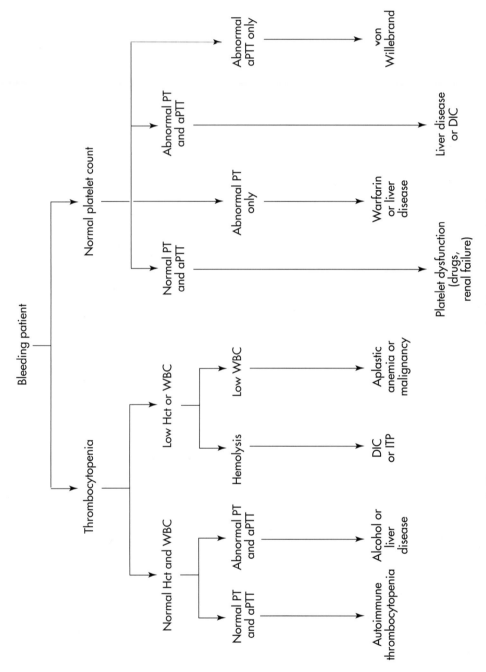

FIGURE **13–4 Approach to the Diagnosis of Common Bleeding Disorders.**

- The choice of therapy is based on the underlying causes as follows:
  - Thrombocytopenia.
    1. Treat underlying disease as appropriate:
       a. Marrow disease: Replace nutritional deficit; discontinue causative medication if possible; avoid toxins.
       b. Autoimmune: HIT should be treated with immediate discontinuation of heparin plus lepirudin or argatroban; ITP should be treated with intravenous immune globulin, corticosteroids and/or splenectomy.
    2. Hematopoietic growth factors (interleukin 3 [IL-3], IL-6, IL-11).
    3. Platelet transfusion: For platelet count ≤10,000/μL; recheck counts at 1 hour and again at 12 to 20 hours after transfusion with a goal of 50,000/μL; single-donor platelets are preferred.
    4. Antifibrinolytic therapy with aminocaproic acid can be effective for patients with chronic mucosal bleeding but who do not require frequent platelet transfusions.
  - Platelet dysfunction.
    1. Hereditary defects are treated with platelet concentrates.
    2. Acquired defects require discontinuation of associated drugs; dialysis for uremia; correction of severe anemia; or treatment of the underlying systemic illness.
  - Hemophilia.
    1. Replacement with recombinant factor VIII or concentrated factor IX for acute hemorrhage; recombinant factor VIIa for those with factor VIII and IX resistance.
    2. Desmopressin (DDAVP) will increase factor VIII in mild cases of hemophilia A.
    3. Antifibrinolytic agents.
    4. Liver transplant is effective but not easily available.
    5. Gene therapy is promising.
  - von Willebrand syndrome.
    1. The goal is to raise the factor VIII and vWF up to 50% of normal levels.
    2. DDAVP indirectly releases vWF from endothelial cell storage sites; it is useful for type I and type II inherited disease and for acquired disease; side effects include facial flushing and headache.
    3. Plasma-derived concentrates are used in patients who have type III or who do not respond to DDAVP. They contain factor VIII concentrates with vWF multimers.
    4. Fibrinolytic inhibitors (e.g., aminocaproic acid) and estrogens (to treat menorrhagia) have been used as adjunctive therapy in some patients.
  - Liver dysfunction.
    1. Discontinuation of alcohol and drugs with hepatic toxicity.
    2. Fresh frozen plasma for acute bleeding and for perioperative treatment.
    3. Vitamin K replacement when indicated.
    4. Recombinant factor VIIa therapy is under investigation.
    5. Antifibrinolytic therapy during hepatic surgery.
  - DIC.
    1. Reverse underlying pathophysiologic condition.
    2. Support circulation, oxygenation and ventilation, and fluid and electrolyte balance.
    3. Avoid transfusion of blood products unless life-threatening exsanguination occurs.
    4. Immediate administration of recombinant human activated protein C (rh-APC) in patients with sepsis-associated DIC.

PATHOPHYSIOLOGY $\longrightarrow$	CLINICAL LINK
What is going on in the disease process that influences how the patient presents and how he or she should be managed?	*What should you do now that you understand the underlying pathophysiology?*
Platelets and vWF are activated by exposure of the vascular subendothelium.	Bleeding from trauma will be excessive and prolonged in both platelet and coagulation factor disorders.
Platelet aggregation is responsible for forming the initial hemostatic barrier; this is subsequently stabilized by fibrin which is derived from the coagulation factor cascade.	In platelet disorders, bleeding will respond easily to local pressure and will not recur. In coagulation factor disorders, bleeding is slow to respond to local pressure and will recur when the pressure is removed.
Thrombocytopenia can result from the inability to produce platelets or from rapid destruction of platelets.	The differential diagnosis of a decreased platelet count includes toxins, marrow disease, and nutritional deficiencies as well as autoimmune diseases and DIC.
Platelet function can be abnormal even when there are adequate quantities of platelets; this is usually the result of uremia or is drug induced.	Patients with bleeding and petechiae should be evaluated for renal disease and for drug use, especially NSAIDs.
Coagulation factor disorders are often inherited (hemophilia and von Willebrand syndrome), resulting in specific factor deficiencies.	Patients with bleeding and an abnormal aPTT as their only laboratory abnormality should have a careful family history and a measurement of serum factor levels.
Ethanol can affect platelet number and function, as well as the production and function of coagulation factors.	In a patient with bleeding and multiple laboratory abnormalities (decreased platelets, increased bleeding time, abnormal PT and aPTT), alcohol abuse and/or liver disease should be suspected.
DIC results in microvascular thrombosis and consumption of platelets and clotting factors. Concurrent lysis of these clots releases fibrin degradation products that are anticoagulant.	Patients with DIC will be thrombocytopenic as well as have increased PT and aPTT. Treatment should begin with control of hemorrhage and rapid administration of recombinant human activated protein C.

SUGGESTED READINGS

Armas-Loughran, B., Kalra, R., & Carson, J. L. (2003). Evaluation and management of anemia and bleeding disorders in surgical patients. *Medical Clinics of North America, 87*, 229-242.

Aster, R. H. (2005). Immune thrombocytopenia caused by glycoprotein IIb/IIIa inhibitors. *Chest, 127*, 53S-59S.

Bartholomew, J. R. (2005). Transition to an oral anticoagulant in patients with heparin-induced thrombocytopenia. *Chest, 127, 27S-34S.*

Bick, R. L. (2003). Disseminated intravascular coagulation current concepts of etiology, pathophysiology, diagnosis, and treatment. *Hematology-Oncology Clinics of North America, 17*, 149-176.

Bishop, P. & Lawson, J. (2004). Recombinant biologics for treatment of bleeding disorders. *Nature Reviews, Drug Discovery, 3*, 684-694.

Caldwell, S. H., Chang, C., & Macik, B. G. (2004). Recombinant activated factor VII (rFVIIa) as a hemostatic agent in liver disease: a break from convention in need of controlled trials. *Hepatology, 39*, 592-598.

Carless, P. A., Henry, D. A., Moxey, A. J., O'Connell, D., McClelland, B., Henderson, K. M., Sly, K., Laupacis, A., & Fergusson, D. (2004). Desmopressin for minimising perioperative allogeneic blood transfusion. *Cochrane Database of Systematic Reviews*, CD001884.

Cattaneo, M. (2003). Inherited platelet-based bleeding disorders. *Journal of Thrombosis & Haemostasis, 1*, 1628-1636.

Chee, Y. L. & Greaves, M. (2003). Role of coagulation testing in predicting bleeding risk. *Hematology Journal, 4*, 373-378.

Chuansumrit, A., McCraw, A., & Preston, E. F. (2004). Essential issues of laboratory investigation for patients with haemophilia and bleeding disorders. *Haemophilia, 10*(suppl 4), 105-108.

Cines, D. B., Bussel, J. B., McMillan, R. B., & Zehnder, J. L. (2004). Congenital and acquired thrombocytopenia. *Hematology*, 390-406.

Clemetson, K. J. (2003). Platelet receptors and their role in diseases. *Clinical Chemistry & Laboratory Medicine, 41*, 253-260.

Cox, G. J. (2005). Diagnosis and treatment of von Willebrand disease. *Hematology-Oncology Clinics of North America, 18*, 1277-1299.

Crowther, M. A. & Wilson, S. (2003). Vitamin K for the treatment of asymptomatic coagulopathy associated with oral anticoagulant therapy. *Journal of Thrombosis & Thrombolysis, 16*, 69-72.

Dempfle, C. E. (2004). Coagulopathy of sepsis. *Thrombosis & Haemostasis, 91*, 213-224.

Drachman, J. G. (2004). Inherited thrombocytopenia: when a low platelet count does not mean ITP. *Blood, 103*, 390-398.

Eilertsen, K. E. & Osterud, B. (2004). Tissue factor: (patho)physiology and cellular biology. *Blood Coagulation & Fibrinolysis, 15*, 521-538.

Favaloro, E. J., Lillicrap, D., Lazzari, M. A., Cattaneo, M., Mazurier, C., Woods, A., Meschengieser, S., Blanco, A., Kempfer, A. C., Hubbard, A., & Chang, A. (2004). von Willebrand disease: laboratory aspects of diagnosis and treatment. *Haemophilia, 10*(suppl 4), 164-168.

Federici, A. B. (2004). Clinical diagnosis of von Willebrand disease. *Haemophilia, 10*(suppl 4), 169-176.

Fourrier, F. (2004). Recombinant human activated protein C in the treatment of severe sepsis: an evidence-based review. *Critical Care Medicine, 32*, S534-S541.

Franchini, M. (2004). Thrombotic complications in patients with hereditary bleeding disorders. *Thrombosis & Haemostasis, 92*, 298-304.

Franchini, M. & Manzato, F. (2004). Update on the treatment of disseminated intravascular coagulation. *Hematology, 9*, 81-85.

George, J. N. (2003). Idiopathic thrombocytopenic purpura: current issues for pathogenesis, diagnosis, and management in children and adults. *Current Hematology Reports, 2*, 381-387.

Hassell, K. (2005). The management of patients with heparin-induced thrombocytopenia who require anticoagulant therapy. *Chest, 127*, 1S-8S.

Hedner, U. (2004). Dosing with recombinant factor VIIa based on current evidence. *Seminars in Hematology, 41*, 35-39.

Hoots, W. K. (2003). Comprehensive care for hemophilia and related inherited bleeding disorders: why it matters. *Current Hematology Reports, 2*, 395-401.

Hoyt, D. B. (2004). A clinical review of bleeding dilemmas in trauma. *Seminars in Hematology, 41*, 40-43.

Ingerslev, J., Hvitfeldt, P. L., & Sorensen, B. (2004). Current treatment of von Willebrand's disease. *Hamostaseologie, 24*, 56-64.

Kelton, J. G. (2005). The pathophysiology of heparin-induced thrombocytopenia: biological basis for treatment. *Chest, 127*, 9S-20S.

Kerr, R. (2003). New insights into haemostasis in liver failure. *Blood Coagulation & Fibrinolysis, 14*(suppl 1), S43-S45.

Kojouri, K., Vesely, S. K., Terrell, D. R., & George, J. N. (2004). Splenectomy for adult patients with idiopathic thrombocytopenic purpura: a systematic review to assess long-term platelet count responses, prediction of response, and surgical complications. *Blood, 104*, 2623-2634.

Kuwana, M. & Ikeda, Y. (2005). The role of autoreactive T-cells in the pathogenesis of idiopathic thrombocytopenic purpura. *International Journal of Hematology, 81*, 106-112.

Levi, M. (2004). Current understanding of disseminated intravascular coagulation. *British Journal of Haematology, 124*, 567-576.

Levi, M., de Jonge, E., & van der Poll, T. (2004). New treatment strategies for disseminated intravascular coagulation based on current understanding of the pathophysiology. *Annals of Medicine, 36*, 41-49.

Levi, M., Keller, T. T., van Gorp, E., & Ten Cate, H. (2003). Infection and inflammation and the coagulation system. *Cardiovascular Research, 60*, 26-39.

Manco-Johnson, M. (2005). Hemophilia management: optimizing treatment based on patient needs. *Current Opinion in Pediatrics, 17*, 3-6.

Mannucci, P. M. (2004). Treatment of von Willebrand's Disease. *New England Journal of Medicine, 351*, 683-694.

Mannucci, P. M., Duga, S., & Peyvandi, F. (2004). Recessively inherited coagulation disorders. *Blood, 104*, 1243-1252.

Matthai, W. H., Jr. (2005). Thrombocytopenia in cardiovascular patients: diagnosis and management. *Chest, 127*, 46S-52S.

Midathada, M. V., Mehta, P., Waner, M., & Fink, L. M. (2004). Recombinant factor VIIa in the treatment of bleeding. *American Journal of Clinical Pathology, 121*, 124-137.

Mohri, H. (2003). Acquired von Willebrand syndrome: its pathophysiology, laboratory features and management. *Journal of Thrombosis & Thrombolysis, 15*, 141-149.

Pipe, S. W. (2004). Coagulation factors with improved properties for hemophilia gene therapy. *Seminars in Thrombosis & Hemostasis, 30*, 227-237.

Ramasamy, I. (2004). Inherited bleeding disorders: disorders of platelet adhesion and aggregation. *Critical Reviews in Oncology-Hematology, 49*, 1-35.

Rick, M. E., Walsh, C. E., & Key, N. S. (2003). Congenital bleeding disorders. *Hematology*, 559-574.

Roberts, H. R., Monroe, D. M., & White, G. C. (2004). The use of recombinant factor VIIa in the treatment of bleeding disorders. *Blood,* 104, 3858-3864.

Saenko, E. L., Ananyeva, N. M., Shima, M., Hauser, C. A., & Pipe, S. W. (2003). The future of recombinant coagulation factors. *Journal of Thrombosis & Haemostasis,* 1, 922-930.

Sandler, S. G. (2004). Review: immune thrombocytopenic purpura: an update for immunohematologists. *Immunohematology,* 20, 112-117.

Scharrer, I. (2004). Women with von Willebrand disease. *Hamostaseologie,* 24, 44-49.

Shankar, M., Lee, C. A., Sabin, C. A., Economides, D. L., & Kadir, R. A. (2004). von Willebrand disease in women with menorrhagia: a systematic review. *BJOG: an International Journal of Obstetrics & Gynaecology,* 111, 734-740.

Silva, M. A., Muralidharan, V., & Mirza, D. F. (2004). The management of coagulopathy and blood loss in liver surgery. *Seminars in Hematology,* 41, 132-139.

Stasi, R. & Provan, D. (2004). Management of immune thrombocytopenic purpura in adults. *Mayo Clinic Proceedings,* 79, 504-522.

Ten Cate, H. (2003). Thrombocytopenia: one of the markers of disseminated intravascular coagulation. *Pathophysiology of Haemostasis & Thrombosis,* 33, 413-416.

Thalheimer, U., Triantos, C. K., Samonakis, D. N., Patch, D., & Burroughs, A. K. (2005). Infection, coagulation, and variceal bleeding in cirrhosis. *Gut,* 54, 556-563.

Virgolini, L. & Marzocchi, V. (2004). Rituximab in autoimmune diseases. *Biomedicine & Pharmacotherapy,* 58, 299-309.

Wada, H. (2004). Disseminated intravascular coagulation. *Clinica Chimica Acta,* 344, 13-21.

Walsh, C. E. (2003). Gene therapy progress and prospects: gene therapy for the hemophilias. *Gene Therapy,* 10, 999-1003.

Warkentin, T. E. (2005). New approaches to the diagnosis of heparin-induced thrombocytopenia. *Chest,* 127, 35S-45S.

Wiklund, R. A. (2004). Preoperative preparation of patients with advanced liver disease. *Critical Care Medicine,* 32, S106-S115.

Winikoff, R., Amesse, C., James, A., Lee, C., & Pollard, D. (2004). The role of haemophilia treatment centres in providing services to women with bleeding disorders. *Haemophilia,* 10(suppl 4), 196-204.

Bleeding Disorders

INITIAL HISTORY

- Patient is a 58-year-old male who has just been transferred in stable condition at 2:15 PM from the operating room to the intensive care unit (ICU) after undergoing an uncomplicated but lengthy (5-hour) right lung decortication procedure.
- Estimated blood loss during the procedure was 550 mL and he received approximately 2500 mL of IV fluid during the surgery.
- Initial drainage amount from his right pleural chest tube on arrival to the ICU is 120 mL.

Question 1.   *What essential information do you want to be sure to receive in the report from the anesthesiologist and surgeon?*

ADDITIONAL HISTORY

- Patient has a medical history significant for a right lower lobectomy for a benign tumor resection, complicated by right empyema.
- 40 pack/year smoking history (quit 3 years ago).
- Otherwise in good health.
- Home medications include only PRN albuterol inhaler use.
- No known medication allergies.
- Surgery progressed with moderate difficulty because the visceral pleura was badly scarred.

INITIAL PHYSICAL EXAMINATION (on arrival to the ICU from the operating room)

- T = 35.8° C rectally; P = 90 and regular.
- No spontaneous respirations on ventilator at intermittent mandatory ventilation (IMV) 10 breaths/minute.
- BP via right radial arterial line = 112/60, correlates with cuff.

Skin
Grossly intact, pale, cool, dry.
3-second capillary refill throughout.
Good turgor.
Right thoracotomy surgical dressing intact with scant bloody drainage present.

□ **Kathryn B. Reid, PhD, RN, CCRN, APRN-BC contributed this case study.**

Pulmonary
- #8.0 oral endotracheal tube, 23 cm at lips
- Fully ventilated with $FIO_2 = 1.00$; IMV = 10; positive end-expiratory pressure (PEEP) = 5; oxygen sat = 100%.
- No spontaneous respirations present.
- Bilateral breath sounds present, slightly diminished in the bases.
- Right lateral pleural chest tube at 20 cm H_2O suction via chest drainage system, with 120 mL bloody drainage present; no air leak.

Cardiovascular
- S_1, S_2 clear; no murmurs or gallops.
- Pulses full throughout.

Gastrointestinal
- Left nasogastric tube to low constant suction, minimal drainage.
- Hypoactive bowel sounds.

Genitourinary
- Urinary catheter draining clear yellow urine.
- Specific gravity 1.010.

Neurologic
- Remains anesthetized and sedated, unable to communicate.
- Glasgow Coma Scale = 2T; PERRL = 2 mm.

ADDITIONAL ASSESSMENTS

- Endotracheal suction reveals scant, thin white secretions.
- Initial arterial blood gas levels: pH = 7.45; $PaCO_2 = 36$; $PaO_2 = 433$.
- ECG monitor lead II shows normal sinus rhythm, no ectopy, rate = 92.

VASCULAR ACCESS

- Right subclavian triple-lumen catheter—proximal port with D_5W at KVO, middle heparin locked, distal with central venous pressure (CVP) monitor and flush per protocol, CVP = 6 mm Hg.
- Bilateral upper extremity IV is with normal saline infusing at KVO from operating room.

POSTOPERATIVE COURSE

- Patient is stable and receives the routine postoperative care and monitoring. He is placed on an FIO_2 of 50% to begin normalizing his arterial blood gases after transport.
- At 2:45 PM (after 30 minutes), patient's chest tube output shows an additional 175 mL.

Question 2.   *What will you evaluate related to his blood loss at this time?*

RAPID ASSESSMENT AND INITIAL LABORATORY RESULTS

- No evidence of hypovolemia.
- Postoperative chest radiograph reveals proper endotracheal tube and chest tube placement, bilateral lung expansion, and no evidence of hemothorax.
- Initial postoperative laboratory results:
  - Hgb = 6.8 mg/dL; Hct = 20%.
  - PLTs = 85,000/mm^3.
  - PT and PTT are normal.
  - Electrolyte levels are within normal limits, except potassium = 3.4 mEq/L and ionized calcium = 3.8 mg/dL.

Question 3.   *What do these values represent?*

Question 4.   *What is your primary concern related to this patient's chest tube drainage?*

Question 5.   *What actions should be taken at this time to attempt to reduce his postoperative hemorrhage?*

FURTHER POSTOPERATIVE COURSE

- At 3 PM, patient has an additional 200 mL of chest tube drainage (postoperative total = 495 mL).
- In addition to the normal postoperative volume resuscitation, patient receives a rapid transfusion of two units packed red blood cells, two units fresh frozen plasma, one unit single-donor platelets, and one ampule of calcium chloride intravenously.

ADDITIONAL POSTOPERATIVE DEVELOPMENTS

- At 4 PM chest drainage = 275 mL (total = 770 mL).
- Results of repeat hematologic studies:
  - Hgb = 7 mg/dL; Hct = 21%.
  - PLTs = 65,000/mm^3.
  - PT = 15 sec; PTT = 42 sec.
- Patient receives additional unit of packed red blood cells and two units of fresh frozen plasma.

Question 6. *What is your assessment of the situation at this time?*

Question 7. *What other laboratory information will guide your decision making at this time?*

FURTHER POSTOPERATIVE COURSE

- At 4:30 PM chest tube drainage = 220 mL (postoperative total = 990 mL). Because of continued excessive bleeding, patient is emergently returned to the operating room for re-exploration.
- While patient is in operating room undergoing re-exploration, his further bloodwork study results return:
  - Hgb = 6.2 mg/dL; Hct = 19%.
  - PLTs – 48,000/mm³.
  - PT = 19 sec; PTT = 47 sec.
  - Fibrinogen = 120 mg/dL.
  - Fibrinogen degradation products = 150 mcg/mL.
  - D-dimer = 220 ng/mL.
  - Ca^{++} = 3.9 mg/dL.

Question 8.   *What do these laboratory results indicate?*

Question 9.   *What are the possible causes for the patient's bleeding problem?*

Question 10.   *Based on this information, what other information do you want to acquire?*

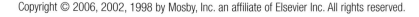

Question 11.   *What are the recommended therapeutic approaches in the management of the patient's DIC-like coagulopathy?*

AFTER RETURNING FROM THE OPERATING ROOM

- At 5:15 PM patient returns from the operating room after his re-exploration procedure.
- Surgeon reports that no single source of bleeding could be identified, and that there was heavy, generalized, diffuse oozing of blood from the chest wall. Surgeon diagnoses the bleeding problem as DIC and orders that administration of all blood products be placed on hold.
- Care of patient's bleeding problem is supportive in nature, with administration of crystalloid fluids as needed to maintain adequate volume status.

FURTHER POSTOPERATIVE CARE

- Over the next 6 hours, patient's chest tube drainage improves from 210 mL/hr to 45 mL/hr.
- Patient does not demonstrate other evidence of a transfusion reaction.
- Hematocrit level reaches a low of 17, and on the first postoperative day he is gently transfused two units of packed red blood cells without complication to bring his hematocrit level higher than 30.
- Patient is placed on an iron supplement and instructed in dietary measures to help improve his postoperative anemia.

Urinary Tract Infection

DEFINITION

- *Urinary tract infection* (UTI) is an inflammation of the urinary tract epithelium in response to a bacterial pathogen that is usually associated with pyuria and bacteriuria.
- *Cystitis* is an infection of the bladder producing characteristic symptoms including dysuria, lower abdominal or suprapubic discomfort, and frequency of urination.
- *Bacteriuria* is the presence of bacteria in the urine; this condition may be associated with UTI symptoms.
- *Pyelonephritis* is an infection of the upper urinary tracts including the renal pelvis and renal parenchyma.
- *Acute pyelonephritis* is a clinical syndrome of chills, fever, and flank pain accompanied by bacteriuria and involving the upper urinary tracts.
- *Chronic pyelonephritis* is a term used to describe a radiographic or surgical finding of a scarred or damaged kidney owing to previous episodes of pyelonephritis that is diagnosed on radiographic or other imaging study. It may be associated with a current urinary tract infection.
- *Urosepsis* is a systemic extension of a pyelonephritis; urine and blood cultures are positive for a common pathogen that can progress to septic shock and death unless successfully treated.
- *Isolated urinary tract infection* is an initial infection or an infection that is remote in time from previous episodes.
- *Recurrent urinary tract infection* is a new infection following successful resolution of previous episode(s).
- *Persistent urinary infection* is lasting bacteriuria caused by inappropriate or incomplete therapy, or arising from bacterial persistence within some focus within the urine, such as a calculus or a foreign object.
- *Nosocomial urinary infection* is a hospital-acquired UTI.
- *Domiciliary urinary tract infection* occurs in people who reside in the community at the time of infection.
- *Complicated urinary tract infection* is associated with hematuria, fever, or an infection in the patient with an indwelling catheter, obstruction, urinary calculus, or anatomic abnormality of the urinary system.

EPIDEMIOLOGY

- 4% to 6% of young adult women have bacteriuria at any given time; the majority are asymptomatic.
- Incidence of symptomatic urinary tract infections among young adult women is approximately 0.2% per month.

□ Mikel Gray, PhD, CUNP, CCCN, FAAN contributed this chapter.

- Spontaneous remission of symptoms after a period of 5 to 7 weeks occurs in only 24%.
- Prevalence of asymptomatic bacteriuria in older adult, community-dwelling women is 20%.
- Patients with an initial UTI are at risk for subsequent infections; for example, 61% of older adult women treated for a UTI will seek treatment for one or more recurrent infections within a decade.
- Prevalence of asymptomatic bacteriuria in women with diabetes mellitus is 26%, including a prevalence of 21% in women with type 1 diabetes mellitus and 29% with type 2 diabetes mellitus.
- Patients with HIV have a higher incidence of UTI when compared with controls.
- Prevalence increases to approximately 20% to community-dwelling older adult women (>65 years of age).
- Incidence of UTI in community-dwelling men is 6 to 8/10,000 men per year.
- The prostate is coinfected in more than 90% of men with a febrile UTI.
- Prevalence of bacteriuria among functionally impaired older adult women and men is 24%, as compared with 12% of nonfunctionally impaired residents.
- Incidence of antimicrobial resistant UTI continues to grow.

PATHOPHYSIOLOGY

- Route of infection: Ascending urethral course is most common.
- The pathogen typically arises from the intestinal bacterial reservoir; postmenopausal women are at higher risk for harboring bacterial pathogens in the vagina.
- Hospital-acquired UTIs are often associated with urethral catheterization and may arise from a cutaneous source.
- *Escherichia coli* is the most common pathogen among domiciliary and hospital-acquired UTI, but enterococci are more common among people with HIV infection.
- Pyelonephritis occurs when bacteria ascend from lower to upper urinary tract via the ureter.
- UTI via a hematogenous route is uncommon; it occasionally occurs with septicemia from *Staphylococcus aureus* from oral infections or from *Candida fungemia*; lymphogenous infection rarely occurs from severe bowel infection or retroperitoneal abscess, particularly when obstruction is present.

Source	Common Pathogen
Community acquired	Intestinal flora
	Escherichia coli (accounts for 85% of all infections)
	Proteus
	Klebsiella
	Enterococcus faecalis
	Staphylococcus saprophyticus
	Cutaneous/vaginal flora
	Staphylococcus epidermidis
	Candida albicans
Nosocomial infections	*Escherichia coli* (accounts for 50% of all infections)
	Klebsiella
	Enterobacter
	Citrobacter
	Pseudomonas aeruginosa
	Providencia
	Enterococcus faecalis
	Staphylococcus epidermidis

- Virulence of pathogen is directly related to its ability to adhere to epithelial cells.
- Adherence is related to host epithelial cell receptivity; a genotypic predisposition that primarily affects women.
- Women with a history of recurring UTI are more likely to be nonsecretors of specific Lewis blood group antigens, leading to increased reservoirs of *E. coli* in vaginal epithelium and greater susceptibility to bacterial adherence.

- Additional risk factors increasing the risk of recurring UTI in young women include using a diaphragm and spermicide during intercourse or a nonlubricated condom.
- Anatomic abnormalities of the upper urinary tracts, visible on ultrasound or radiographic imaging studies, are uncommon among adult women with first-time or recurring UTI.
- Anatomic abnormalities of the upper urinary tract are comparatively common among men who experience febrile UTI, or who fail to respond to empiric or sensitivity-guided antimicrobial therapy, affecting approximately 25%.
- Use of antibiotics within 15 to 28 days increases the risk of a subsequent UTI in young women.
- Risk factors for recurring UTI in postmenopausal women include incomplete bladder emptying, cystocele, urinary incontinence, history of UTI prior to menopause and nonsecretor status.
- Urine osmolality, urea concentration, and pH influence bacterial reproduction; a dilute urine or a concentrated urine with a low pH is bacteriostatic.
- Glucosuria associated with diabetes may increase bacterial reproduction and urinary tract infection risk.
- The average urinary pH of a pregnant woman tends to favor bacterial reproduction more than the average urinary pH of a nonpregnant woman.
- Pregnancy exacerbates the risk of progression of asymptomatic bacteriuria to clinically relevant UTI and increases the risk of preterm delivery.
- Pyelonephritis leads to immunoglobulin synthesis and antibodies in the urine; cystitis produces little or no detectable serologic response.
- Adult women are more likely to require hospitalization for acute pyelonephritis than men, but men who require hospitalization are at a significantly higher risk for death. The risk of mortality also increases with age, recent invasive procedures, and multiple comorbidities.
- Obstruction and vesicoureteral reflux increase the risk of febrile urinary infection.
- Constipation increases the perianal and vaginal bacterial reservoir and has been associated with urinary tract infections in children.
- Voiding dysfunction (particularly detrusor sphincter dyssynergia) increases risk of cystitis and fever.

PATIENT PRESENTATION

History
Previous urinary tract infection; history of "gastroenteritis" as child; congenital defect of urinary system; urinary retention; recent onset of sexual activity (women).

Symptoms
Lower abdominal discomfort or nausea in child; dysuria, urinary frequency, lower abdominal, or suprapubic discomfort in young adult; lower abdominal discomfort or urinary incontinence in older adult; symptoms of cystitis and flank pain with chills and sweating, nausea, and vomiting with pyelonephritis; urine may or may not be odorous or cloudy.

Examination
Suprapubic discomfort or no physical findings with cystitis, costovertebral angle tenderness, fever, dehydration with pyelonephritis.

DIFFERENTIAL DIAGNOSIS

- Vaginitis.
- Urethritis.
- Interstitial cystitis.
- Pelvic pain.
- Prostatitis.
- Gastroenteritis (particularly in children with pyelonephritis).

- Urinary calculus.
- Urinary system tumor (may be confused with hemorrhagic cystitis).

KEYS TO ASSESSMENT

- Urine specimen collection: Clean-catch urine adequate for community-dwelling patients; catheterized specimen for patients with complicated infection, persistent bacteriuria, immobile patient, individual with urinary or fecal incontinence requiring incontinence undergarments.
- Centrifuge urine for 5 minutes at 2000 rpm before dipstick urinalysis and microscopic examination.
- Urine culture and sensitivity if:
    - Patient with first febrile infection, recurrent afebrile infection (more than 1 per year), complicated urinary tract infection, history of urinary system conditions including congenital defect, urinary calculi.
    - The dipstick urinalysis shows nitrates and leukocytes.
    - Bacteriuria and pyuria are seen on microscopic examination.
- An ultrasound and voiding cystourethrogram for an infant or child with first febrile urinary tract infection or recurrent cystitis.
- Imaging study in otherwise healthy adult with febrile UTI, persistent bacteriuria, or suspicion of foreign body or obstruction.

KEYS TO MANAGEMENT

- Prevention.
    - Avoid dehydration; the recommended daily allowance (RDA) for fluids in the active adult living in a moderate climate is approximately 30 mL/kg/day.
    - Avoid constipation (encourage fluids, dietary fiber, and recreational exercise).
    - Manage urinary retention, urinary incontinence, or bladder outlet obstruction.
    - Consider repair of cystocele in a postmenopausal woman with incomplete bladder emptying and recurring UTI.
    - Teach women about proper hygiene after toileting and urination after intercourse.
    - Encourage community-dwelling women to ingest daily or twice daily intake of cranberry or blueberry products, such as cranberry juice, to reduce the risk of UTI.
    - Treat infections early, particularly in patients with compromised immune function or those with urinary retention, or voiding dysfunction.
    - Remove indwelling catheter and treat patients with voiding dysfunction with an alternative management program such as bladder retraining, pharmacotherapy for urinary incontinence, intermittent catheterization, and/or scheduled voiding.
- Acute urinary tract infection.
    - Empiric treatment is adequate for first-time infection in otherwise healthy young women; begin empiric treatment before the culture and sensitivity results for complicated or febrile urinary tract infection.
    - Antipyretics and hospitalization with intravenous fluids is necessary if pyelonephritis is associated with significant nausea and vomiting or urosepsis.
    - Select an antibiotic according to the culture and sensitivity report (when indicated), frequency of administration, risk of associated vaginitis, cost to the patient, and risk of promoting bacterial resistance (Table 14-1).
    - Emphasize adherence to antibiotic course; treatment of an uncomplicated infection for 3 days is expected to produce symptomatic relief; treatment for 5 to 10 days is required in order to eradicate bacteriuria. Treatment for 7 to 14 days may be needed to eradicate bacteriuria in complicated UTI.
    - Supplement antibiotic treatment with urinary analgesic (pyridium is available as over-the-counter medication) or a prescriptive combination agent such as Urised.

TABLE **14-1** Common Antibiotic Choices for UTI

Antibiotic	Typical Dosage and Administration Schedule	Implications
Trimethoprim-sulfamethoxazole (TMP-SMX)	1 double-strength tablet po bid	Relatively inexpensive Risk of secondary vaginitis
Nitrofurantoin (Macrodantin or Macrobid)	Macrodantin given as 50-100 mg po qid; Macrobid given as 1 capsule po bid	More expensive than TMP-SMX Risk of vaginitis negligible May be used for *Enterococcus* infection; may be effective when managing vancomycin-resistant *Enterococcus* in certain patients
Ampicillin	500 mg qid	qid dosage may reduce compliance Relatively inexpensive Risk of secondary vaginitis
Amoxicillin	500 mg po tid	tid dosage may reduce compliance Relatively inexpensive compared with TMP-SMX, other penicillins
Cephalexin	500 mg po qid	qid dosage may reduce compliance Relatively expensive when compared to penicillins, TMP-SMX Risk of secondary vaginitis
Levofloxacin	500 mg po daily	Daily dosage promotes compliance Relatively expensive Risk of secondary vaginitis Reserved for complicated infections
Ciprofloxacin	500 mg po bid	bid dosage promotes compliance Relatively expensive Risk of secondary vaginitis Reserved for complicated infections
Norfloxacin	400 mg po bid	bid dosage promotes compliance Relatively expensive Risk of secondary vaginitis Reserved for complicated infections

- Begin prophylactic treatment using an antifungal cream for woman with a history of vaginitis when receiving antibiotic therapy, unless nitrofurantoin is administered.
- Encourage adequate fluid intake.
- Prevention of recurrent infection.
  - Obtain a culture and sensitivity with persistent symptoms.
  - Obtain an imaging study (ultrasound, kidneys/ureter/bladder [KUB], intravenous pyelogram) when hematuria persists, when hematuria is found in isolation of a UTI, or refer the patient to a urologist.
  - Refer to urologist if infection with *Proteus, Klebsiella,* or *Pseudomonas* spp. or obtain imaging study to rule out urinary calculi.
  - Rule out bacterial prostatitis in men.
  - Refer to a urologist when an explanation of persistent bacteriuria is not identified.
  - Obtain upper urinary tract imaging (ultrasonography) with febrile urinary tract infection.
  - Consider low-dose, suppressive therapy for recurrent, febrile infections.
  - Consider self-start, intermittent therapy (in which the patient is taught to obtain a culture with a dip-slide device followed by empiric treatment).
  - Consider postintercourse suppressive antibiotic therapy when the relation between intercourse and UTI is established.

PATHOPHYSIOLOGY $\longrightarrow$	CLINICAL LINK
What is going on in the disease process that influences how the patient presents and how he or she should be managed?	*What should you do now that you understand the underlying pathophysiology?*
Bacterial adherence is influenced by genotypic epithelial cell receptivity. $\longrightarrow$	There is a risk for recurrent urinary tract infections, particularly among otherwise healthy adult women.
Ascending urethral course is the most common route of bacterial invasion. $\longrightarrow$	Risk of recurrent infection is increased with sexual intercourse; teach the patient to urinate immediately following intercourse and to have proper hygiene following urination. Consider postcoital suppression antibiotic therapy.
Dilute urine is bacteriostatic. $\longrightarrow$	Adequate fluid intake.
Gastrointestinal flora account for the majority of pathogens in the community-dwelling population. $\longrightarrow$	Maintain proper hygiene following urination and avoid constipation, which increases intestinal bacterial reservoir.
Risk of pyelonephritis is greater in patients with voiding dysfunction, foreign object in urinary system (including indwelling catheter), vesicoureteral reflux, and diabetes. $\longrightarrow$	Identify and manage risk factors. Treat UTI promptly in the at-risk patient; treat complicated infection for 7 days and febrile UTI for 14 days.
Enterococcus is predominant pathogen in patients with HIV infection. $\longrightarrow$	Nitrofurantoin is often effective in the treatment of an enterococcal UTI, and it may be effective in cases of vancomycin-resistant *Enterococcus* provided the infection is limited to the lower urinary tract.
The incidence and prevalence of UTI with antimicrobial resistant pathogens continue to rise. $\longrightarrow$	Suppressive or prophylactic treatment of UTI increases the risk of infection with antimicrobial-resistant pathogens. Fluoroquinolones and related agents should be reserved for complicated infections.
Pregnancy increases the risk of asymptomatic bacteriuria progressing to cystitis and the risk of preterm delivery. $\longrightarrow$	Consult the obstetrician concerning treatment of asymptomatic bacteriuria in a pregnant woman.
Pathogenic flora may colonize the vaginal vault, particularly following menopause. $\longrightarrow$	Intravaginal estrogens may be administered to reduce the risk of recurring UTI in older adult women.

SUGGESTED READINGS

Barry, H. C., Ebell, M. H., & Hickner, J. (1997). Evaluation of suspected urinary tract infection in ambulatory women: a cost utility analysis of office-based strategies. *Journal of Family Practice, 44*, 49-60.

Bjornson, D. C., Rovers, J. P., Burian, J. A., & Hall, N. L. (1997). Pharmacoepidemiology of urinary tract infection in Iowa medicaid patients in long-term care facilities. *Annals of Pharmacotherapy, 31*, 837-841.

Childs, S. J. & Egan, R. J. (1996). Bacteriuria and urinary infections in the elderly. *Urologic Clinics of North America, 23*, 45-54.

Cockerill, F. R. & Edson, R. S. (1991). Trimethoprim-sulfamethoxazole. *Mayo Clinic Proceedings, 66*, 1249-1251.

Connolly, A. & Throp, J. M. (1999). Urinary tract infections in pregnancy. *Urologic Clinics of North America, 26*, 779-787.

Ferry, S. A., Holm, S. E., Stenlund, H., Lundholm, R., & Monsen, T. J. (2004). The natural course of uncomplicated lower urinary tract infection in women illustrated by a randomized placebo controlled study. *Scandinavian Journal of Infectious Diseases, 36*(4), 296-301.

Finer, G. & Landau, D. (2004). Pathogenesis of urinary tract infections with normal female anatomy. *The Lancet Infectious Diseases, 4*(10), 631-635, 2004.

Foxman, B. (2003). Epidemiology of urinary tract infections: incidence, morbidity, and economic costs. *Disease-A-Month, 49*(2), 53-70.

Foxman, B., Marsh, J., Gillespie, B., Rubin, M., Koopman, J. S., & Spear, S. (1997). Condom use and first time urinary tract infection. *Epidemiology, 8*, 612-614.

Geerlings, S. E., Stolk, R. P., Camps, M. J., Netten, P. M., Hoekstra, J. B., Bouter, K. P., Bravenboer, B., Collet, J. T., Jansz, A. R., & Hoepelman, A. I. (2000). Asymptomatic bacteriuria may be considered a complication in women with diabetes. *Diabetes Care, 23*, 744-749.

Goettsch, W., van Pelt, W., Kagelkerke, N., Hendrix, M. G., Buiting, A. G., Sabbe, L. J., van Griethuysen, J. A., & de Neeling, A. J. (2000). Increasing resistance to fluoro-quinolones in *Escherichia coli* from urinary tract infections in the Netherlands. *Journal of Antimicrobial Therapy, 46*, 223-228.

Goldstein, F. W. (2000). Antibiotic susceptibility of bacterial strains from patients with community-acquired urinary tract infections in France. *European Journal of Clinical Microbiology & Infectious Diseases, 19*, 112-117.

Gray, M. (2002). Are cranberry juice or cranberry products effective in the prevention or management of urinary tract infection? *Journal of Wound Ostomy & Continence Nursing, 29*, 122-126.

Hassay, K. A. (1995). Effective management of urinary discomfort. *Nurse Practitioner, 20*, 36, 39-40, 41-44.

Jepson, R. G., Mihaljevic, L., & Craig, J. (2003). Cranberries for preventing urinary tract infections. Cochrane Renal Group. *Cochrane Database of Systematic Reviews.* Last substantive update November 2003.

Karlowsky, J. A., Kelly, L. J., Thornsberry, C., Jones, M. E., & Sahm, D. F. (2002).Trends in antimicrobial resistance among urinary tract infection isolates of *Escherichia coli* from female outpatients in the United States. *Antimicrobial Agents & Chemotherapy, 46*(8), 2540-2545.

Kau, A. L., Hunstad, D. A., & Hultgren, S. J. (2005). Interaction of uropathogenic *Escherichia coli* with host uroepithelium. *Current Opinion in Microbiology, 8*(1), 54-59.

Leiner, S. (1995). Recurrent urinary tract infection in otherwise healthy adult women. Rational strategies for work-up and management. *Nurse Practitioner, 20*, 48, 51-52, 54-56.

Liss, P. E., Aspevall, O., Karlsson, D., & Forsum, U. (2003). Terms used to describe urinary tract infections—the importance of conceptual clarification. *APMIS, 111*(2), 291-299.

Loening-Bacucke, V. (1997). Urinary incontinence and urinary tract infection and their resolution with treatment of chronic constipation of childhood. *Pediatrics, 100*, 228-232.

Milo, G., Katchman, E. A., Paul, M., Christiaens, T., Baerheim, A., & Leibovici, L. Duration of antibacterial treatment for uncomplicated urinary tract infection in women. Cochrane Renal Group *Cochrane Database of Systematic Reviews.* Most recent substantial update February 2005.

Molander, U., Arvidsson, L., Milsom, I., & Sandberg, T. (2000). A longitudinal study of elderly women with urinary tract infection. *Maturitas, 34*, 127-131.

Morgan, K. L. (2004). Management of UTIs during pregnancy. *MCN, American Journal of Maternal Child Nursing, 29*(4), 254-258.

Perfetto, E. M., Keating, K., Merchant, S., & Nichols, B. R. (2004). Acute uncomplicated UTI and *E. coli* resistance: implications for first-line empirical antibiotic therapy. *Journal of Managed Care Pharmacy, 10*(1), 17-25.

Raz, R., Gennesin, Y., Wasser, J., Stolzer, Z., Rosenfeld, S., Rottensterich, E., & Stamm, W. E. (2000). Recurrent urinary tract infections in postmenopausal women. *Clinical Infectious Diseases, 30*, 152-156.

Rozenberg, S., Pastijn, A., Gevers, R., & Murillo, D. (2004). Estrogen therapy in older patients with recurrent urinary tract infections: a review. *International Journal of Fertility & Women's Medicine, 49*(2), 71-74.

Schaeffer, A. J. (2002). Urinary tract infections. In Gillenwater, J. Y., Grayuhack, J. T., Howards, S. S., & Duckett, J. D. (Eds.). *Adult and pediatric urology,* ed 4, St. Louis, Mosby, 211-272.

Schaeffer, A. J. (2002). Infections of the urinary tract. In Walsh, P. C., Retik, A. B., Vaughan, E. D., & Wein, A. J. (Eds.). *Campbell's urology,* ed 8, Philadelphia, Saunders, 515-602.

Schonwald, S., Begovac, J., & Skerek, V. (1999). Urinary tract infections in HIV disease. *International Journal of Antimicrobial Agents, 11*, 309-311.

Stamm, W. E. & Raz, R. (1999). Factors contributing to susceptibility of postmenopausal women to recurrent urinary tract infections. *Clinical Infectious Diseases, 28*, 723-725.

Stapleton, A. (1999). Host factors in susceptibility to urinary tract infections. *Advances in Experimental Medicine and Biology, 462*, 351-358.

Stern, J. A., Hsieh, Y. C., & Schaeffer, A. J. (2004). Residual urine in an elderly female population: novel implications for oral estrogen replacement and impact on recurrent urinary tract infection. *Journal of Urology, 171*(2 Pt 1), 768-770.

Ulleryd, P. (2003). Febrile urinary tract infection in men. *International Journal of Antimicrobial Agents, 22*(suppl 2), 89-93.

Urinary Tract Infection

INITIAL HISTORY

- 27-year-old female complaining of symptoms of urgency to urinate, frequent urination, and urethral burning during urination persisting for 48 hours.
- Patient awoke from sleep with urgency and suprapubic discomfort 2 nights ago.
- Urine now has strong odor and cloudy appearance.

Question 1. *What is your differential diagnosis based on the information you have now?*

Question 2. *What other questions would you like to ask now?*

ADDITIONAL HISTORY

- Recurring urinary tract infections since she married at age 22 years.
- Prior UTI associated with similar symptoms.
- Denies history of febrile or hemorrhagic UTI.
- Three episodes over past 2 years.
- May be associated with strenuous physical exertion and sexual intercourse.
- No other medical history.
- She reports an allergy to penicillin which causes a "rash" and "trouble breathing."

Question 3. *Now what do you think of her history?*

□ **Mikel Gray, PhD, CUNP, CCCN, FAAN contributed this case study.**

PHYSICAL EXAMINATION

- Well-nourished female experiencing mild discomfort.
- Tenderness on palpation of abdominal pelvic area; physical examination otherwise unremarkable.
- T = 98.6 °C orally; BP = 114/64; P = 68; RR = 12.

Question 4.   *What laboratory studies are indicated in this patient?*

LABORATORY RESULTS

- Dipstick urinalysis:
  - Color: Dark yellow; specific gravity = 1.030; pH = 6.5.
  - Protein: Negative; glucose: negative; ketones: negative; bilirubin: negative.
  - Trace occult blood.
  - Leukocytes: Large amount.
  - Nitrates: Positive; urobilinogen: negative.
- Microscopic examination:
  - WBC: Too numerous to count (TNTC)/HPF (high-power field).
  - Bacteria: TNTC.
  - RBC: 3 or 4/HPF.
  - Casts: Negative.
- Urine culture:
  - *E. coli:* >104 CFU/mL.
  - Organism sensitive to ampicillin, nitrofurantoin, trimethoprim-sulfamethoxazole (TMP-SMX), ciprofloxacin, cephalexin.

Question 5.   *What additional studies are indicated in this patient?*

Question 6.   *Based on these findings, what therapy would you initiate?*

Question 7.   *What measures would you recommend to reduce the risk of a recurrence?*

Peptic Ulcer Disease

DEFINITION

- Peptic ulcer disease (PUD) is defined as defects in the gastrointestinal mucosa extending through the muscularis mucosae occurring in the esophagus, stomach, or duodenum.
- Peptic ulcers are associated with a number of conditions; however, most are associated with *Helicobacter pylori (H. pylori)* infection and/or nonsteroidal anti-inflammatory drug (NSAID) intake.
- Other less common forms occur with acid hypersecretory syndromes (gastrinoma, mastocytosis), herpes simplex virus [HSV] type 1, cytomegalovirus [CMV], duodenal obstruction, vascular insufficiency, and radiation and chemotherapy-associated ulcers.

EPIDEMIOLOGY

- Lifetime prevalence of PUD is 3% to 10%; there is increasing risk with age.
- Duodenal ulcer (DU) is more common than gastric ulcer (GU) and occurs in younger patients; it affects males more often than females.
- Gastric ulcers (GU) have a peak incidence in individuals ages 55 to 65 and are rare before age 40; they occur in men at the same rate as women.
- Hospitalization rates for PUD are declining, but complication rates (perforation, hemorrhage, death) are relatively stable. Hemorrhage from PUD results in mortality rates of 7% to 10%.
- *H. pylori* infection can be identified in 95% of DU and 80% to 85% of GU.
  - In developed countries, seroprevalence (30% to 40% overall in United States and western Europe) is directly correlated with increasing age and is inversely correlated with socioeconomic status. Prevalence is 70% to 90% in Central and South America, Africa, and Asia.
  - Direct transmission from person to person via exposure to vomitus, saliva, or feces is common in developed countries, although transmission rates are decreasing in recent decades. In developing countries, contaminated water and unsanitary conditions provide transmission.
  - In addition to increasing the risk of PUD, *H. pylori* infection confers up to a ninefold increase in risk for gastric adenocarcinoma. *H. pylori* also increases the risk for gastric lymphoma (mucosa-associated lymphoid tissue [MALT] lymphoma).
  - Recently *H. pylori* has been implicated in non-ulcer dyspepsia, gastroesophageal reflux disease, iron deficiency anemia, and idiopathic thrombocytopenic purpura.
- In the United States NSAID use is estimated to cause 100,000 hospitalizations and 10,000 to 20,000 deaths per year due to NSAID-related gastrointestinal complications. The risk of gastric and duodenal ulceration ranges from 11% to 30% for patients on daily NSAIDs; it is much higher if patients are also on corticosteroids; also increases risk for upper gastrointestinal bleeding fourfold, particularly in older adults.

- Psychologic stress has been associated with increased gastric acid secretion, acute gastric erosions, and PUD.
- Cigarette smoking is a risk factor for PUD and has been shown to decrease gastric mucus production.
- Other risk factors include type O blood group, alcohol, chronic pulmonary disease, reflux esophagitis, cirrhosis, and renal failure and transplantation.

PATHOPHYSIOLOGY

- *Genetics:* Several gene polymorphisms have been linked to PUD, including:
  - Genes that influence pathophysiologic responses to *H. pylori* infection including the interleukin genes IL-1RN*2 and IL-8, the epithelial cell antigen genes Lewis and Secretor, FcγRIIa, and the duodenal ulcer promoting gene A (dupA).
  - Genes that affect mucosal defenses such as the histamine *N*-methyltransferase gene.
  - Genes that influence the effectiveness of medications such as the *CYP2C19*, which affects the metabolism of proton pump inhibitors and IL-β511, which affects the ability of triple therapy to eradicate *H. pylori.*
- Ulcers form when there is a breakdown in the mucosal defense and repair mechanisms that normally protect the stomach and duodenum from the acid and peptic environment of the upper gastrointestinal tract.
- Defense mechanisms.
  - A layer of mucus and bicarbonate over the surface of the mucosa provides a buffer and prevents pepsin diffusion into the mucosal layer.
  - A mucosal barrier of tight cellular junctions, growth factors, and membrane transport systems removes excess ions, preventing back-diffusion of hydrogen ions into the mucosa.
  - A vigorous supply of blood to the mucosa removes excess hydrogen ion and maintains nutrient flow for normal cellular function and repair.
- *H. pylori* and NSAIDs cause tissue injury, resulting in defects in one or more of these defense mechanisms with subsequent exposure of the mucosa to acid and pepsin. *H. pylori* and NSAIDs are synergistic in their negative effects on the gastric and duodenal mucosa.
- *H. pylori* causes tissue injury by the following mechanisms:
  - The bacterium attaches to gastric and duodenal epithelial cells via adhesion molecules. It then produces lipopolysaccharide (LPS, endotoxin) and other toxic proteins such as the secreted exotoxin VacA.
  - Macrophages, neutrophils, and lymphocytes are recruited to the area of infection and release numerous inflammatory mediators (IL-1, IL-8, tumor necrosis factor [TNF]). Lymphocytes also produce autoantibodies that attack the gastric and duodenal epithelial cells and enduce apoptosis.
  - Active gastritis is followed by
    1. Chronic antral-predominant gastritis and duodenal ulceration.
    2. Persistent nonatrophic gastritis.
    3. Corpus-predominant atrophic gastritis with gastric ulceration. Atrophic gastritis and ulceration increase the risk for increasing dysplastic changes and gastric cancer (Figure 15-1).
  - Persistent asymptomatic infection is common.
- NSAIDs cause cyclooxygenase-1 (COX-1) inhibition resulting in decreased synthesis of the prostaglandins responsible for gastrointestinal mucosal protection (the selective cyclooxygenase-2 [COX-2] inhibitors cause less GI toxicity). Risk for PUD is increased because NSAIDs:
  - Inhibit bicarbonate secretion from the gastric and duodenal mucosa.
  - Decrease mucus cell secretion.
  - Inhibit mucosal proliferation and healing.
  - Cause microvascular ischemia.
  - Inhibit physiologic regulation of acid secretion.
  - Stimulate neutrophil adhesion to the splanchnic endothelium.
  - Trap hydrogen ions in mucosal cells.

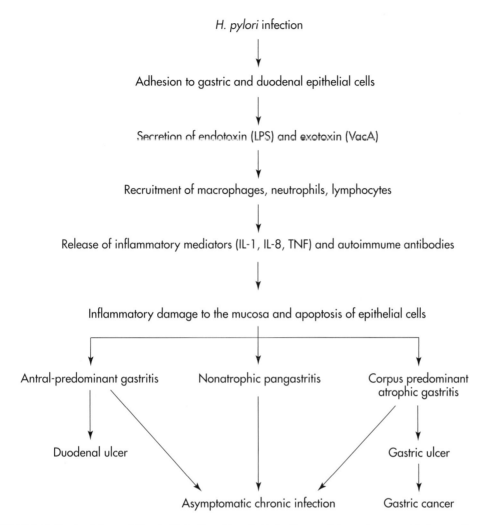

FIGURE **15-1 Pathophysiology of *H. pylori* Infection.** *H. pylori* infection and the subsequent inflammation of gastric and duodenal mucosa can lead to acute ulceration, chronic gastritis and infection, and gastric cancer. (Adapted from Suerbaum, S. & Michetti, P. [2002]. *Helicobacter pylori* infection. *New England Journal of Medicine,* 347[15], 1175-1186.)

- • Promote gastric and pepsin penetration through the gastric mucous lining.
- • Gastric ulcers can occur in the absence of hyperacidity, whereas duodenal ulcers commonly occur in association with hyperacidity and are associated with both increased basal and postprandial acid secretion.
- • Gastric hypermotility and duodenal hypomotility have been implicated in DU, whereas gastric hypomotility and pyloric reflux have been associated with GU.
- • PUD can be complicated by bleeding, perforation and peritonitis, penetration into surrounding tissues such as pancreas and colon, and pyloric obstruction.

PATIENT PRESENTATION

History

Family history of PUD; smoking; alcohol; stress; older age; low socioeconomic status; NSAID use; chronic pulmonary, hepatic, or renal disease.

Uncomplicated Symptoms

Epigastric burning or "hunger" sensation occurring 2 to 3 hours after meals and at night, temporarily relieved with antacids, food, and milk; occasionally the epigastric discomfort is exacerbated rather than relieved by eating; "irritable stomach" to certain foods; belching; bloating; nausea; vomiting; regurgitation; fatty food intolerance; early satiety; weight loss or weight gain.

Complicated Symptoms

Severe unremitting pain; pain radiating to the back; projectile vomiting; hematemesis; melena; fever; hypotension.

Examination

The examination results are often nonspecific and unrevealing in uncomplicated PUD with only epigastric tenderness; guarding, decreased bowel sounds, fever, heme-positive stools indicate complications.

DIFFERENTIAL DIAGNOSIS

- Gastroesophageal reflux disease (GERD).
- Esophageal spasm.
- Drug-induced dyspepsia.
- Cholelithiasis/cholecystitis.
- Gastric carcinoma.
- Pancreatitis.
- Ischemic heart disease.
- Diverticulitis.
- Appendicitis.
- Intestinal ischemia.
- Infectious gastritis (herpes simplex virus [HSV], cytomegalovirus [CMV], tuberculosis, strongyloidiasis, giardiasis).

KEYS TO ASSESSMENT

- Complete blood count, liver function tests (LFTs), amylase, bilirubin, and chemistries including calcium, and stool guaiac.
- Assessment should follow two basic pathways:
  - Patients younger than 50 years with dyspepsia and no history of NSAID use should undergo noninvasive *H. pylori* testing and therapy if indicated.
    1. Urea breath test and fecal antigen tests document active infection for primary diagnosis and can be used for follow-up 4 to 8 weeks after completion of *H. pylori* eradication therapy.
    2. Serum serology testing should be done in a certified laboratory and may be positive in the absence of active infection (false positive) and cannot be used for follow-up to therapy.
  - Patients older than the age of 50 or any patient with "alarm" markers (anemia, gastrointestinal bleeding, anorexia, early satiety, weight loss) should undergo upper gastrointestinal endoscopy with biopsy and rapid urease test. This is highly sensitive and specific for *H. pylori* infection and allows for differentiation of gastric and duodenal ulcer and between benign and malignant gastric ulceration.

KEYS TO MANAGEMENT

- Prevention.
  - Smoking cessation; decrease alcohol consumption.
  - Avoid milk and foods that give dyspeptic symptoms (does not induce or prevent ulcers but decreases symptoms). A diet high in fruits and vegetables and vitamin A appears to be helpful in reducing the risk for duodenal ulcer.

- Avoid NSAIDs if possible; if not, add a proton pump inhibitor (PPI) (e.g., omeprazole), which has been shown to be more effective than misoprostol in reducing NSAID-induced ulcers. Selective cyclooxygenase-2 inhibitors (celecoxib, valdecoxib) cause less ulceration than older NSAIDs but high cost and the risk of other complications (e.g., cardiac ischemic events) must be considered. New COX-inhibiting nitric oxide donors (CINODs) that may be safer are being explored.
- Pharmacologic management of PUD.
    - Indications for *H. pylori* treatment include gastric or duodenal ulceration, lymphoma, atrophic gastritis, gastric cancer, first-degree relative with gastric cancer, functional dyspepsia, gastroesophageal reflux disease, and the use of NSAIDs.
    - Currently, triple-drug therapy is recommended and can result in eradication of the *H. pylori* in 78% to 90% of patients.
    - The most effective therapies include a combination of a proton pump inhibitor (PPI) (omeprazole, lansoprazole, esomeprazole, pantoprazole, rabeprazole) plus two antibiotics (e.g., clarithromycin, amoxicillin, tetracycline, or metronidazole) for 10 to 14 days.
    - Other possible therapies include a histamine-2 (H_2) receptor blocker (cimetidine, ranitidine, famotidine, nizatidine) plus an antibiotic followed by bismuth citrate, or a combination of bismuth citrate plus two antibiotics.
    - Ulcer recurrence rates in cases in which *H. pylori* has been eradicated are as low as 4% to 20%, compared with 60% to 70% of patients who remain positive for the organism.
- Treatment of ulcer complications.
    - Acute upper gastrointestinal bleeding from PUD requires rapid patient stabilization and possible transfusion while preparing for:
        1. Endoscopy with electrocoagulation, heater probe application, or injection tamponade.
        2. Intravenous PPI administration.
        3. Possible surgery for uncontrolled bleeding.
        4. Treatment for *H. pylori*, which reduces the risk for recurrent bleeding.
    - PUD perforation or penetration is a surgical emergency. Surgery for complicated or refractory ulcers includes vagotomy (truncal or selective), and a variety of gastric and duodenal resection procedures; complications include gastric hypomotility, reflux esophagitis, dumping syndrome, and diarrhea.

PATHOPHYSIOLOGY $\longrightarrow$	CLINICAL LINK
What is going on in the disease process that influences how the patient presents and how he or she should be managed?	*What should you do now that you understand the underlying pathophysiology?*
H. pylori and NSAID use cause defects in the mucosal defense mechanisms and must be treated directly; however, healing can be facilitated by reducing gastric and duodenal acidity. $\longrightarrow$	In addition to antibiotics for *H. pylori* and discontinuing NSAID use, management should include PPIs or H$_2$ blockers.
The majority of PUD is associated with *H. pylori* infection and associated mucosal injury. $\longrightarrow$	Patients with dyspepsia must be evaluated for *H. pylori*, and adequate management must include triple-drug therapy.
Prostaglandins are important for maintaining GI mucosal defense mechanisms. These cytokines are produced primarily via the cyclooxygenase-1 (COX-1) pathway of arachidonate metabolism. $\longrightarrow$	Traditional NSAIDs block both COX-1 and COX-2 and cause mucosal tissue injury with the associated risk of PUD. Selective COX-2 inhibitors are less damaging to the GI mucosa but have other risks. New COX-inhibiting nitric oxide donors (CINODs) may be safer.
NSAID use is widespread in the United States and is frequently employed in situations in which it is not truly indicated or necessary. $\longrightarrow$	Patients who do not need to take NSAIDs should be encouraged to stop, and those that must continue their use should be considered for alternative therapies or the addition of a PPI to the regimen.
H. pylori infection is common in the population and is a risk factor for gastric cancer and lymphoma. $\longrightarrow$	Detection and treatment of *H. pylori* infection may reduce the risk for gastric cancer and lymphoma. In older individuals, or for those with "alarm" symptoms, endoscopy is indicated to evaluate for the possibility of gastric carcinoma or lymphoma.
PUD can be complicated by hemorrhage, perforation, pyloric obstruction, or penetration. $\longrightarrow$	Increasing symptoms such as melena, hematemesis, back pain, fever, or hypotension require immediate and aggressive evaluation and possible emergent surgical intervention.

SUGGESTED READINGS

Akarca, U. S. (2005). Gastrointestinal effects of selective and non-selective non-steroidal anti-inflammatory drugs. *Current Pharmaceutical Design,* 11, 1779-1793.

Asaka, M. & Dragosics, B. A. (2004). *Helicobacter pylori* and gastric malignancies. *Helicobacter,* 9(suppl 1), 35-41.

Barkun, A. N., Herba, K., Adam, V., Kennedy, W., Fallone, C. A., & Bardou, M. (2004). The cost-effectiveness of high-dose oral proton pump inhibition after endoscopy in the acute treatment of peptic ulcer bleeding. *Alimentary Pharmacology & Therapeutics,* 20, 195-202.

Behm, B. W. & Stollman, N. (2004). Endoluminal therapies for gastroesophageal reflux disease. *Journal of Clinical Gastroenterology,* 38, 209-217.

Behrman, S. W. (2005). Management of complicated peptic ulcer disease. *Archives of Surgery,* 140, 201-208.

Bergman, M. P., Vandenbroucke-Grauls, C. M., Appelmelk, B. J., D'Elios, M. M., Amedei, A., Azzurri, A., Benagiano, M., & Del Prete, G. (2005). The story so far: *Helicobacter pylori* and gastric autoimmunity. *International Reviews of Immunology,* 24, 63-91.

Blaser, M. J. & Atherton, J. C. (2004). *Helicobacter pylori* persistence: biology and disease. *Journal of Clinical Investigation,* 113, 321-333.

Bumann, D., Jungblut, P. R., & Meyer, T. F. (2004). *Helicobacter pylori* vaccine development based on combined subproteome analysis. *Proteomics,* 4, 2843-2848.

Bytzer, P. (2004). Diagnostic approach to dyspepsia. *Best Practice & Research in Clinical Gastroenterology,* 18, 681-693.

Chan, F. K. (2005). NSAID-induced peptic ulcers and *Helicobacter pylori* infection: implications for patient management. *Drug Safety,* 28, 287-300.

Chey, W. D. & Moayyedi, P. (2004). Review article: uninvestigated dyspepsia and non-ulcer dyspepsia—the use of endoscopy and the roles of *Helicobacter pylori* eradication and antisecretory therapy. *Alimentary Pharmacology & Therapeutics,* 19(suppl 1), 1-8.

Conway, B. R. (2005). Drug delivery strategies for the treatment of *Helicobacter pylori* infections. *Current Pharmaceutical Design,* 11, 775-790.

Cover, T. L. & Blanke, S. R. (2005). *Helicobacter pylori* VacA, a paradigm for toxin multifunctionality. *Nature Reviews, Microbiology,* 3, 320-332.

Crowe, S. E. (2005). *Helicobacter* infection, chronic inflammation, and the development of malignancy. *Current Opinion in Gastroenterology,* 21, 32-38.

Del Giudice, G. & Michetti, P. (2004). Inflammation, immunity and vaccines for *Helicobacter pylori. Helicobacter,* 9(suppl 1), 23-28.

D'Elios, M. M., Bergman, M. P., Amedei, A., Appelmelk, B. J., & Del Prete, G. (2004). *Helicobacter pylori* and gastric autoimmunity. *Microbes & Infection,* 6, 1395-1401.

Ford, A., Delaney, B., Forman, D., & Moayyedi, P. (2004). Eradication therapy for peptic ulcer disease in *Helicobacter pylori* positive patients. *Cochrane Database of Systematic Reviews,* CD003840.

Gisbert, J. P. & Pajares, J. M. (2004). Stool antigen test for the diagnosis of *Helicobacter pylori* infection: a systematic review. *Helicobacter,* 9, 347-368.

Gisbert, J. P., Khorrami, S., Carballo, F., Calvet, X., Gene, E., & Dominguez-Munoz, E. (2004). Meta-analysis: *Helicobacter pylori* eradication therapy vs. antisecretory non-eradication therapy for the prevention of recurrent bleeding from peptic ulcer. *Alimentary Pharmacology & Therapeutics,* 19, 617-629.

Goldstein, J. L. (2004). Challenges in managing NSAID-associated gastrointestinal tract injury. *Digestion,* 69(suppl 1), 25-33.

Gyires, K. (2005). Gastric mucosal protection: from prostaglandins to gene-therapy. *Current Medicinal Chemistry,* 12, 203-215.

Hatakeyama, M. (2004). Oncogenic mechanisms of the *Helicobacter pylori* CagA protein. *Nature Reviews, Cancer,* 4, 688-694.

Hawkey, C. J. (2004). Non-steroidal anti-inflammatory drugs: who should receive prophylaxis? *Alimentary Pharmacology & Therapeutics,* 20(suppl 2), 59-64.

Holtmann, G. & Howden, C. W. (2004). Review article: management of peptic ulcer bleeding—the roles of proton pump inhibitors and *Helicobacter pylori* eradication. *Alimentary Pharmacology & Therapeutics,* 19(suppl 1), 66-70.

Holtmann, G., Maldonado-Lopez, E., & Haag, S. (2004). Heartburn in primary care: problems below the surface. *Journal of Gastroenterology,* 39, 1027-1034.

Jakobs, R. & Riemann, J. F. (2004). cagA-positive *Helicobacter pylori* strains and gastro-oesophageal reflux disease: still puzzling. *European Journal of Gastroenterology & Hepatology,* 16, 635-637.

Janssen, M. J., Laheij, R. J., de Boer, W. A., & Jansen, J. B. (2005). Meta-analysis: the influence of pre-treatment with a proton pump inhibitor on *Helicobacter pylori* eradication. *Alimentary Pharmacology & Therapeutics,* 21, 341-345.

Kabir, S. (2004). Detection of *Helicobacter pylori* DNA in feces and saliva by polymerase chain reaction: a review. *Helicobacter,* 9, 115-123.

Kato, S. & Sherman, P. M. (2005). What is new related to *Helicobacter pylori* infection in children and teenagers? *Archives of Pediatrics & Adolescent Medicine,* 159, 415-421.

Kripke, C. (2005). Comparison of short-term treatments for GERD. *American Family Physician,* 71, 1303-1304.

Laine, L. (2004). Proton pump inhibitor co-therapy with nonsteroidal anti-inflammatory drugs—nice or necessary? *Reviews in Gastroenterological Disorders,* 4(suppl 4), S33-S41.

Leontiadis, G. I., McIntyre, L., Sharma, V. K., & Howden, C. W. (2004). Proton pump inhibitor treatment for acute peptic ulcer bleeding. *Cochrane Database of Systematic Reviews,* CD002094.

Leontiadis, G. I., Sharma, V. K., & Howden, C. W. (2005). Systematic review and meta-analysis of proton pump inhibitor therapy in peptic ulcer bleeding. *British Medical Journal,* 330, 568.

Makristathis, A., Hirschl, A. M., Lehours, P., & Megraud, F. (2004). Diagnosis of *Helicobacter pylori* infection. *Helicobacter,* 9(suppl 1), 7-14.

Malfertheiner, P. & Peitz, U. (2005). The interplay between *Helicobacter pylori,* gastro-oesophageal reflux disease, and intestinal metaplasia. *Gut,* 54(suppl 1), i13-i20.

Marshall, B. J. & Windsor, H. M. (2005). The relation of *Helicobacter pylori* to gastric adenocarcinoma and lymphoma: pathophysiology, epidemiology, screening, clinical presentation, treatment, and prevention. *Medical Clinics of North America,* 89, 313-344.

McLoughlin, R., Racz, I., Buckley, M., O'Connor, H. J., & O'Morain, C. (2004). Therapy of *Helicobacter pylori. Helicobacter,* 9(suppl 1), 42-48.

Megraud, F. (2004). Basis for the management of drug-resistant *Helicobacter pylori* infection. *Drugs,* 64, 1893-1904.

Metz, D. C. (2005). Preventing the gastrointestinal consequences of stress-related mucosal disease. *Current Medical Research & Opinion,* 21, 11-18.

Meyer, T. K., Olsen, E., & Merati, A. (2004). Contemporary diagnostic and management techniques for extraesophageal reflux disease. *Current Opinion in Otolaryngology & Head & Neck Surgery,* 12, 519-524.

Moayyedi, P. & Hunt, R. H. (2004). *Helicobacter pylori* public health implications. *Helicobacter,* 9(suppl 1), 67-72.

Moayyedi, P., Soo, S., Deeks, J., Delaney, B., Harris, A., Innes, M., Oakes, R., Wilson, S., Roalfe, A., Bennett, C., & Forman, D. (2005). Eradication of *Helicobacter pylori* for non-ulcer dyspepsia *Cochrane Database of Systematic Reviews* CD002096.

Modlin, I. M., Moss, S. F., Kidd, M., & Lye, K. D. (2004). Gastroesophageal reflux disease: then and now. *Journal of Clinical Gastroenterology,* 38, 390-402.

Nakajima, S., Bamba, N., & Hattori, T. (2004). Histological aspects and role of mast cells in *Helicobacter pylori*-infected gastritis. *Alimentary Pharmacology & Therapeutics,* 20(suppl 1), 165-170.

Ong, S. P. & Duggan, A. (2004). Eradication of *Helicobacter pylori* in clinical situations. *Clinical & Experimental Medicine,* 4, 30-38.

Orlando, R. C. (2005). Pathogenesis of reflux esophagitis and Barrett's esophagus. *Medical Clinics of North America,* 89, 219-241.

Perini, R., Fiorucci, S., & Wallace, J. L. (2004). Mechanisms of nonsteroidal anti-inflammatory drug-induced gastrointestinal injury and repair: a window of opportunity for cyclooxygenase-inhibiting nitric oxide donors. *Canadian Journal of Gastroenterology,* 18, 229-236.

Peura, D. A. (2004). Prevention of nonsteroidal anti-inflammatory drug-associated gastrointestinal symptoms and ulcer complications. *American Journal of Medicine,* 117(suppl 5A), 63S-71S.

Pisegna, J. R. & Martindale, R. G. (2005). Acid suppression in the perioperative period. *Journal of Clinical Gastroenterology,* 39, 10-16.

Raghunath, A. S., Hungin, A. P., Wooff, D., & Childs, S. (2004). Systematic review: the effect of *Helicobacter pylori* and its eradication on gastro-oesophageal reflux disease in patients with duodenal ulcers or reflux oesophagitis. *Alimentary Pharmacology & Therapeutics,* 20, 733-744.

Rieder, G., Fischer, W., & Haas, R. (2005). Interaction of *Helicobacter pylori* with host cells: function of secreted and translocated molecules. *Current Opinion in Microbiology,* 8, 67-73.

Ryan-Harshman, M. & Aldoori, W. (2004). How diet and lifestyle affect duodenal ulcers. Review of the evidence. *Canadian Family Physician,* 50, 727-732.

Saad, R., & Chey, W. D. (112). A clinician's guide to managing *Helicobacter pylori* infection. *Cleveland Clinic Journal of Medicine,* 72, 109-110.

Spirt, M. J. (2004). Stress-related mucosal disease: risk factors and prophylactic therapy. *Clinical Therapeutics,* 26, 197-213.

Stoicov, C., Saffari, R., Cai, X., Hasyagar, C., & Houghton, J. (2004). Molecular biology of gastric cancer: *Helicobacter* infection and gastric adenocarcinoma: bacterial and host factors responsible for altered growth signaling. *Gene,* 341, 1-17.

Vakil, N. (2004). Review article: new pharmacological agents for the treatment of gastro-oesophageal reflux disease. *Alimentary Pharmacology & Therapeutics,* 19, 1041-1049.

van Pinxteren, B., Numans, M. E., Bonis, P. A., & Lau, J. (2004). Short-term treatment with proton pump inhibitors, H2-receptor antagonists and prokinetics for gastro-oesophageal reflux disease–like symptoms and endoscopy negative reflux disease. *Cochrane Database of Systematic Reviews,* CD002095.

Wollner, T. (2004). Eradicate *H. pylori* with effective treatment regimens. *Nurse Practitioner,* 29, 40-44.

Peptic Ulcer Disease

INITIAL HISTORY

- 58-year-old male complaining of 3-week history of increasing epigastric pain.
- Has had dyspepsia in the past for which he took Tums, but this is much worse and only partially relieved with chewable antacids.

Question 1.   *What is your differential diagnosis based on this limited history?*

Question 2.   *What questions would you like to ask this patient about his symptoms?*

ADDITIONAL HISTORY

- Pain has a burning quality.
- Relieved with eating, especially drinking milk, but recurs about 2 hours later.
- Denies radiation to his back, melena, hematemesis, or fever.
- Denies early satiety, anorexia, or weight loss.

- Denies fatty food intolerance or change in stools.
- Denies jaundice, increasing abdominal girth, or easy bruising.
- Denies shortness of breath or pain with exercise.

Question 3. *What questions would you like to ask about his recent and past medical history?*

MORE HISTORY

- Has been taking ibuprofen for the past 2 months for a sore knee.
- Drinks approximately 3 mixed drinks each day.
- Smokes 1 pack of cigarettes a day.
- Has had recent job change with a great deal of stress.
- Has been feeling a little tired lately but no recent illnesses or hospitalization.
- Has a history of mild hypertension treated with diet.
- No medications or known allergies.

PHYSICAL EXAMINATION

- Thin white male in no acute distress.
- T = 37° C orally; P = 90 and regular; RR = 16 and unlabored; BP = 148/96 right arm (sitting).

HEENT, Neck
- PERRLA, fundi without vascular changes.
- Pharynx clear.
- No thyromegaly.
- No bruits.
- No adenopathy.

Lungs, Cardiac
- Lungs clear to auscultation and percussion.
- Cardiac with RRR without murmurs or gallops.

Abdomen
- Abdomen not distended.
- Bowel sounds present.
- Liver percusses to 8 cm at the midclavicular line, one fingerbreadth below the right costal margin.
- Epigastric tenderness without rebound or guarding.
- Spleen not palpable.

Rectal
- No hemorrhoids seen or felt.
- Prostate not enlarged and soft.
- Stool grossly normal but weakly heme positive.

Extremities, Neurologic
- No edema.
- Pulses full, no bruits.
- Oriented ×4.
- Normal strength, sensation, and DTR.

Question 4.   *What are the pertinent positives and negatives on the physical examination?*

Question 5.   *What initial diagnostic tests would you obtain now?*

LABORATORY RESULTS

- Chemistries including calcium and BUN/Cr normal.
- WBC = 9000 with normal differential.
- Hct = 45%.
- Liver function test including bilirubin normal.
- Serum and urine amylase and lipase normal.
- ECG = normal sinus rhythm without evidence of ischemic changes.

Question 6.   *What test should be chosen to best evaluate for peptic ulcer disease in this patient?*

ENDOSCOPY RESULTS

- Normal esophageal mucosa.
- Gastric mucosa with superficial gastritis without ulceration.
- 0.5-cm duodenal ulcer with evidence of recent bleeding, but no acute hemorrhage and no visible vessels in the ulcer crater.
- Biopsy reveals acute inflammation without dysplasia or malignancy. *H. pylori* rapid urease testing positive.

Question 7.   *What management would you recommend?*

Hepatitis B and C

DEFINITION

- Inflammation of the liver due to viral infection with hepatitis B or hepatitis C virus.
- Epidemiology, pathophysiology, and clinical manifestations depend on the causative virus and the host inflammatory and immunologic response to infection.

EPIDEMIOLOGY

Hepatitis B (HBV)

- More than 350 million people in the world are infected with HBV; nearly 10% have chronic infection.
- There are approximately 78,000 new cases of HBV in the United States each year. More than 1.25 million people in the United States have chronic HBV infection; overall prevalence of HBV infection is 0.5% to 1% (prevalence is significantly greater in Alaskan Native population and in blacks).
- Incidence of acute infection has decreased 67% over the past 10 years (in the United States, vaccination for hepatitis B is recommended for all infants).
- HBV is spread by parenteral transmission of virus via blood or blood products, sexual contact, or prenatal exposure. Most infected individuals report no known exposures.
- High-risk groups include intravenous (IV) drug users, first-generation immigrants from endemic areas such as Southeast Asia, men having sex with men, household contacts and sexual partners of HBV carriers, heterosexuals with multiple partners, people requiring hemodialysis, patients in custodial institutions, and health care workers.
- 30% to 40% of cases have no known risk factors.
- Risk of developing chronic HBV infection varies inversely with age at infection (90% of infants infected at birth, 50% of these infected as infants, 20% of those infected as children, and 2% to 3% of those infected as adults become chronically infected).

Hepatitis C (HCV)

- Worldwide, more than 200 million people are chronically infected with HCV. Asia and Africa have the highest infection rates.
- It is estimated that 3 to 4 million Americans are chronically infected with HCV, the prevalence is greatest in urban areas.
- HCV is the most common blood-borne infection in the United States, surpassing alcoholic cirrhosis as the predominant chronic liver disease in this country.
- HCV is spread by direct parenteral inoculation, sexual contact, transplantation of an infected organ, or perinatal exposure. Most infected individuals report no known exposures.
- HCV infection is associated with IV drug use, multiple transfusions, individuals with needlestick injury, people with hemophilia, people requiring hemodialysis, health care workers,

HIV infected patients, liver and renal transplant patients, and household and sexual contacts of chronically infected people.

- It is estimated that nearly 30% to 50% of IV drug users with human immunodeficiency virus (HIV) infection also have HCV infection; coinfection exacerbates both diseases.
- 40% of cases have no known risk factors.
- Chronic infection occurs in 70% to 80% of cases; 20% of those individuals with chronic infection will develop cirrhosis, and 4% will develop hepatocellular carcinoma.

PATHOPHYSIOLOGY

Genetics

Host genetic markers of increased susceptibility to hepatitis B and C include polymorphisms of both humoral and cellular immunity. These include genes for IL-4, MHC II, MHC I, and CD8 activity.

Hepatitis B

- Hepatitis B is 100 times more infectious than HIV and can live outside the body in dried blood for longer than a week.
- HBV consists of six genotypes labeled A through F that affect infectivity and prognosis.
    - HBV has an envelope and surface antigens and a neocapsid "core" that contains double-stranded deoxyribonucleic acid (DNA). It also has an enzyme that functions as both a DNA polymerase and a reverse transcriptase to make ribonucleic acid (RNA) replicas.
    - HBV virions bind to surface receptors and are brought into the hepatocyte.
    - Viral core particles migrate to the hepatocyte nucleus, where they form a circular DNA (cccDNA) that is the template for viral messenger RNA (mRNA) transcription.
    - Viral mRNA is translated into viral components and undergoes reverse transcriptase activity to make more viral DNA.
    - Viral components reassemble and then the virus buds from the endoplasmic reticulum ready to infect other cells.
- Hepatocyte injury is mediated by the host immune response to the infection rather than by direct cytopathic effects by the virus.
    - Once HBV has entered the body, macrophages, dendritic cells, and B lymphocytes present viral antigen on their surfaces, which activates CD4 lymphocytes to make interferons and interleukins (especially IL-2).
    - These cytokines contribute to cellular immunity by activating CD8 lymphocytes and macrophages.
        1. Infected hepatocytes present viral antigen on their surfaces that can be recognized by CD8 lymphocytes, which then release perforins and other toxic substances that cause necrosis and apoptosis of the hepatocytes.
        2. Macrophages release inflammatory cytokines such as tumor necrosis factor-alpha (TNF-α) and interferon gamma (INF-γ), which are vital to clearance of HBV.
    - A vigorous immune response will increase symptoms and cause more hepatocellular necrosis, but is crucial to clearing the virus. Patients with less effective immune responses are less symptomatic with the acute infection, but are more likely to develop chronic infection.
    - Circulating antigen-antibody complexes may result in a serum sickness–like syndrome with angioneurotic edema, polyarteritis nodosa, systemic vasculitis with bowel ischemia, renal disease, neuropathy, and arthritis.
- Although most acute infections resolve without sequelae, approximately 5% to 10% of patients will develop chronic infection with varying degrees of ongoing hepatocyte injury (Figure 16-1). There are three clinical categories of chronic infection:
    - Chronic active hepatitis, characterized by active viral replication, widespread inflammation, and sustained increases in alanine aminotransferase (ALT); nearly 50% of these patients will develop cirrhosis by 10 years after infection.
    - Chronic persistent hepatitis, in which the inflammation is limited to portal areas and ALT is only slightly elevated; long-term prognosis is very good.

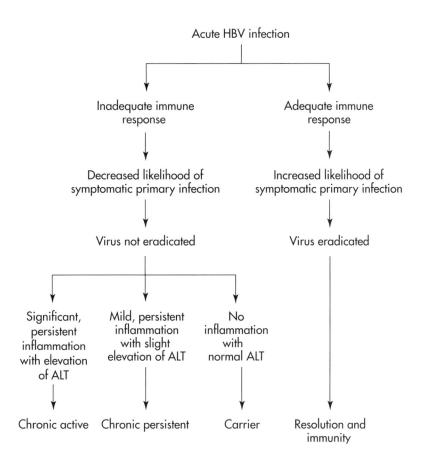

FIGURE **16-1 Natural History of HBV Infection.** The clinical outcome of HBV infection depends on the adequacy of the immune response in eradicating the virus. An adequate immune response is associated with an increased likelihood for both acute symptoms and viral eradication. An inadequate immune response may lead to chronic infection with varying degrees of persistent hepatic inflammation.

- True carrier state, characterized by normal liver enzymes and normal liver histology; only about 2% of these patients will develop progressive disease.
- The mechanism of long-term asymptomatic carrier state is believed to be immunologic tolerance to the virus so that the virus is not cleared but hepatocyte injury is minimal and the carrier state is lifelong; this is especially common in infants in whom the immune system is immature and unable to eradicate the virus.
- Chronic HBV infection is associated with a 10- to 100-fold risk of hepatocellular carcinoma.

Hepatitis C
- HCV is a small envelope virus containing RNA. There are six genotypes with some subcategories; genotype 1b is most common in the United States and Canada.
- Direct viral cytopathicity is the primary mode of hepatocyte injury, and the viral load positively correlates with the amount of inflammation seen on liver biopsy.
- CD8 lymphocyte–mediated cellular destruction of infected cells is the primary means of effective immune response to HCV but is effective in eradicating the virus in only 15% to 30% of cases. The virus can evade humoral immunity by its rapid mutation rate, thus it quickly develops resistant strains to antibodies.
- Further liver damage results from autoimmune hepatitis which is commonly associated with HCV infection. This is characterized by the development of anti–liver-kidney microsomal antibodies that can destroy uninfected hepatocytes. There is also release of inflammatory mediators such as IL-2, TNF-α, and INF-γ, which further contribute to liver damage.
- The autoimmune component of HCV can also result in multiple extrahepatic manifestations of the disease including membranous glomerulonephritis, cryoglobulinemia, vasculitis, dermatitis, pulmonary fibrosis, and rheumatoid arthritis.

- Recent studies suggest that only 15% to 30% of infected patients are able to completely eradicate the virus. Rapid viral mutation and suppression of dendritic and natural killer cells and lymphocyte function have been implicated in viral persistence.
- Approximately 70% to 75% of infected individuals will develop chronic hepatitis; disease progression is usually clinically silent and characterized by ongoing inflammation.
- Cirrhosis occurs in 20% of chronic HCV infections, and may be evident as early as 15 months after the acute infection, although the average time to cirrhosis is 20 years. Cofactors in the development of cirrhosis include increasing age, alcoholism, coinfection with HIV, and coinfection with HBV.
- Hepatocellular carcinoma (HCC) occurs in approximately 20% of untreated and 4% of treated patients with chronic HCV infection. The pathogenesis of HCC is related to the high level of hepatocellular regeneration seen with chronic HCV hepatitis (mitogenesis), as well as possible mutagenic effects of the virus.

PATIENT PRESENTATION

History

Needlestick injury; hemodialysis; blood transfusion; organ transplant; homosexual contact with an infected individual; alcohol abuse.

Symptoms

Acute infection is often asymptomatic with both HBV and HCV (50% to 80%); incubation periods from time of exposure to development of symptoms can be 5 to 8 weeks or as long as 6 months; if acute symptoms occur, they include fatigue, fever, myalgias and arthralgias, jaundice, anorexia, abdominal discomfort, and nausea; some cases of acute HBV infection will present with fulminant hepatic failure, including encephalitis, coagulopathy, and ascites; symptoms of chronic infection are most common in HCV and include fatigue, nausea, anorexia, coagulopathy, ascites, encephalopathy, and gastrointestinal bleeding; extrahepatic manifestations of both HBV and HCV may occur including rashes, severe abdominal pain, renal dysfunction, dyspnea, joint pain, and Raynaud phenomenon.

Examination

The examination is often normal in the absence of significant hepatic failure; when liver dysfunction is severe, exam findings may include asterixis, decreased mental status, jaundice, ecchymoses, ascites, edema, pectoral alopecia, palmar erythema, spider angiomata, gynecomastia, and heme-positive stools; evidence of extraarticular disease may be seen including skin lesions, arthritic changes, pulmonary crackles, and corneal ulcers.

DIFFERENTIAL DIAGNOSIS

- Hepatitis A, D, E, or G.
- Hepatitis due to other viruses (Epstein-Barr [EBV], cytomegalovirus [CMV], herpes, coxsackievirus).
- Alcoholic hepatitis or cirrhosis.
- Autoimmune hepatitis.
- α_1-antitrypsin deficiency.
- Biliary cirrhosis.
- Toxins or drugs (isoniazid, rifampin, acetaminophen).
- Hemochromatosis.
- Sclerosing cholangitis.

KEYS TO ASSESSMENT

- History of exposures is important, but the incubation period is long and the acute infection is usually asymptomatic so that even a careful history may not pinpoint the time or source of initial infection.

- The examination may be relatively unrevealing until late in the course of the disease; diagnosis before hepatic failure depends on serologic testing.
- Serologic testing.
  - HBV.
    1. Four viral antigens (viral DNA, HBsAg, HBcAg, and HBeAg) and three antibodies (anti-HBs, anti-HBc [IgM or IgG], and anti-HBe) can be detected.
    2. In acute infection, HBsAg is positive, but could represent a previous carrier state; the diagnosis of acute HBV infection is confirmed with a positive HBeAg and IgM anti-HBc antibody.
    3. Chronic infection is diagnosed by the presence of HBsAg in serum for 6 months or longer after initial detection; IgG anti-HBc are usually present at low levels; and anti-HBs and anti-HBe are present in most, but not all, cases and may take months to become detectable. Severity of chronic infection (chronic active or chronic persistent) is determined by ALT levels.
    4. HBV DNA by polymerase chain reaction (PCR) testing is available and can detect active viral replication in both acute and chronic infection; it is used to follow response to treatment for research protocols.
  - HCV.
    1. HCV screening is indicated for (a) people who received blood products prior to 1991, (b) people with hemophilia, (c) dialysis patients, (d) children born to HCV-positive mothers, (e) IV drug users, and (f) donors for transplants.
    2. Antibody HCV testing has evolved rapidly and the "second- and third-generation" testing techniques have fewer problems with specificity and sensitivity than did the older assays; antibody titers become detectable weeks to months after the original infection.
    3. PCR testing for viral RNA detects presence of the virus (acute or chronic)—not widely available and expensive.
- Serum ALT and aspartate aminotransferase (AST) levels usually rise 2 to 3 months after the initial infection.
- Diagnosis of liver failure is evidenced by increased bilirubin, prolonged coagulation times, decreased albumin, and evidence of ascites and portal hypertension with the possibility of finding esophageal varices on endoscopy.

KEYS TO MANAGEMENT

- Prevention.
  - HBV.
    1. Behavior changes in sexual practices, discontinuation of IV drug use and standard precautions in health care.
    2. Passive immunoprophylaxis.
       a. Recommended for perinatal exposure to an infected mother, prolonged contact of a younger than 12-month-old infant with an infected primary care deliverer, needlestick from an infected patient, sexual exposure to an infected individual, and organ transplant if infected prior to transplantation.
       b. Hepatitis B immunoglobulin (HBIG) is given within 12 hours of delivery or 14 days of other exposures followed by the three-dose vaccination series. Prevents infection in nearly 80% of cases.
    3. Active immunoprophylaxis is recommended for all children and for other high-risk groups such as health care workers and IV drug users.
       a. A three-dose regimen at 0, 1, and 6 months results in 95% of patients developing antibody with a subsequent rate of HBV infection of 3.2% compared with 26% in controls.
       b. Follow-up measurement of antibody response should be done in infants born to infected mothers, dialysis patients, immunocompromised individuals, sexual partners of chronically infected individuals, and people with occupational exposure risk.

- HCV
  1. Behavior changes in sexual practices, discontinuation of IV drug use and the use of standard precautions in health care.
  2. If there has been a known exposure, testing for antibody at 6 months is indicated, but there is no prevention available at this time, and trials of passive immunoprophylaxis have been ineffective thus far.
  3. Vaccine development is difficult due to the high mutation rate of the virus.
- Pharmacologic treatment.
  - HBV.
    1. Indicated for patients with chronic active disease.
    2. Pegylated interferon-alpha (INF-α) plus lamivudine or adefovir; combined regimen has higher response rates than either drug alone.
    3. Side effects are frequent and include an influenza-like illness with fever, chills, myalgias, and headache 4 to 8 hours after injection; fatigue; myalgias; anorexia; weight loss; bone marrow suppression; nephrotoxicity psychologic side effects such as anxiety, depression, and irritability; and autoimmune phenomena such as autoimmune thyroiditis, hemolytic anemia, and collagen vascular disease.
    4. Patients with HBV may experience a "flare" of their disease with interferon treatment characterized by a dramatic rise in ALT. This is a good prognostic sign indicating an increased likelihood of response; this is not seen with HCV.
  - HCV.
    1. Indicated for patients with acute or chronic HCV infection, including those with cirrhosis.
    2. Pegylated INF-α plus ribavirin; combined regimen has higher response rates than either drug alone.
    3. Approximately half of treated individuals will achieve a sustained response, and some will actually achieve significant improvement in established cirrhosis.
    4. Decreased response rates are found in older males, those who are immunosuppressed (especially HIV-positive individuals), and those who abuse alcohol.
    5. Side effects similar to HBV regimen.
    6. Contraindicated in patients with severe depression, active alcoholism or substance abuse, severe autoimmune disease, or severe pancytopenia; controversial use in HIV-positive patients or those with normal serum ALT.
    7. New therapies include synthetic interferon (Infrogen), protease inhibitors, RNA polymerase inhibitors, and DNA vaccines.
- Liver transplant.
  - Indications include severe symptoms, decreased quality of life, and sustained jaundice and coagulopathy.
  - Living, related donor liver transplantation is the norm; survival rates are now 70% to 85% at 5 years.
  - HBV accounts for 5% to 10% of liver transplants in the United States. It is associated with a high risk of recurrence after transplantation (approximately 75%) unless the recipient is also treated with interferon and lamivudine or adefovir before and after transplantation, and HBIG plus lamivudine after transplantation which reduces reinfection rates to less than 10%.
  - HCV accounts for the majority of all liver transplants performed in the United States. Postoperative survival is excellent although relapse of infection occurs in nearly 100% of patients, with 70% developing recurrent chronic liver disease requiring antiviral treatment.

PATHOPHYSIOLOGY	→	CLINICAL LINK
What is going on in the disease process that influences how the patient presents and how he or she should be managed?		*What should you do now that you understand the underlying pathophysiology?*
HBV causes liver injury primarily through immune-dependent mechanisms rather than through direct viral cytopathicity.	→	Patients with an effective immune response are less likely to become carriers but will present with a more fulminant acute clinical presentation and a high ALT.
Some patients are immunologically tolerant to HBV and will have persistent viral replication and chronic hepatitis.	→	HBV carrier state occurs in approximately 5% of patients and is associated with persistent infectivity, chronic liver damage, and a risk of hepatocellular carcinoma.
Treatment of HBV with pegylated INF-α and lamivudine may result in a transient flare in immunologic activity that indicates effective HBV killing.	→	Patients may experience an increase in ALT and a flulike illness after therapy.
Both active and passive immuno-prophylaxis for HBV are effective in preventing infection.	→	Postexposure HBIG and vaccination with the three-dose regimen are effective in preventing active infection.
HCV mutates rapidly and can avoid the immune system and can develop resistance to vaccines.	→	Chronic HCV infection is common, and both passive and active immunoprophylaxis have been ineffective so far.
HCV has direct cytopathicity to the hepatocytes with significant hepatocellular injury and necrosis.	→	HCV is associated with a significant risk of cirrhosis and hepatocellular carcinoma.
HCV is associated with autoantibodies that can attack the kidney, the skin, joints, and the thyroid.	→	HCV infection may be associated with membranous glomerulonephritis, rashes, collagen vascular disease, and an autoimmune thyroiditis.

SUGGESTED READINGS

Akuta, N. & Kumada, H. (2005). Influence of hepatitis B virus genotypes on the response to antiviral therapies. *Journal of Antimicrobial Chemotherapy*, 55, 139-142.

Andre, F. (2004). Hepatitis B: a comprehensive prevention, diagnosis, and treatment program—past, present, and future. *Journal of Gastroenterology & Hepatology*, 19(suppl), S1-S4.

Arbuthnot, P., Carmona, S., & Ely, A. (2005). Exploiting the RNA interference pathway to counter hepatitis B virus replication. *Liver International*, 25, 9-15.

Atkins, M. & Nolan, M. (2005). Sexual transmission of hepatitis B. *Current Opinion in Infectious Diseases*, 18, 67-72.

Balasubramanian, S. & Kowdley, K. V. (2005). Effect of alcohol on viral hepatitis and other forms of liver dysfunction. *Clinics in Liver Disease*, 9, 83-101.

Brok, J., Mellerup, M. T., Krogsgaard, K., & Gluud, C. (2004). Glucocorticosteroids for viral hepatitis C. *Cochrane Database of Systematic Reviews* CD002904.

Cacoub, P. (2005). Treatment of hepatitis C in HIV/hepatitis C co-infected patients: what is the evidence? *International Journal of STD & AIDS*, 16, 1-4.

Castera, L., Chouteau, P., Hezode, C., Zafrani, E. S., Dhumeaux, D., & Pawlotsky, J. M. (2005). Hepatitis C virus-induced hepatocellular steatosis. *American Journal of Gastroenterology*, 100, 711-715.

Chan, H. L., Leung, N. W., Hui, A. Y., Wong, V. W., Liew, C. T., Chim, A. M., Chan, F. K., Hung, L. C., Lee, Y. T., Tam, J. S., Lam, C. W., & Sung, J. J. (2005). A randomized, controlled trial of combination therapy for chronic hepatitis B: comparing pegylated interferon-α2b and lamivudine with lamivudine alone. *Annals of Internal Medicine*, 142, 240-250.

Chou, R., Clark, E. C., Helfand, M., & U.S. Preventive Services Task Force (2004). Screening for hepatitis C virus infection: a review of the evidence for the U.S. Preventive Services Task Force. *Annals of Internal Medicine*, 140, 465-479.

Daniel, S. (2005). Chronic hepatitis C treatment patterns in African American patients: an update. *American Journal of Gastroenterology*, 100, 716-722.

Darling, J. M. & Wright, T. L. (2004). Immune responses in hepatitis C: is virus or host the problem? *Current Opinion in Infectious Diseases*, 17, 193-198.

De Clercq, E. (2004). Antiviral drugs in current clinical use. *Journal of Clinical Virology*, 30, 115-133.

Ganem, D. & Prince, A. M. (2004). Hepatitis B virus infection—natural history and clinical consequences. *New England Journal of Medicine*, 350, 1118-1129.

Gowans, E. J., Jones, K. L., Bharadwaj, M., & Jackson, D. C. (2004). Prospects for dendritic cell vaccination in persistent infection with hepatitis C virus. *Journal of Clinical Virology*, 30, 283-290.

Hayashi, P. H. & Di Bisceglie, A. M. (2005). The progression of hepatitis B- and C-infections to chronic liver disease and hepatocellular carcinoma: epidemiology and pathogenesis. *Medical Clinics of North America*, 89, 371-389.

Hnatyszyn, H. J. (2005). Chronic hepatitis C and genotyping: the clinical significance of determining HCV genotypes. *Antiviral Therapy*, 10, 1-11.

Kanwal, F., Gralnek, I. M., Martin, P., Dulai, G. S., Farid, M., & Spiegel, B. M. R. (2005). Treatment alternatives for chronic hepatitis B virus infection: a cost-effectiveness analysis. *Annals of Internal Medicine*, 142, 821-831.

Keating, G. M. & Plosker, G. L. (2005). Peginterferon alpha-2a (40KD) plus ribavirin: a review of its use in the management of patients with chronic hepatitis C and persistently "normal" ALT levels. *Drugs*, 65, 521-536.

Kumar, R. & Agrawal, B. (2004). Novel treatment options for hepatitis B virus infection. *Current Opinion in Investigational Drugs*, 5, 171-178.

Lavanchy, D. (2004). Hepatitis B virus epidemiology, disease burden, treatment, and current and emerging prevention and control measures. *Journal of Viral Hepatitis*, 11, 97-107.

Lee, J. M., Botteman, M. F., Xanthakos, N., & Nicklasson, L. (2005). Needlestick injuries in the United States. Epidemiologic, economic, and quality of life issues. *AAOHN Journal*, 53, 117-133.

Lessells, R. & Leen, C. (2004). Management of hepatitis B in patients coinfected with the human immunodeficiency virus. *European Journal of Clinical Microbiology & Infectious Diseases*, 23, 366-374.

Lin, K. W. & Kirchner, J. T. (2004). Hepatitis B. *American Family Physician*, 69, 75-82.

Locarnini, S. (2005). Therapies for hepatitis B: where to from here. *Gastroenterology*, 128, 789-792.

Lonardo, A., Adinolfi, L. E., Loria, P., Carulli, N., Ruggiero, G., & Day, C. P. (2004). Steatosis and hepatitis C virus: mechanisms and significance for hepatic and extrahepatic disease. *Gastroenterology*, 126, 586-597.

Lutchman, G. & Ghany, M. (2005). Pushing the treatment envelope for chronic hepatitis C—is more necessarily better? *Hepatology*, 41, 234-236.

Manns, M. P., Hadem, J., & Wedemeyer, H. (2004). Hepatitis B virus: where are we and where are we going? *Methods in Molecular Medicine*, 96, 415-443.

Marrero, J. A. & Lok, A. S. (2004). Occult hepatitis B virus infection in patients with hepatocellular carcinoma: Innocent bystander, cofactor, or culprit. *Gastroenterology*, 126, 347-350.

McCaughan, G. W., Koorey, D. J., & Strasser, S. I. (2005). Liver transplantation for viral hepatitis. *Hospital Medicine (London)*, 66, 8-12.

McMahon, B. J., Bruden, D. L., Petersen, K. M., Bulkow, L. R., Parkinson, A. J., Nainan, O., Khristova, M., Zanis, C., Peters, H., & Margolis, H. S. (2005). Antibody levels and protection after hepatitis B vaccination: results of a 15-year follow-up. *Annals of Internal Medicine*, 142, 333-341.

Mohanty, S. R. & Cotler, S. J. (2005). Management of hepatitis B in liver transplant patients. *Journal of Clinical Gastroenterology*, 39, 58-63.

Moreno-Otero, R. (2005). Therapeutic modalities in hepatitis C: challenges and development. *Journal of Viral Hepatitis*, 12, 10-19.

Neumann-Haefelin, C., Blum, H. E., Chisari, F. V., & Thimme, R. (2005). T cell response in hepatitis C virus infection. *Journal of Clinical Virology*, 32, 75-85.

Omata, M. & Yoshida, H. (2004). Prevention and treatment of hepatocellular carcinoma. *Liver Transplantation*, 10, S111-S114.

Pachiadakis, I., Pollara, G., Chain, B. M., & Naoumov, N. V. (2005). Is hepatitis C virus infection of dendritic cells a mechanism facilitating viral persistence? *The Lancet Infectious Diseases*, 5, 296-304.

Pawlotsky, J. M. (2004). Pathophysiology of hepatitis C virus infection and related liver disease. *Trends in Microbiology*, 12, 96-102.

Pearlman, B. L. (2004). Hepatitis C infection: a clinical review. *Southern Medical Journal*, 97, 364-373.

Penin, F., Dubuisson, J., Rey, F. A., Moradpour, D., & Pawlotsky, J. M. (2004). Structural biology of hepatitis C virus. *Hepatology*, 39, 5-19.

Pineda, J. A. & Macias, J. (2005). Progression of liver fibrosis in patients coinfected with hepatitis C virus and human immunodeficiency virus undergoing antiretroviral therapy. *Journal of Antimicrobial Chemotherapy*, 55, 417-419.

Rawls, R. A. & Vega, K. J. (2005). Viral hepatitis in minority America. *Journal of Clinical Gastroenterology*, 39, 144-151.

Rehermann, B. & Nascimbeni, M. (2005). Immunology of hepatitis B virus and hepatitis C virus infection. *Nature Reviews, Immunology*, 5, 215-229.

Rockstroh, J. K. & Spengler, U. (2004). HIV and hepatitis C virus co-infection. *The Lancet Infectious Diseases, 4,* 437-444.

Rockstroh, J. K. & Vogel, M. (2004). Therapy of hepatitis C in HIV-coinfection. *European Journal of Medical Research, 9,* 304-308.

Sansonno, D. & Dammacco, F. (2005). Hepatitis C virus, cryoglobulinaemia, and vasculitis: immune complex relations. *The Lancet Infectious Diseases, 5,* 227-236.

Schaefer, S. (2005). Hepatitis B virus: significance of genotypes. *Journal of Viral Hepatitis, 12,* 111-124.

Shimada, M., Fujii, M., Morine, Y., Imura, S., Ikemoto, T., & Ishibashi, H. (2005). Living-donor liver transplantation: present status and future perspective. *Journal of Medical Investigation, 52,* 22-32.

Soriano, V., Puoti, M., Sulkowski, M., Mauss, S., Cacoub, P., Cargnel, A., Dieterich, D., Hatzakis, A., & Rockstroh, J. (2004). Care of patients with hepatitis C and HIV co-infection. *AIDS, 18,* 1-12.

Spiegel, B. M., Younossi, Z. M., Hays, R. D., Revicki, D., Robbins, S., & Kanwal, F. (2005). Impact of hepatitis C on health related quality of life: a systematic review and quantitative assessment. *Hepatology, 41,* 790-800.

Sprengers, D. & Janssen, H. L. (2005). Immunomodulatory therapy for chronic hepatitis B virus infection. *Fundamental & Clinical Pharmacology, 19,* 17-26.

Taylor, J. A. & Naoumov, N. V. (2005). The potential of RNA interference as a tool in the management of viral hepatitis. *Journal of Hepatology, 42,* 139-144.

The Global Burden of Hepatitis. (2004). Global burden of disease (GBD) for hepatitis C. *Journal of Clinical Pharmacology, 44,* 20-29.

Thomson, B. J. & Finch, R. G. (2005). Hepatitis C virus infection. *Clinical Microbiology & Infection, 11,* 86-94.

Triantos, C., Samonakis, D., Stigliano, R., Thalheimer, U., Patch, D., & Burroughs, A. (2005). Liver transplantation and hepatitis C virus: systematic review of antiviral therapy. *Transplantation, 79,* 261-268.

Trujillo-Murillo, K. C., Garza-Rodriguez, M. I., Martinez-Rodriguez, H. G., Barrera-Saldana, H. A., Bosques-Padilla, F., Ramos-Jimenez, J., & Rivas-Estilla, A. M. (2004). Experimental models for hepatitis C virus (HCV): new opportunities for combating hepatitis C. *Annals of Hepatology, 3,* 54-62.

Weber, B. (2005). Genetic variability of the S gene of hepatitis B virus: clinical and diagnostic impact. *Journal of Clinical Virology, 32,* 102-112.

Weber, B. (2005). Recent developments in the diagnosis and monitoring of HBV infection and role of the genetic variability of the S gene. *Expert Review of Molecular Diagnostics, 5,* 75-91.

Wedemeyer, H., Jackel, E., Wiegand, J., Cornberg, M., & Manns, M. P. (2004). Whom? When? How? Another piece of evidence for early treatment of acute hepatitis C. *Hepatology, 39,* 1201-1203.

Wheeler, M. (2005). Ethanol and HCV-induced cytotoxicity: the perfect storm. *Gastroenterology, 128,* 232-234.

Hepatitis B and C

INITIAL HISTORY

- 37-year-old male IV drug user.
- Several days of increasing fatigue and anorexia.
- Now with fever, abdominal discomfort, and myalgias.

Question 1.   *What questions would you like to ask this patient about his symptoms?*

ADDITIONAL HISTORY

- Discomfort is dull and located over the right upper quadrant.
- Patient denies jaundice, easy bruising, increasing abdominal girth, edema, or confusion.
- Stools are normal; no bloody or dark stools.
- No rashes; no hot, swollen joints.
- No dyspnea; no decrease in urination.

Question 2.   *What questions would you like to ask this patient about his life-style or past medical history?*

MORE HISTORY

- Patient lived in Philadelphia and has used IV drugs for years; he was in a needle exchange program.
- Moved to this area 6 months ago; no needle exchange program is available here.
- Lives alone; has not had a sexual encounter since moving here.
- Does not know of anyone who has had hepatitis.
- No dyspnea; no decrease in urination.
- Denies history of significant illnesses or any hospitalizations except for drug rehabilitation.
- Drinks alcohol "occasionally."
- On no medications; no known allergies.

PHYSICAL EXAMINATION

- Ill-appearing, alert male in mild distress.
- T = 38° C orally; P = 90 and regular; RR = 18 and unlabored; BP = 128/82 right arm (sitting).

HEENT, Neck, Skin
- PERRLA, fundi without lesions.
- Nares clear.
- No mouth lesions.
- Pharynx clear without erythema or exudate.
- No thyromegaly.
- No adenopathy.
- Nonicteric.
- No rashes; no petechiae or ecchymoses.

Lungs, Cardiac
- Lungs clear to auscultation and percussion.
- Cardiac examination with regular rate and rhythm without murmurs or gallops.

Abdomen
- Nondistended.
- Bowel sounds present.
- Liver percusses to 12 cm at the midclavicular line.
- Tenderness over the right upper quadrant without guarding or rebound.
- Spleen not palpable.

Rectal
- No hemorrhoids felt.
- Prostate not enlarged or tender.
- Stool heme negative.

Extremities
- No edema.
- No joint swelling or erythema.

Neurologic
- Alert and oriented.
- No sensory or motor deficits.
- DTR 2+ and symmetric.

Question 3. *What are the pertinent positives and negatives on examination?*

Question 4.   *What is the differential diagnosis based on the history and physical examination?*

Question 5.   *What laboratory assessment would you do now?*

LABORATORY RESULTS

- WBC = 15,000 with a mild increase in lymphocytes.
- Chemistries normal, including albumin.
- PT and PTT normal.
- ALT >700 and AST >300 international units/L.
- Total bilirubin upper limit of normal, alkaline phosphatase mildly elevated.
- Serum ferritin normal.
- HBsAg positive, IgM anti-HBc positive, HBeAg positive.
- IgM anti-HAV negative, HCV RNA negative by polymerase chain reaction (PCR) testing.
- HIV RNA by PCR negative, anti-HIV ELISA negative.

Question 6.   *What do these laboratory results mean?*

Question 7. *What should you do for the patient now?*

PATIENT'S RETURN VISIT (8 months later)

- Patient states he recovered slowly without therapy; finally feeling back to "normal" 3 months after his initial visit.
- Did not see why he needed to return for follow-up (as instructed) until now.
- Heard he might still be infectious and wants to be checked.
- Has no complaints at this time; has been sexually active for the past 2 months.

Question 8. *What tests would you do now?*

LABORATORY RESULTS

- AST and ALT upper limit of normal.
- Total bilirubin normal.
- HIV ELISA negative.
- HBsAg still positive.
- HBV DNA (PCR) low level.

Question 9. *What does this mean and what should you tell the patient?*

Chapter 17

Alcoholic Hepatic Cirrhosis and Portal Hypertension

DEFINITION

- Alcoholic cirrhosis.
  - A chronic disease of the liver caused by alcohol intake characterized by steatosis (fatty infiltration), inflammation, and fibrosis.
  - Destroys normal hepatic architecture and results in fibrous bands of connecting tissue separating lobules with nodules of regenerating liver cells unrelated to the normal vasculature.
- Portal hypertension.
  - Increased pressure in the portal system due to increased portal blood flow and increased resistance to hepatic perfusion.
  - Results in dilation of collateral veins and is associated with liver dysfunction, splenomegaly, and fluid and electrolyte imbalances.

EPIDEMIOLOGY

- There are an estimated 15.3 million alcoholics in the United States.
- In the United States, alcoholic cirrhosis has been surpassed recently by chronic hepatitis C infection as the most common cause of chronic liver disease.
- Cirrhosis requires a cumulative intake of approximately 600 kg of ethanol for men and 150 to 300 kg for women; however, of those who consume this much alcohol, only 40% develop cirrhosis.
- Additional cofactors for alcoholic cirrhosis include genetic polymorphisms of the enzymes responsible for ethanol metabolism, female gender (although males tend to have a more rapid progression of their cirrhosis once it is established), poor nutrition, body mass index, and viral hepatitis (hepatitis B or C).
- In the United States, portal hypertension is most commonly the result of alcoholic cirrhosis, followed by chronic viral hepatitis (especially hepatitis C).
- In patients with alcoholic cirrhosis and portal hypertension, 30% will bleed from esophageal varices with a mortality of nearly 50%; if the patient survives the first episode, there is a 70% chance of recurrence within a year.

PATHOPHYSIOLOGY

Genetics

- Many genes have been identified that are associated with alcoholism, but fewer have been directly linked to alcoholic cirrhosis. Genes that have been implicated include those that affect the metabolism of alcohol and those that regulate vascular tone including nitric oxide synthetase, angiotensinogen, endothelin, angiotensin-converting enzyme, and angiotensin II receptors.

Tissue Effects

- Alcoholic cirrhosis.
    - Ethanol is metabolized by several enzymes. When alcohol intake is excessive, these enzymatic reactions result in the release of toxic oxygen radicals. In addition, alcohol intake reduces the activity of endogenous antioxidants (vitamins E and A, glutathione). Oxygen radicals cause hepatocyte lipid peroxidation and deoxyribonucleic acid (DNA) damage.
    - Ethanol increases intestinal permeability leading to alcohol-associated endotoxemia (translocation of gram-negative bacteria and endotoxin from the gut into the bloodstream) and further inflammation of the liver with recruitment of polymorphonucleocytes (PMNs). Hepatocyte apoptosis and degeneration with PMN infiltration is common.
    - Hepatic injury stimulates production of inflammatory cytokines including interleukin (IL)-1, IL-6, IL-8, and tumor necrosis factor (TNF)-α, which contribute to more hepatocyte injury.
    - Ethanol also directly affects mitochondria with intrahepatocyte accumulation of microvesicular fat described as alcoholic foamy steatosis. This process is reversible with discontinuation of alcohol intake and does not necessarily lead to cirrhosis.
    - One of the major metabolites of ethanol is acetaldehyde, which affects protein synthesis and can stimulate hepatic fibrosis.
    - In addition, fibrinogenic inflammatory cytokines such as transforming growth factor (TGF)-β_1, angiotensin II, and leptin activate hepatic stellate cells, which proliferate and produce large amounts of collagen, resulting in fibrosis.
    - The pathologic characteristics of established alcoholic cirrhosis include steatosis, ballooning degeneration of hepatocytes, Mallory bodies (crescent-shaped bunches of intracellular filaments), neutrophilic inflammation, and pericellular fibrosis.
    - Cirrhosis causes loss of the normal hepatic functions, resulting in the risk for many complications including jaundice, ascites, coagulopathy, pancytopenia, hypoalbuminemia (with resultant edema), and hyperestrinism (decreased estrogen metabolism leads to increased circulating estrogen levels). Hepatic encephalopathy is an important complication that occurs due to the accumulation of toxic metabolites (especially ammonia) leading to an increase in neuronal gamma-aminobutyric acid (GABAergic) tone, neurologic dysfunction, and mental status changes.
- Portal hypertension.
    - Increased portal pressure results from resistance to portal flow into the liver, and from increased portal blood flow.
    - Increased resistance.
        1. Alcoholic cirrhosis with inflammation causes hepatocyte swelling and collagen deposition with obstruction of the hepatic sinusoids.
        2. Myofibroblasts (found in cirrhotic livers) have some contractile function; their constriction further obstructs portal inflow to the sinusoids (and provides some response to vasodilator therapy).
        3. Intrahepatic vasoactive mediators such as endothelin and nitric oxide cause further changes in hepatic resistance to portal blood flow.
    - Increased portal blood flow.
        1. A complex interaction of neurohumoral factors (sympathetic nervous system, glucagon, serotonin, adenosine, angiotensin, atrial natriuretic factor, and nitric oxide) results in splanchnic vasodilation and increased portal blood flow.
        2. This causes a fall in effective systemic arterial volume and decreases systemic blood pressure.
        3. Compensatory responses include tachycardia, release of antidiuretic hormone (ADH), and activation of the renin angiotensin aldosterone (RAA) system with water and sodium retention.

- The result of all of these interactions is increased pressure in the portal system, with a systemic hyperdynamic state (increased cardiac output and tachycardia but decreased systemic arterial pressure).
- Once portal pressure exceeds a level of 10 to 12 mm Hg greater than the pressure in the hepatic vein, portal collaterals begin shunting portal blood.
    1. Portal hypertension persists due to further increases in portal flow and increases in collateral resistance modulated by serotonin and nitric oxide.
    2. The major portal collaterals include those around the esophagus, stomach, rectum, and umbilicus; patients that have undergone previous abdominal surgery may also have collaterals around the intestines.
    3. Dilation of these collaterals (esophageal and gastric varices, and hemorrhoids) results in considerable risk for serious hemorrhage.
- Ascites.
    - Multiple factors contribute to the formation of ascites in individuals with cirrhosis and portal hypertension (Figure 17-1).
        1. Portal hypertension increases splanchnic intravascular hydrostatic pressure with translocation of intravascular volume into the peritoneum.
        2. Nitric oxide–mediated systemic vasodilation further contributes decreased effective systemic arterial volume which in turn causes the release of ADH and the activation of the RAA, leading to salt and water retention. Decreased hepatic metabolism of ADH and aldosterone leads to further increases in salt and water retention.
        3. Decreased hepatic synthesis of albumin, along with hypersplenism-associated pancytopenia, result in decreased intravascular oncotic pressure and translocation of fluid out of the vessels and into the tissues and peritoneal space.

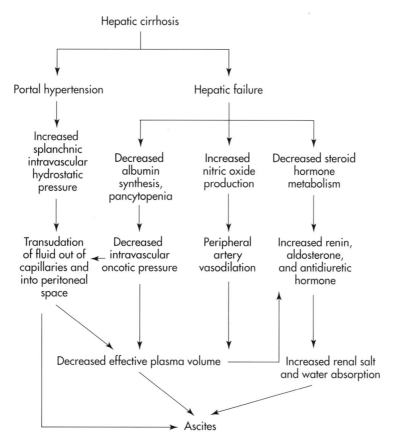

FIGURE **17-1 Pathophysiology of Ascites.**

- Decreased intravascular volume and neurohumoral perturbations can lead to hepatorenal syndrome (combined hepatic and renal failure), which has a very high mortality.
- Ascites and relative immune compromise (decreased T-cell activity) from cirrhosis and portal hypertension create a risk for urinary and pulmonary infections and for spontaneous bacterial peritonitis (SBP). The incidence of infection in patients admitted with cirrhosis is approximately 33% compared with 6% for general hospital admissions. SBP is monomicrobial in 92% of cases (usually *Escherichia coli* or *Klebsiella* spp.) and is a major cause of hepatorenal syndrome and mortality in cirrhosis.

PATIENT PRESENTATION

History

Alcohol abuse (40 to 80 g of ethanol a day, or about 2 to 4 drinks); female gender; poor diet; history of hepatitis.

Symptoms

Confusion; coma; jaundice; easy bruising; increasing abdominal girth; decreased exercise tolerance; hematemesis; hematochezia; melena; anorexia; weight loss; edema.

Examination

Hepatomegaly; hard nodular surface to the liver; splenomegaly; jaundice; ascites; encephalopathy; asterixis; fever; edema; ecchymoses; gynecomastia; palmar erythema; testicular atrophy; spider nevi; caput medusae; hemorrhoids; heme-positive stools.

DIFFERENTIAL DIAGNOSIS

- Viral or toxic hepatitis.
- Nonalcoholic steatohepatitis (NASH).
  - Parenteral nutrition.
  - Obesity.
  - Diabetes.
  - Diethylstilbestrol.
  - Glucocorticoids.
  - Amiodarone.
- Hemochromatosis.
- Primary biliary fibrosis.
- Hepatic carcinoma.
- Portal vein thrombosis.
- Polycystic liver.

KEYS TO ASSESSMENT

- Laboratory findings include macrocytic anemia, leukocytosis, modest elevations in aspartate aminotransferase (AST) and alanine aminotransferase (ALT) with an AST/ALT ratio >2, increased bilirubin, elevated prothrombin time (PT) and partial thromboplastin time (PTT), and decreased albumin.
- Although AST and ALT are called "liver function tests," they actually indicate acute hepatocyte damage, and therefore may normalize as liver fibrosis supercedes acute hepatic inflammation late in the course of cirrhosis. Newer tests that are being used in some centers are called the "quantitative liver function tests" and include aminopyrine breath test, galactose elimination capacity, sorbitol, and indocyanine green clearance. The clinical utility of these tests is still being evaluated.
- Measurement of renal function (blood urea nitrogen [BUN] and creatinine [Cr]) and urinary sodium and protein is indicated.

- Ascitic fluid should be tested (paracentesis) for cell count, bacterial culture, and measurement of total protein. A PMN count >250 cells/mm^3 ascitic fluid is considered diagnostic for SBP.
- Other markers of alcoholic cirrhosis include laminin, hyaluronan, type III procollagen, type IV collagen, tissue inhibitor of metalloproteinase, and prolyl hydroxylase (these are not used clinically at this time).
- The Child-Pugh classification of liver failure suggests that patients at high risk for early mortality can be identified by assessing prothrombin time and bilirubin levels. If 4.6 × [PT(seconds) – control] + bilirubin (mg/dL) is greater than 32, the 1-month mortality is 50%.
- Ultrasound and pulsed Doppler are used to evaluate biliary tree and portal vein blood flow. Direct portal vein pressure measurements of the portal circulation are rarely needed, but can be done in selected cases prior to surgical intervention. Magnetic resonance angiography can further evaluate the portal vein for surgery.
- If portal hypertension is present, endoscopy is indicated to evaluate for varices.
- Abdominal computed tomography (CT) should be considered for evaluation of possible hepatocellular carcinoma.
- Liver biopsy is indicated for clinical evidence of cirrhosis with a minimal alcohol intake.
- Clinical assessment for the presence of hepatic encephalopathy often misses mild cases (which may respond to conservative therapy). Serum ammonia levels may be suggestive but are not specific. The use of electrophysiologic data can improve sensitivity and specificity for diagnosis.

KEYS TO MANAGEMENT

Management of Cirrhosis

- Abstinence is the most important intervention and can improve survival in most patients, but it does not guarantee improvement.
- Malnutrition is correlated with poor prognosis in alcoholic cirrhosis, and although nutritional supplementation has not been clearly shown to improve outcomes, it is reasonable to provide some nutritional support to malnourished and anorexic patients. Protein supplements are important to raise albumin levels, but must be given with caution in patients with a history of encephalopathy.
- Bed rest with *careful* administration of diuretics (e.g., spironolactone) can improve edema and ascites; however, high doses of diuretics can result in worsening intravascular hypovolemia, hypotension, and renal toxicity (hepatorenal syndrome).
- Pharmacologic intervention can include propylthiouracil, corticosteroids, colchicine, and antioxidants in an effort to reduce hepatic inflammation and fibrosis. All of these have been shown in a few studies to have some benefit in alcoholic cirrhosis, but results are not dramatic and side effects are common.
- Liver transplant for alcoholic cirrhosis requires evaluation for strict preoperative criteria including 6 months' confirmed abstinence; survival rates after transplant are equivalent for nonalcoholic liver disease, and recidivism is less than 10%.
- Hepatic encephalopathy ranges from mild confusion to deep coma and is often precipitated by associated insults such as gastrointestinal bleeding or surgery. Management includes protein-restricted diet, nonabsorbable disaccharides (e.g., lactulose) and nonabsorbable antibiotics (e.g., neomycin, rifaximin). The benzodiazepine receptor antagonist flumazenil has been documented to improve symptoms.

Management of Portal Hypertension and Its Complications

- Propranolol improves portal pressures and decreases the risk of variceal bleeding. Carvedilol has both β-antagonist and α$_1$-receptor antagonist properties and may be superior to propranolol. Nitrates can be tried in patients that are intolerant of β-blockade. Thalidomide, which inhibits endotoxin-induced TNF-α, has been shown to reduce portal pressures in early studies, but further evaluation is needed.

- Ascites.
  - Bed rest (decreases activity of the renin-angiotensin-aldosterone system).
  - Salt restriction to 1500 mg/day.
  - Fluid restriction to 1000 mL/day in patients with dilutional hyponatremia.
  - Spironolactone or amiloride can be administered carefully to further induce diuresis (low-dose furosemide can also be added in patients who have low urinary sodium concentrations) to achieve no more than a weight loss of 500 g/day (more rapid fluid excretion can cause hepatorenal syndrome).
  - Therapeutic paracentesis or higher-dose diuretics is reserved for patients with tense ascites.
- If spontaneous bacterial peritonitis is suspected, rapid paracentesis for diagnosis and prompt administration of empiric antibiotics are crucial. In patients with variceal bleeding or low protein concentrations in the ascitic fluid (<15 g/L) but without SBP, prophylactic antibiotics (e.g., norfloxacin or ciprofloxacin) can be given to reduce the risk for SBP.
- Hepatorenal syndrome can result from portal hypertension, overly aggressive diuresis, and or spontaneous bacterial peritonitis. Intravenous albumin helps to prevent this syndrome and improves survival in selected patients.
- Endoscopic prophylactic ligation (banding) of esophageal varices with or without β-blockade has been shown in some studies to be superior to propranolol alone in preventing variceal bleeding in selected patients.
- Management of acute variceal hemorrhage requires emergent endoscopy and banding combined with administration of terlipressin, somatostatin, or octreotide (or vasopressin plus nitroglycerin). Emergent transjugular or surgical portosystemic shunting can also be considered (see following).
- Balloon tamponade can be used to control bleeding until the patient can undergo one of several surgical interventions such as esophageal devascularization or splenorenal shunt.
- A transjugular intrahepatic portosystemic shunt (TIPS) can be placed percutaneously for prevention and control of variceal bleeding, but this procedure is associated with significant risk of encephalopathy, accelerated liver failure, and restenosis and has a 15% mortality at 1 month.
- Surgical devascularization (e.g., proximal gastrectomy) can reduce the risk of recurrent variceal bleeding in selected patients.
- Studies suggest that if the individual is eligible, liver transplant should be considered as soon as ascites develops. Artificial and bioartificial support systems can improve survival and serve as a bridge to transplantation.

PATHOPHYSIOLOGY ⟶	CLINICAL LINK
What is going on in the disease process that influences how the patient presents and how he or she should be managed?	*What should you do now that you understand the underlying pathophysiology?*
Ethanol is directly toxic to hepatocytes and results in the release of inflammatory and fibrinogenic cytokines.	Abstinence from alcohol can reduce inflammation and fibrosis in many individuals. Unfortunately, anti-inflammatory and antifibrotic medications generally have been disappointing so far.
Edema of the gut mucosa with translocation of gram-negative bacteria into the bloodstream is a key step in the pathophysiology of cirrhosis.	In addition to infection contributing to cirrhosis itself, spontaneous bacterial peritonitis and other infections are common, and prompt diagnosis and management of these infections is essential to survival.
Hepatic dysfunction due to cirrhosis results in inability to excrete bilirubin, inability to make coagulation factors, inability to make albumin, inability to metabolize ADH and estrogen, and suppresses bone marrow.	Patients with severe cirrhosis may present with jaundice, coagulopathy, edema and ascites, feminization, and anemia.
Increased portal pressure is not only due to increased hepatic resistance to perfusion by the portal vein but also to sustained increases in portal blood flow.	Therapy for portal hypertension includes shunting procedures and drugs that influence the neurohumorally mediated increases in portal blood flow (e.g., propranolol, carvedilol).
Increased portal pressure dilates collateral veins around the esophagus, stomach, rectum, and umbilicus.	Dilated collaterals form esophageal and gastric varices, hemorrhoids, and caput medusae; varices and hemorrhoids can bleed spontaneously, with considerable morbidity and mortality.
Portal hypertension is associated with systemic hemodynamic changes such as decreased peripheral resistance, increased cardiac output, and decreased arterial pressure.	Although the patient may have considerable edema and ascites, he or she is often intravascularly depleted and may respond to diuretics with hypotension and oliguria; overdiuresis can lead to hepatorenal syndrome.

SUGGESTED READINGS

Abraldes, J. G., Dell'Era, A., & Bosch, J. (2004). Medical management of variceal bleeding in patients with cirrhosis. *Canadian Journal of Gastroenterology*, 18, 109-113.

Ahboucha, S. & Butterworth, R. F. (2004). Pathophysiology of hepatic encephalopathy: a new look at GABA from the molecular standpoint. *Metabolic Brain Disease*, 19, 331-343.

Als-Nielsen, B., Gluud, L. L., & Gluud, C. (2004). Benzodiazepine receptor antagonists for hepatic encephalopathy. *Cochrane Database of Systematic Reviews*, CD002798.

Als-Nielsen, B., Gluud, L. L., & Gluud, C. (2004). Dopaminergic agonists for hepatic encephalopathy. *Cochrane Database of Systematic Reviews*, CD003047.

Als-Nielsen, B., Gluud, L. L., & Gluud, C. (2004). Nonabsorbable disaccharides for hepatic encephalopathy. *Cochrane Database of Systematic Reviews*, CD003044.

Als-Nielsen, B., Gluud, L. L., & Gluud, C. (2004). Nonabsorbable disaccharides for hepatic encephalopathy: systematic review of randomised trials. *British Medical Journal*, 328, 1046.

Austin, A. S., Mahida, Y. R., Clarke, D., Ryder, S. D., & Freeman, J. G. (2004). A pilot study to investigate the use of oxpentifylline (pentoxifylline) and thalidomide in portal hypertension secondary to alcoholic cirrhosis. *Alimentary Pharmacology & Therapeutics*, 19, 79-88.

Baker, D. E. (2005). Rifaximin: a nonabsorbed oral antibiotic. *Reviews in Gastroenterological Disorders*, 5, 19-30.

Bataller, R. & Brenner, D. A. (2005). Liver fibrosis. *Journal of Clinical Investigation*, 115, 209-218.

Blei, A. T. (2004). Infection, inflammation and hepatic encephalopathy, synergism redefined. *Journal of Hepatology*, 40, 327-330.

Bosch, J. & Abraldes, J. G. (2004). Management of gastrointestinal bleeding in patients with cirrhosis of the liver. *Seminars in Hematology*, 41, 8-12.

Boyer, T. D. (2004). Changing clinical practice with measurements of portal pressure. *Hepatology*, 39, 283-285.

Boyer, T. D. (2005). Primary prophylaxis for variceal bleeding: are we there yet? *Gastroenterology*, 128, 1120-1122.

Boyer, T. D., Haskal, Z. J., & American Association for the Study of Liver Diseases. (2005). The role of transjugular intrahepatic portosystemic shunt in the management of portal hypertension. *Hepatology*, 41, 386-400.

Coto, E., Rodrigo, L., Alvarez, R., Fuentes, D., Rodriguez, M., Menendez, L. G., Ciriza, C., Gonzalez, P., & Alvarez, V. (2004). Variation at the angiotensin-converting enzyme and endothelial nitric oxide synthase genes is associated with the risk of esophageal varices among patients with alcoholic cirrhosis. *Journal of Cardiovascular Pharmacology*, 38, 833-839.

D'Amico, G. (2004). The role of vasoactive drugs in the treatment of oesophageal varices. *Expert Opinion on Pharmacotherapy*, 5, 349-360.

de Franchis, R. (2004). Review article: definition and diagnosis in portal hypertension—continued problems with the Baveno consensus? *Alimentary Pharmacology & Therapeutics*, 20(suppl 3), 2-6.

de Franchis, R. (2004). Somatostatin, somatostatin analogues and other vasoactive drugs in the treatment of bleeding oesophageal varices. *Digestive & Liver Disease*, 36(suppl 1), S93-S100.

de Franchis, R., Dell'Era, A., & Iannuzzi, F. (2004). Diagnosis and treatment of portal hypertension. *Digestive & Liver Disease*, 36, 787-798.

Farnsworth, N., Fagan, S. P., Berger, D. H., & Awad, S. S. (2004). Child-Turcotte-Pugh versus MELD score as a predictor of outcome after elective and emergent surgery in cirrhotic patients. *American Journal of Surgery*, 188, 580-583.

Fiorucci, S., Antonelli, E., Tocchetti, P., & Morelli, A. (2004). Treatment of portal hypertension with NCX-1000, a liver-specific NO donor. A review of its current status. *Cardiovascular Drug Reviews*, 22, 135-146.

Ford, J. M., Shah, H., Stecker, M. S., & Namyslowski, J. (2004). Embolization of large gastric varices using vena cava filter and coils. *Cardiovascular & Interventional Radiology*, 27, 366-369.

Garcia-Tsao, G. & Wiest, R. (2004). Gut microflora in the pathogenesis of the complications of cirrhosis. *Best Practice & Research in Clinical Gastroenterology*, 18, 353-372.

Gines, P., Cardenas, A., Arroyo, V., & Rodes, J. (2004) Management of cirrhosis and ascites. *New England Journal of Medicine*, 350, 1646-1654.

Gotzsche, P. C. & Hrobjartsson, A. (2005). Somatostatin analogues for acute bleeding oesophageal varices. *Cochrane Database of Systematic Reviews*, CD000193.

Grange, J. D. & Amiot, X. (2004). Nitric oxide and renal function in cirrhotic patients with ascites: from physiopathology to practice. *European Journal of Gastroenterology & Hepatology*, 16, 567-570.

Hausegger, K. A., Karnel, F., Georgieva, B., Tauss, J., Portugaller, H., Deutschmann, H., & Berghold, A. (2004). Transjugular intrahepatic portosystemic shunt creation with the Viatorr expanded polytetrafluoroethylene-covered stent-graft. *Journal of Vascular & Interventional Radiology*, 15, 239-248.

Hemstreet, B. A. (2004). Evaluation of carvedilol for the treatment of portal hypertension. *Pharmacotherapy*, 24, 94-104.

Hsieh, J. S., Wang, W. M., Perng, D. S., Huang, C. J., Wang, J. Y., & Huang, T. J. (2004). Modified devascularization surgery for isolated gastric varices assessed by endoscopic ultrasonography. *Surgical Endoscopy*, 18, 666-671.

Ito, K. & Mitchell, D. G. (2004). Imaging diagnosis of cirrhosis and chronic hepatitis. *Intervirology*, 47, 134-143.

Kamath, P. S. (2005). Esophageal variceal bleeding: primary prophylaxis. *Clinical Gastroenterology & Hepatology*, 3, 90-93.

Kassem, A. M. (2004). Gastrointestinal bleeding. *Endoscopy*, 36, 947-949.

Khuroo, M. S., Khuroo, N. S., Farahat, K. L., Khuroo, Y. S., Sofi, A. A., & Dahab, S. T. (2005). Meta-analysis: endoscopic variceal ligation for primary prophylaxis of oesophageal variceal bleeding. *Alimentary Pharmacology & Therapeutics*, 21, 347-361.

Kiyosue, H., Matsumoto, S., Yamada, Y., Hori, Y., Okino, Y., Okahara, M., & Mori, H. (2004). Transportal intravariceal sclerotherapy with N-butyl-2-cyanoacrylate for gastric varices. *Journal of Vascular & Interventional Radiology*, 15, 505-509.

Le Lan, C., Ropert, M., Laine, F., Medevielle, M., Jard, C., Pouchard, M., Le Treut, A., Moirand, R., Loreal, O., & Brissot, P. (2004). Serum ceruloplasmin and ferroxidase activity are not decreased in hepatic failure related to alcoholic cirrhosis: clinical and pathophysiological implications. *Alcoholism: Clinical & Experimental Research*, 28, 775-779.

Leevy, C. B. & Elbeshbeshy, H. A. (2005). Immunology of alcoholic liver disease. *Clinics in Liver Disease*, 9, 55-66.

Lefkowitch, J. H. (2005). Morphology of alcoholic liver disease. *Clinics in Liver Disease*, 9, 37-53.

Liu, J. P., Gluud, L. L., Als-Nielsen, B., & Gluud, C. (2004). Artificial and bioartificial support systems for liver failure. *Cochrane Database of Systematic Reviews*, CD003628.

Lockwood, A. H. (2004). Blood ammonia levels and hepatic encephalopathy. *Metabolic Brain Disease*, 19, 345-349.

Lozeva-Thomas, V. (2004). Serotonin brain circuits with a focus on hepatic encephalopathy. *Metabolic Brain Disease*, 19, 413-420.

Madoff, D. C., Wallace, M. J., Ahrar, K., & Saxon, R. R. (2004). TIPS-related hepatic encephalopathy: management options with novel endovascular techniques. *Radiographics,* 24, 21-36.

Moller, S. & Henriksen, J. H. (2004). Review article: pathogenesis and pathophysiology of hepatorenal syndrome—is there scope for prevention? *Alimentary Pharmacology & Therapeutics,* 20(suppl 3), 31-41.

Montagnese, S., Amodio, P., & Morgan, M. Y. (2004). Methods for diagnosing hepatic encephalopathy in patients with cirrhosis: a multidimensional approach. *Metabolic Brain Disease,* 19, 281-312.

Morgan, T. R., Mandayam, S., & Jamal, M. M. (2004). Alcohol and hepatocellular carcinoma. *Gastroenterology,* 127, S87-S96.

Mullen, K. D. & Dasarathy, S. (2004). Protein restriction in hepatic encephalopathy: necessary evil or illogical dogma. *Journal of Hepatology,* 41, 147-148.

Parsi, M. A., Atreja, A., & Zein, N. N. (2004). Spontaneous bacterial peritonitis: recent data on incidence and treatment. *Cleveland Clinic Journal of Medicine,* 71, 569-576.

Rossle, M. & Grandt, D. (2004). TIPS: an update. *Best Practice & Research in Clinical Gastroenterology,* 18, 99-123.

Ryan, B. M., Stockbrugger, R. W., & Ryan, J. M. (2004). A pathophysiologic, gastroenterologic, and radiologic approach to the management of gastric varices. *Gastroenterology,* 126, 1175-1189.

Saadeh, S. & Davis, G. L. (2004). Management of ascites in patients with end-stage liver disease. *Reviews in Gastroenterological Disorders,* 4, 175-185.

Sivayokan, T. & Dillon, J. F. (2004). Cirrhotic ascites: a review of management. *Hospital Medicine (London),* 65, 22-26.

Solga, S. F. & Diehl, A. M. (2004). Gut flora-based therapy in liver disease? The liver cares about the gut. *Hepatology,* 39, 1197-1200.

Talwalkar, J. A. & Kamath, P. S. (2004). An evidence-based medicine approach to beta-blocker therapy in patients with cirrhosis. *American Journal of Medicine,* 116, 759-766.

Thalheimer, U., Mela, M., Patch, D., & Burroughs, A. K. (2004). Targeting portal pressure measurements: a critical reappraisal. *Hepatology,* 39, 286-290.

Thalheimer, U., Triantos, C. K., Samonakis, D. N., Patch, D., & Burroughs, A. K. (2005). Infection, coagulation, and variceal bleeding in cirrhosis. *Gut,* 54, 556-563.

Toftengi, F. & Larsen, F. S. (2004). Management of patients with fulminant hepatic failure and brain edema. *Metabolic Brain Disease,* 19, 207-214.

Zhang, F. K., Zhang, J. Y., & Jia, J. D. (2005). Treatment of patients with alcoholic liver disease. *Hepatobiliary & Pancreatic Diseases International,* 4, 12-17.

Alcoholic Cirrhosis and Portal Hypertension

INITIAL HISTORY

- 59-year-old male.
- Brought into the emergency department by wife who noticed increased confusion over the past 3 days.
- Dark stools all week.
- Increased abdominal girth and tenderness.

Question 1.   *What is your differential diagnosis based on initial information?*

Question 2.   *What additional history would you obtain?*

ADDITIONAL HISTORY (via wife)

- No recent infections, fever, illnesses, falls.
- Drinks 8 to 12 beers per day and more on weekends (± 25 years); had last beer 2 days ago.
- Smoking: 20 pack/year history.
- Has had a "beer belly" for about 10 years, getting bigger over the past month (tender for 3 to 4 days).

□ **Suzanne M. Burns, RN, MSN, ACNP, CCRN contributed this case study.**

- Confusion over the past 3 to 4 days.
- Occasional use of Advil or Tylenol for headache; no known use of prescription or illicit drugs.
- No history to suggest prior cardiac or gallbladder disease; no history of hepatitis.

Question 3.   *Now what do you think?*

PHYSICAL EXAMINATION

- Confused; knows his name and his wife's name; restless in bed, lying on side.
- T = 36.7° C orally; P = 120 and regular; RR = 24, slightly labored; BP = 138/80 lying, 120/75 sitting.

HEENT, Skin, Neck
- Slight scleral icterus.
- No bruises, masses, deformities on head.
- Nystagmus with lateral gaze.
- Pupils 3 mm, reactive to light.
- Funduscopy without lesions.
- Ears: cerumen in left ear canal.
- Spider angiomas over upper chest and abdomen.
- Palmar erythema.
- Slightly diaphoretic.
- Mild jaundice.
- Several bruises on lower extremities.
- Supple neck.
- No adenopathy, thyromegaly, bruits.

Lungs, Chest
- Clear to auscultation.
- Poor diaphragmatic excursions (rapid, shallow breathing pattern).
- Gynecomastia.

Cardiac
- Tachycardia.
- Grade II systolic ejection murmur.
- No gallops, rubs, or clicks.

Abdomen
- Large, distended.
- Hyperactive bowel sounds (has just passed large, dark maroon stool, and vomited about 100 mL bright red blood).
- Diffusely tender to palpation.
- No aortic, iliac, renal bruits.
- Positive fluid wave, shifting dullness, difficult to ascertain liver border.
- Splenomegaly.

Extremities
- Good capillary refill.
- Trace to +1 edema of feet.

Neurologic
- Oriented to person only; confused, muttering.
- Cranial nerves: II through XII grossly intact (exception noted cranial nerve VI).
- Sensory: extremities grossly intact to pinprick and light touch.
- Reflexes: hyperreflexic.
- Asterixis.

Rectal
- Hemorrhoids (no visible bleeding).
- Passing dark maroon stool.

Question 4. *What are the pertinent positives and significant negatives on the examination and what do they suggest?*

Question 5. *What diagnostic studies and/or therapeutic interventions do you think are indicated now?*

LABORATORY RESULTS

- SaO_2 = 89%, ABGs: pH = 7.43, $PaCO_2$ = 33 mm Hg, PaO_2 = 58 mm Hg on room air.
- CBC: Hgb/Hct = 9/27, WBC = 12,000, PLTs = 75,000.
- Electrolytes = Na, K, Mg, and phosphate decreased.
- Bilirubin (direct) slightly increased.
- AST and ALT both elevated (ratio >2:1), alkaline phosphatase = normal.
- PT = 20, PTT = 32, INR = 2 (all elevated).
- Serum ammonia = elevated.
- Albumin = low; cholesterol = low.
- Chest radiograph = normal, although poor inspiration noted.
- ECG = sinus tachycardia.

Question 6. *Which laboratory studies are most important for you to act on now and what will you do?*

Question 7. *Do other laboratory studies suggest the etiology of this patient's internal bleeding?*

STATUS UPON ICU TRANSFER

- The patient is transferred to ICU.
- Continues to pass maroon-colored stools.
- Started on octreotide.
- The patient is still confused and is intubated for airway protection prior to variceal banding procedure.
- GI consult service performs endoscopy, which demonstrates both esophageal and gastric varices; four esophageal varices (which appear to be the sites of active bleeding) are banded.

Question 8.   *Why is octreotide used?*

Question 9.   *Following endoscopy and the banding procedure, the patient is more stable (appears to have stopped bleeding). Despite being confused, he is able to protect his airway and is extubated. What other management do you want to consider now?*

HOSPITAL COURSE

- The patient does well and is transferred from the ICU to a medical floor within 48 hours of admission.
- PT is corrected; bleeding has stopped.
- Mental status has improved.
- Has not experienced delirium tremens.
- Spontaneous bacterial peritonitis is ruled out.

Question 10.   *Now what should the plan be?*

DAY 4 ON MEDICAL FLOOR (hospitalization day 6)

- The patient is ready to be discharged in the care of his wife.
- Tired but alert and oriented.
- No further bleeding.

Question 11.   *What instructions and medications should go home with Mr. Z. and his wife?*

Headache

DEFINITION

- Primary headaches are defined as those that fit the diagnostic criteria for one of four categories of primary headache as described by the 2004 International Classification of Headache Disorders. There are several subcategories under each of the four types of primary headache:
  - Migraine.
    1. Without aura.
    2. With aura.
    3. Childhood periodic syndromes that are common precursors of migraine.
    4. Retinal migraine.
    5. Complications of migraine.
    6. Probable migraine.
  - Tension-type headache (TTH).
    1. Episodic TTH.
    2. Frequent episodic TTH.
    3. Chronic TTH.
    4. Probable TTH.
  - Cluster headache and other trigeminal autonomic cephalalgias.
    1. Cluster headache.
    2. Paroxysmal hemicrania.
    3. Short-lasting unilateral neuralgiform headache attacks with conjunctival injection and tearing.
  - Other primary headaches.
    1. Stabbing.
    2. Cough.
    3. Exertional.
    4. Associated with sexual activity.
    5. Hypnotic.
    6. Thunderclap.
    7. Hemicrania.
    8. New daily persistent.
- There are eight categories of secondary headaches: those that are associated with (1) head or neck trauma, (2) vascular disorders, (3) nonvascular intracranial disorders, (4) substance use or withdrawal, (5) infection, (6) bleeding, (7) disorders of cranial, facial, or sensory organ structures, or (8) psychiatric disorders.
- Medication-overuse headache (MOH) is a form of secondary headache that affects up to 1% of the U.S. population.

EPIDEMIOLOGY

- 90% to 95% of the people in the United States have unprovoked headaches annually, and an estimated 4% overuse analgesics such as aspirin, triptans, nonsteroidal anti-inflammatory drugs, and caffeine contributing to the prevalence of MOH.
- Migraine.
    - The World Health Organization ranks migraine among the world's most disabling illnesses.
    - Prevalence is 18% for females and 6% for males. Migraine is the most common reason for patient visits for headache treatment.
    - Onset is often in the teens; peak prevalence is between ages 35 to 45.
    - More than 70% of migraine patients have a positive family history, with a possible association with mitochondrial deoxyribonucleic acid (DNA) and chromosome 19.
    - Chronic daily headache (CDH) is an important complication of migraine and is defined as headache that meets the criteria for migraine and occurs on 15 or more days per month for 3 or more months in the absence of medication overuse.
- Tension-type headache.
    - It is the most common type of primary headache; overall prevalence of episodic headache is 38.3%, including 47% of women ages 30 to 39; incidence increases with educational level.
    - Episodic TTH describes fewer than 15 attacks per month; chronic TTH describes 15 or more attacks per month.
- Cluster headache.
    - The most painful primary headache affecting 0.1% of the population.
    - The male-to-female ratio is approximately 2:1, with peak incidence in the 40- to 50-year age-group.
    - First-degree relatives have a 5- to 18-times greater risk of developing cluster headaches.

PATHOPHYSIOLOGY

Genetics

- Migraine: P/Q-type calcium channel gene (*CACNA1A*—mediates 5-HT and excitatory neurotransmitter release), sodium-potassium pump gene *(ATP1A2)*, methylenetetrahydrofolate reductase *(MTHFR)* gene, and susceptibility loci on chromosomes 4, 11, 14, and 6.
- Tension-type headache: Although there is some familial tendency in TTH, genetics are felt to play a very minor role in the pathogenesis of TTH and environment is considered to have far greater effect.
- Cluster headache: Mitochondrial transfer *RNAleu* gene.

Mechanisms

- Migraine.
    - Triggers include fasting, alcohol intake, oral contraceptives, menstruation, hormone replacement, stress, caffeine withdrawal, sleep disturbance, bright lights, scents, smoke, certain foods (chocolate, aged cheese, nitrites, aspartame, citrus), and trauma.
    - An estimated 20% to 60% of patients experience symptoms of mood change, headache, difficulty concentrating, stiff neck, hunger, or drowsiness during the 24 hours prior to headache, and the onset of headache is often associated with circadian rhythms, thus suggesting a central site for initiation of migraine near the hypothalamus.
    - Preceding the headache, there is a reduction in blood flow (oligemia) and resultant cortical depression that spreads across the hemicortex at a rate of 2 to 3 mm/minute. Transient increases in potassium, nitric oxide, and glutamate also spread across the cortex. This may or may not be associated with the symptoms of an aura including scintillating scotomata, paresthesias, blurred vision, or other focal neurologic signs.

- Neurons that arise in the trigeminal ganglion produce a variety of neurohumoral cytokines (e.g., substance P and calcitonin gene-related peptide [CGRP]) that cause perivascular neurogenic inflammation, mast cell degranulation, platelet aggregation, and changes in serotonin receptor function that further promote migraine progression.
  - Decreased serotonin receptor activity appears to be important in migraine pathogenesis. Triptans are serotonin agonists and cause vasoconstriction, reduce neurogenic inflammation, and reduce pain transmission through the trigeminal system.
  - As the headache progresses, trigeminal ganglion sensitization and stimulation by inflammatory cytokines appears to be an important step in migraine pathogenesis causing intracerebral and extracerebral vasodilation.
  - Blood flow in the brainstem increases; in unilateral migraine, contralateral brainstem blood flow increases.
  - Other proposed mechanisms for migraine pathogenesis include dopamine receptor hypersensitivity and parasympathetic hypofunction.
  - In premenopausal women, cyclic estrogen withdrawal contributes to changes in serotonin and other neurotransmitters and causes a rise in serum prostaglandins that promotes migraine pathogenesis (menstrual migraine).
  - Migraines are associated with strokes in four ways: (1) migrainous infarcts (very rare), (2) migraine and stroke sharing a common cause (migraine-like headache due to vascular, blood, cardiac disorder), (3) migraines triggered by stroke, and (4) migraine as a risk factor for stroke (relative risk 2 to 4).
- Tension-type headache.
  - There has been a long-standing appreciation for the presence of pericranial muscle spasm and headache in many patients, but it is clear that most patients who fit the criteria for tension-type headache do not have these muscle spasms.
  - In those patients who do have pericranial muscle spasms, there is increased electromyographic activity in pericranial muscles, decreased blood flow, and muscle ischemia especially of the temporalis muscle, and tenderness of the head and neck muscles.
  - It has been postulated that there are several possible central mechanisms for tension-type headaches that are not associated with pericranial muscle spasms, but these are poorly understood. Sensitization of peripheral nociceptors (increased myofascial pain response) has been implicated, as has altered brainstem control of masseter and temporalis muscle contraction. Recent evidence shows that serotonin levels are reduced in patients with chronic tension-type headache.
- Cluster headache.
  - In susceptible individuals, alterations in seasonal photoperiod may contribute to "cluster periods" lasting 2 to 4 months and affecting hypothalamic function.
  - Hypothalamic dysfunction leads to changes in chemoreceptor responses to hypoxemia, impaired autoregulation, and neuroendocrine dysfunction (luteinizing hormone, cortisol, growth hormone, and prolactin alterations).
  - Several mechanisms are shared with migraine, including cranial autonomic activation in cluster headache that is believed to be centrally mediated through the same pathways that are activated during migraine. Changes in CGRP levels in cluster headaches are analogous to the changes seen in migraine, and it is believed the trigeminal system is activated in a way similar to migraine.
  - With "triggering" (hypoxemia, alcohol, histamine, vasodilators), unilateral extra and intracranial vasodilation occurs with increased intracerebral blood flow resulting in compression of the sympathetic plexus and release of serotonin and histamine.
  - Patients may exhibit nasal stuffiness, lacrimation, rhinorrhea, miosis, ptosis, sweating, and eyelid edema.

PATIENT PRESENTATION

- Criteria for diagnosis of each type and subtype of primary headache were established by the 2004 International Classification of Headache Disorders. Diagnostic criteria for selected types of primary headache are listed in Box 18-1. Common classic features are described as follows:
    - Migraine: Unilateral (can be bilateral in up to 40%), pulsating headache of severe intensity associated with nausea, photophobia, phonophobia, and aggravated by physical activity lasting 4 to 72 hours; some will be preceded (less than 1 hour before onset of headache) by one or more fully reversible aura symptoms indicating focal cerebral cortical or brainstem dysfunction (e.g., visual blurring or scotoma, paresthesias, focal weakness, or numbness); common in women in their 30s and 40s (e.g., often in association with menses); often a positive family history of migraine can be elicited.

BOX **18-1** International Classification of Headache Disorders, second edition (First Revision 2005)

1.1 MIGRAINE WITHOUT AURA

A. At least 5 attacks fulfilling criteria B to D
B. Headache attacks lasting 4 to 72 hours (untreated or unsuccessfully treated)
C. Headache has two or more of the following characteristics:
  1. Unilateral location
  2. Pulsating quality
  3. Moderate or severe pain intensity
  4. Aggravation by or causing avoidance of routine physical activity (e.g., walking, climbing stairs)
D. During headache one or more of the following:
  1. Nausea and/or vomiting
  2. Photophobia and phonophobia
E. Not attributed to another disorder

1.2.1 TYPICAL AURA WITH MIGRAINE HEADACHE

A. At least 2 attacks fulfilling criteria B to D
B. Aura consisting of one or more of the following, but no motor weakness:
  1. Fully reversible visual symptoms including positive and/or negative features
  2. Fully reversible sensory symptoms including positive and/or negative features
  3. Fully reversible dysphasic speech disturbance
C. At least two of the following:
  1. Homonymous visual symptoms and/or unilateral sensory symptoms
  2. At least one aura symptom develops gradually over more than 5 minutes and/or different aura symptoms occur in succession over more than 5 minutes
  3. Each symptom lasts more than 5 minutes and less than 60 minutes
D. Headache fulfilling criteria B to D for 1.1 *Migraine without aura* begins during the aura or follows aura within 60 minutes
E. Not attributed to another disorder

2.1 INFREQUENT EPISODIC TTH

A. At least 10 episodes occurring on fewer than 1 day per month or 12 days per year and fulfilling criteria B to D
B. Headache lasting from 30 minutes to 7 days
C. Headache has two or more of the following characteristics:
  1. Bilateral location
  2. Pressing/tightening (non-pulsating) quality
  3. Mild or moderate intensity
  4. Not aggravated by routine physical activity
D. Both of the following:
  1. No nausea or vomiting (anorexia may occur)
  2. No more than one of photophobia or phonophobia
E. Not attributed to another disorder

2.2 FREQUENT EPISODIC TTH

As 2.1 except:
A. At least 10 episodes occurring on more than 1 but fewer than 15 days per month for more than 3 months (more than 12 and less than 180 days per year) and fulfilling criteria B to D

3.1 CLUSTER HEADACHE

A. At least 5 attacks fulfilling criteria B to D
B. Severe or very severe unilateral orbital, supraorbital, and/or temporal pain lasting 15 minutes to 3 hours if untreated
C. Headache is accompanied by more than one of the following:
  1. Ipsilateral conjunctival injection and/or lacrimation
  2. Ipsilateral nasal congestion and/or rhinorrhea
  3. Ipsilateral eyelid edema
  4. Ipsilateral forehead and facial sweating
  5. Ipsilateral miosis and/or ptosis
  6. A sense of restlessness or agitation
D. Attacks have a frequency from half a day to eight per day
E. Not attributed to another disorder

Adapted from Headache Classification Subcommittee of the International Headache Society (2004). The international classification of headache disorders, ed 2, *Cephalalgia*, 24(suppl 1), 1-150.

- Tension-type headache: Episodic or chronic nonpulsating mild to moderate headache with or without pericranial and neck muscle pain and tenderness that is bilateral and is not aggravated by routine physical activity and not associated with nausea, photophobia, or phonophobia.
- Cluster headache: Episodic clustered attacks of excruciating unilateral periorbital headache with associated conjunctival injection, lacrimation, nasal congestion and rhinorrhea, facial sweating, miosis, and ptosis, occurring up to eight times a day lasting 15 to 180 minutes, and often awakening the patient from sleep; more common in men and may be triggered by alcohol, histamine, or vasodilators.

DIFFERENTIAL DIAGNOSIS

Primary headache must be differentiated from secondary headaches, which fall into eight categories:
- Head or neck trauma (e.g., posttraumatic headache after concussion).
- Vascular disorders (e.g., stroke, temporal arteritis, arteriovenous malformation, hypertension).
- Nonvascular intracranial disorders (e.g., tumor).
- Substance use or withdrawal (alcohol, MOH).
- Infection (e.g., meningitis, encephalitis).
- Bleeding (e.g., chronic subdural hematoma, subarachnoid hemorrhage) .
- Disorders of cranial, facial, or sensory organ structures (e.g., sinusitis, temporomandibular joint disorder, eyestrain, diplopia, glaucoma, otitis media, toothache).
- Psychiatric disorders (e.g., depression).

KEYS TO ASSESSMENT

History

- History should identify the pattern of symptoms that may help identify the cause.
  - Onset.
  - Frequency/duration.
  - Intensity.
  - Location.
  - Quality.
  - Precipitators and exacerbators.
  - Ameliorators.
  - Associated symptoms.
  - Neurologic accompaniments.
- Medical history about childhood and adult illnesses, injuries, immunizations, medications, and allergies.
  - Family history.
  - Life-style and social history.
  - Systems review.

Examination

- General appearance and activity (e.g., migraine patients usually lie still, cluster patients are often restless).
- Look for fever and hypertension.
- Do a careful physical examination for signs of infection, neoplasm, or vascular disease.
- Perform a head examination for scalp or facial tenderness and vascular bruits.
- Check the eyes, ears, and temporomandibular joints.
- Check the neck for mobility and tenderness.
- Perform a careful neurologic examination for focal neurologic findings.

Diagnostics

- If the patient has a normal examination and history is consistent with primary headache, no more studies may be indicated.
- Further studies would be indicated based on any specific findings on the physical examination.
- Magnetic resonance imaging (MRI) or computed tomography (CT) is indicated for focal neurologic signs, altered consciousness, nuchal rigidity, severe headache or first headache in a person older than age 50, worsening headache while under observation, or inconsistent pattern.
- If meningitis or subarachnoid hemorrhage is suspected, lumbar puncture (LP) is indicated.
- Other suspected causes of secondary headache should be evaluated as appropriate (e.g., routine blood tests, C-reactive protein).
- *Acute diagnosis* (taken from Cortelli et al in a consensus statement in *Headache*, 2004):
  - Severe headache with acute onset (thunderclap), neurologic signs, vomiting, or syncope → (1) Immediate head CT or MRI. (2) If CT or MRI negative, do LP. (3) If LP negative, a neurologist should be consulted within 24 hours.
  - Severe headache with fever and/or stiff neck → (1) If no evidence of focal neurologic signs or increased intracranial pressure, then do immediate LP. (2) If evidence is present, perform CT prior to LP.
  - Headache of recent onset (days or weeks), progressively worsening headache, or persistent headache (weeks or months) → (1) CT and routine blood tests including C-reactive protein. (2) If negative a neurologist should be consulted within 7 days.
  - Headache similar to previous headaches in terms of intensity, duration, and associated symptoms → No further studies needed acutely beyond physical examination.

KEYS TO MANAGEMENT

- Migraine.
  - Avoid precipitating factors.
    1. Modify diet (e.g., decrease caffeine, highly seasoned foods, and chocolate).
    2. Maintain a regular sleeping schedule.
    3. Avoid alcohol.
    4. Maximize stress coping mechanisms.
    5. Avoid oral contraceptives.
    6. Avoid medication overuse.
- Acute migraine headache.
  - Triptans (sumatriptan, zolmitriptan, naratriptan, rizatriptan, fovatriptan, eletriptan, almotriptan) are serotonin agonists that provide effective and rapid relief (>80% respond) and are well tolerated. Contraindications include coronary artery disease, Prinzmetal angina, uncontrolled hypertension, liver disease, or neurologic deficits with the headache.
  - Dihydroergotamine (DHE) intravenous (IV) or intramuscular (IM) injection gives rapid and effective relief (up to 90% respond) but may require repeated injections. Indicated if patient does not respond to sumatriptan; but may cause coronary spasm (less so than ergotamine).
  - Ergotamine (usually in combination with caffeine) effectiveness is lower, with less than 50% of individuals responding; also carries a significant risk for coronary spasm.
  - Opioids are effective but should be used no more than twice a week in patients with refractory migraine due to the risks of opioid dependence.
  - Nonsteroidal anti-inflammatory drugs (NSAIDs) (ibuprofen, ketorolac, etc.) may be adequate for mild to moderate headache.
  - Dexamethasone is sometimes given for very severe headache.
  - Others: Intranasal lidocaine; intravenous chlorpromazine or prochlorperazine; narcotics.
  - Future: CGRP inhibitors, substance P antagonists, and nitric oxide synthetase inhibitors.
- Migraine prophylaxis is indicated when attack frequency is between two and eight per month and are severe enough to impair normal life, or when patient is intolerant to abortive therapies due to side effects.

- β-blockers (propranolol, metoprolol, atenolol, nadolol, and timolol) are the first choice, with 10% to 15% of patients having side effects.
- Amitriptyline and nortriptyline are useful in patients with both migraine and tension-type headaches, but have significant side effects.
- Calcium antagonists (verapamil, flunarizine) may be helpful in selected patients.
- Valproate, gabapentin, topiramate, and divalproex sodium are effective, but have frequent side effects.
- NSAIDs are useful in some patients who do not tolerate β-blockers.
- Methysergide should be used only for severe refractory cases due to high risk of serious side effects such as abdominal pain, nausea, and retroperitoneal fibrosis.
- Botulinum toxin A has been demonstrated to be effective in several clinical trials; more studies are pending.
- The herb feverfew is used by many patients, but has not been shown to be effective in a large meta-analysis. Other complementary therapies are being evaluated.
- Tension-type headache.
  - Episodic headaches can usually be managed with over-the-counter (OTC) drugs such as aspirin, acetaminophen, or nonsteroidal anti-inflammatory agents in combination with caffeine. MOH is a concern with frequent or chronic TTH.
  - Chronic headache should be treated with antidepressants—tricyclic antidepressants have the longest track record. Selective serotonin reuptake inhibitors (SSRIs) are used effectively in many patients.
  - Physical therapy including proper attention to posture (especially at work) and daily exercises to loosen up the neck and shoulder muscles can be very helpful.
  - Stress management and relaxation therapy can also be effective, sometimes in combination with biofeedback or percutaneous electrical nerve stimulation (PENS).
  - Obtain a referral for a psychologic evaluation if indicated.
- Cluster headache.
  - Avoidance of triggers.
    1. Avoid alcohol, histamine, and vasodilators.
    2. Avoid prolonged contact with solvents, gasoline, and oil-based paints.
    3. Prophylaxis prior to airplane or high-altitude travel (see following).
  - Acute cluster headache.
    1. Oxygen inhalation (aborts 90% of attacks) should be started immediately at 7 L/minute for 15 minutes.
    2. Parenteral or intranasal sumatriptan.
    3. Intranasal lidocaine, dihydroergotamine, and capsaicin are also used with some success.
  - Cluster headache prophylaxis.
    1. Verapamil daily (70% respond).
    2. Lithium.
    3. Prednisone.
    4. Anticonvulsant (divalproex, topiramate).
    5. Ergotamine daily.
    6. Methylergonovine and melatonin can be tried.
    7. Microvascular decompression of the fifth cranial nerve can be helpful in refractory cases.

PATHOPHYSIOLOGY ⟶	CLINICAL LINK
What is going on in the disease process that influences how the patient presents and how he or she should be managed?	*What should you do now that you understand the underlying pathophysiology?*
Genes implicated in migraine pathogenesis affect neurotransmitter and electrolyte function in neurons. ⟶	Management of migraine is now focused on medications that affect neurotransmitter function and neuronal transmission.
Migraines are associated with vasoconstriction followed by vasodilation and inflammation with activation of the trigeminal ganglion and disturbances in neurotransmitters, especially serotonin. ⟶	Many migraines are preceded by an aura of neurologic symptoms such as scotoma or paresthesias, followed by severe pulsating headache; serotonin agonists and vasoconstrictor medications can be used to abort an attack, and anti-inflammatories help some patients.
Estrogen withdrawal just prior to menses is associated with changes in neurotransmitters in the central nervous system (CNS), especially serotonin. ⟶	Migraines are often associated with the menstrual cycle or the use of exogenous hormones.
Tension-type headaches are sometimes associated with pericranial muscle spasms, but most are not and there appears to be a central mechanism that may also be related to serotonin. ⟶	Some tension-type headaches are associated with poor posture and stress-related muscle tension and will respond to physical therapy and relaxation techniques; other patients have features of both tension-type and migraine and may respond to antidepressants and/or serotonin agonists.
Cluster headaches are associated with hypothalamic dysfunction, cerebral hypoxemia, and neuroendocrine dysfunction with release of histamine; intracranial vasodilation may compress the sympathetic plexus. ⟶	Seasonal "clusters" of headaches are related to changes in photoperiod; headaches are associated with nasal stuffiness and lacrimation as well as miosis and ptosis.
There are many structures in the head that can cause cranial pain such as sinuses, eyes, ears, mouth, etc., but most are associated with positive findings on physical examination. ⟶	The differential diagnosis of headache is extensive, but a primary headache is common, and patients with a normal examination do not require extensive diagnostic testing.

SUGGESTED READINGS

Aguggia, M. (2004). Neurophysiological tests in primary headaches. *Neurological Sciences, 25*(suppl 3), S203-S205.

Ashina, M. (2004). Neurobiology of chronic tension-type headache. *Cephalalgia, 24,* 161-172.

Balbisi, E. A. (2004). Frovatriptan succinate, a 5-HT1B/1D receptor agonist for migraine. *International Journal of Clinical Practice, 58,* 695-705.

Beck, E., Sieber, W. J., & Trejo, R. (2005). Management of cluster headache [see comment]. *American Family Physician, 71,* 717-724.

Bigal, M. E., Lipton, R. B., & Krymchantowski, A. V. (2004). The medical management of migraine. *American Journal of Therapeutics, 11,* 130-140.

Blumenfeld, A. M., Dodick, D. W., & Silberstein, S. D. (2004). Botulinum neurotoxin for the treatment of migraine and other primary headache disorders. *Dermatologic Clinics, 22,* 167-175.

Bogduk, N. (2004). The neck and headaches. *Neurologic Clinics, 22,* 151-171.

Chronicle, E. & Mulleners, W. (2004). Anticonvulsant drugs for migraine prophylaxis. *Cochrane Database of Systematic Reviews,* CD003226.

Colman, I., Brown, M. D., Innes, G. D., Grafstein, E., Roberts, T. E., & Rowe, B. H. (2005). Parenteral dihydroergotamine for acute migraine headache: a systematic review of the literature. *Annals of Emergency Medicine, 45,* 393-401.

Colombo, B., Annovazzi, P. O., & Comi, G. (2004). Therapy of primary headaches: the role of antidepressants. *Neurological Sciences, 25*(suppl 3), S171-S175.

Cortelli, P., Cevoli, S., Nonino, F., Baronciani, D., Magrini, N., Re, G., De Berti, G., Manzoni, G. C., Querzani, P., Vandelli, A., & Multidisciplinary Group for Nontraumatic Headache in the Emergency Department. (2004). Evidence-based diagnosis of nontraumatic headache in the emergency department: a consensus statement on four clinical scenarios. *Headache, 44,* 587-595.

Cutrer, F. M. & Boes, C. J. (2004). Cough, exertional, and sex headaches. *Neurologic Clinics, 22,* 133-149.

D'Andrea, G., Perini, F., Terrazzino, S., & Nordera, G. P. (2004). Contributions of biochemistry to the pathogenesis of primary headaches. *Neurological Sciences, 25*(suppl 3), S89-S92.

Davenport, R. (2004). Diagnosing acute headache. *Clinical Medicine, 4,* 108-112.

Diamond, M. & Cady, R. (2005). Initiating and optimizing acute therapy for migraine: the role of patient-centered stratified care. *American Journal of Medicine, 118*(suppl 1), 18S-27S.

Diener, H. C. (2004). Advances in the field of headache 2003/2004. *Current Opinion in Neurology, 17,* 271-273.

Diener, H. C. (2004). Important advances in headache. *Lancet Neurology, 3,* 12.

Diener, H. C. & Limmroth, V. (2004). Medication-overuse headache: a worldwide problem. *Lancet Neurology, 3,* 475-483.

Dodick, D., Lipton, R. B., Martin, V., Papademetriou, V., Rosamond, W., MaassenVanDenBrink, A., Loutfi, H., Welch, K. M., Goadsby, P. J., Hahn, S., Hutchinson, S., Matchar, D., Silberstein, S., Smith, T. R., Purdy, R. A., Saiers, J., & Triptan Cardiovascular Safety Expert Panel. (2004). Consensus statement: cardiovascular safety profile of triptans (5-HT agonists) in the acute treatment of migraine. *Headache, 44,* 414-425.

Dowson, A. J., Bradford, S., Lipscombe, S., Rees, T., Sender, J., Watson, D., & Wells, C. (2004). Managing chronic headaches in the clinic. *International Journal of Clinical Practice, 58,* 1142-1151.

Durham, P. L. (2004). CGRP receptor antagonists: a new choice for acute treatment of migraine? *Current Opinion in Investigational Drugs, 5,* 731-735.

Edvinsson, L. (2004). Blockade of CGRP receptors in the intracranial vasculature: a new target in the treatment of headache. *Cephalalgia, 24,* 611-622.

Estevez, M., & Gardner, K. L. (2004). Update on the genetics of migraine. *Human Genetics, 114,* 225-235.

Etminan, M., Takkouche, B., Isorna, F. C., & Samii, A. (2005). Risk of ischaemic stroke in people with migraine: systematic review and meta-analysis of observational studies. *British Medical Journal, 330,* 63.

Evans, R. W. (2004). Post-traumatic headaches. *Neurologic Clinics, 22,* 237-249.

Frediani, F. (2004). Anticonvulsant drugs in primary headaches prophylaxis. *Neurological Sciences, 25*(suppl 3), S161-S166.

Freitag, F. G. (2004). Cluster headache. *Primary Care; Clinics in Office Practice, 31,* 313-329.

Gladstone, J. P. & Dodick, D. W. (2004). Revised 2004 International Classification of Headache Disorders: new headache types. *Canadian Journal of Neurological Sciences, 31,* 304-314.

Goadsby, P. J. (2004). The future of headache. *Journal of Neurology, 251,* 630-636.

Gobel, H. (2004). Botulinum toxin in migraine prophylaxis. *Journal of Neurology, 251*(suppl 1), I8-11.

Headache Classification Subcommittee of the International Headache Society (2004). The international classification of headache disorders; ed 2, *Cephalalgia, 24*(suppl 1), 1-150.

Hutchinson, S. (2004). Chronic daily headache. *Primary Care; Clinics in Office Practice, 31,* 353-367.

Kors, E. E., Vanmolkot, K. R., Haan, J., Frants, R. R., van den Maagdenberg, A. M., & Ferrari, M. D. (2004). Recent findings in headache genetics. *Current Opinion in Neurology, 17,* 283-288.

Krusz, J. C. (2004). Tension-type headaches: what they are and how to treat them. *Primary Care; Clinics in Office Practice, 31,* 293-311.

Lainez, M. (2004). Clinical benefits of early triptan therapy for migraine. *Cephalalgia, 24*(suppl 2), 24-30.

Landy, S. (2004). Migraine throughout the life cycle: treatment through the ages. *Neurology, 62,* S2-S8.

Landy, S. H. (2004). Challenging or difficult headache patients. *Primary Care; Clinics in Office Practice, 31,* 429-440.

Lawrence, E. C. (2004). Diagnosis and management of migraine headaches. *Southern Medical Journal, 97,* 1069-1077.

Lenaerts, M. E. (2004). Alternative therapies for tension-type headache. *Current Pain & Headache Reports, 8,* 484-488.

Lenssinck, M. L., Damen, L., Verhagen, A. P., Berger, M. Y., Passchier, J., & Koes, B. W. (2004). The effectiveness of physiotherapy and manipulation in patients with tension-type headache: a systematic review. *Pain, 112,* 381-388.

Linde, K. & Rossnagel, K. (2004). Propranolol for migraine prophylaxis. *Cochrane Database of Systematic Reviews,* CD003225.

Lipton, R. B. & Bigal, M. E. (2005). The epidemiology of migraine. *American Journal of Medicine, 118*(suppl 1), 3S-10S.

Lipton, R. B., Bigal, M. E., & Goadsby, P. J. (2004). Double-blind clinical trials of oral triptans vs other classes of acute migraine medication—a review. *Cephalalgia, 24,* 321-332.

Lipton, R. B., Bigal, M. E., Steiner, T. J., Silberstein, S. D., & Olesen, J. (2004). Classification of primary headaches. *Neurology, 63,* 427-435.

Lipton, R. B. & Dodick, D. W. (2004). CGRP antagonists in the acute treatment of migraine. *Lancet Neurology, 3,* 332.

Maizels, M. (2004). The patient with daily headaches. *American Family Physician, 70,* 2299-2306.

Manzoni, G. C. & Torelli, P. (2004). Headache screening and diagnosis. *Neurological Sciences, 25* Suppl 3, S255-S257.

Martin, V. T. & Goldstein, J. A. (2005). Evaluating the safety and tolerability profile of acute treatments for migraine. *American Journal of Medicine,* 118(suppl 1), 36S-44S.

Mathew, N. T. & Loder, E. W. (2005). Evaluating the triptans. *American Journal of Medicine,* 118 Suppl 1, 28S-35S.

Montagna, P. (2004). The physiopathology of migraine: the contribution of genetics. *Neurological Sciences,* 25(suppl 3), S93-S96.

Morillo, L. E. (2004). Migraine headache. *Clinical Evidence,* 1696-1719.

Moskowitz, M. A., Bolay, H., & Dalkara, T. (2004). Deciphering migraine mechanisms: clues from familial hemiplegic migraine genotypes. *Annals of Neurology,* 55, 276-280.

Narbone, M. C., Abbate, M., & Gangemi, S. (2004). Acute drug treatment of migraine attack. *Neurological Sciences,* 25(suppl 3), S113-S118.

Papademetriou, V. (2004). Cardiovascular risk assessment and triptans. *Headache,* 44(suppl 1), S31-S39.

Parsons, A. A. (2004). Cortical spreading depression: its role in migraine pathogenesis and possible therapeutic intervention strategies. *Current Pain & Headache Reports,* 8, 410-416.

Peters, K. S. (2004). Secondary headache and head pain emergencies. *Primary Care; Clinics in Office Practice,* 31, 381-393.

Pittler, M. H. & Ernst, E. (2004). Feverfew for preventing migraine. *Cochrane Database of Systematic Reviews,* CD002286.

Pryse-Phillips, W. (2005). Assessment and management of disability in chronic daily headache. *Current Pain & Headache Reports,* 9, 53-58.

Rapoport, A. M. & Bigal, M. E. (2004). Preventive migraine therapy: what is new. *Neurological Sciences,* 25(suppl 3), S177-S185.

Rapoport, A. M., Bigal, M. E., Tepper, S. J., & Sheftell, F. D. (2004). Intranasal medications for the treatment of migraine and cluster headache. *CNS Drugs,* 18, 671-685.

Recober, A. & Geweke, L. O. (2005). Menstrual migraine. *Current Neurology & Neuroscience Reports,* 5, 93-98.

Rothrock, J. F. (2000). Headaches due to vascular disorders. *Neurologic Clinics,* 22, 21-37.

Rozen, T. D. (2005). Cluster headache: diagnosis and treatment. *Current Neurology & Neuroscience Reports,* 5, 99-104.

Russell, M. B. (2004). Epidemiology and genetics of cluster headache. *Lancet Neurology,* 3, 279-283.

Ryan, R. E., Jr. & Pearlman, S. H. (2004). Common headache misdiagnoses. *Primary Care; Clinics in Office Practice,* 31, 395-405.

Sadovsky, R., & Dodick, D. W. (2005). Identifying migraine in primary care settings. *American Journal of Medicine,* 118(suppl 1), 11S-17S.

Sanchez-del-Rio, M. & Reuter, U. (2004). Migraine aura: new information on underlying mechanisms. *Current Opinion in Neurology,* 17, 289-293.

Schim, J. (2004). Effect of preventive treatment with botulinum toxin type A on acute headache medication usage in migraine patients. *Current Medical Research & Opinion,* 20, 49-53.

Schoenen, J. & Sandor, P. S. (2004). Headache with focal neurological signs or symptoms: a complicated differential diagnosis. *Lancet Neurology,* 3, 237-245.

Schreiber, C. P. (2004). The pathophysiology of primary headache. *Primary Care; Clinics in Office Practice,* 31, 261-276.

Silberstein, S. D. (2000). Headaches due to nasal and paranasal sinus disease. *Neurologic Clinics,* 22, 1-19.

Silberstein, S. D. (2004). Headaches in pregnancy. *Neurologic Clinics,* 22, 727-756.

Silberstein, S. D. (2004). Migraine pathophysiology and its clinical implications. *Cephalalgia,* 24(suppl 2), 2-7.

Smith, T. R. (2004). Epidemiology and impact of headache: an overview. *Primary Care; Clinics in Office Practice,* 31, 237-241.

Steinberg, J. (2005). Anticonvulsant medications for migraine prevention. *American Family Physician,* 71, 1699-1700.

Taylor, F. R. (2005). Migraine headache: options for acute treatment. *Current Neurology & Neuroscience Reports,* 5, 86-92.

Tepper, S. J. (2004). New thoughts on sinus headache. *Allergy & Asthma Proceedings,* 25, 95-96.

Tsushima, Y. & Endo, K. (2005). MR imaging in the evaluation of chronic or recurrent headache. *Radiology,* 235, 575-579.

Ward, T. N. (2004). Medication overuse headache. *Primary Care; Clinics in Office Practice,* 31, 369-380.

Wessman, M., Kaunisto, M. A., Kallela, M., & Palotie, A. (2004). The molecular genetics of migraine. *Annals of Medicine,* 36, 462-473.

Young, W. B. (2004). Drug-induced headache. *Neurologic Clinics,* 22, 173-184.

Headache

INITIAL HISTORY

- 24-year-old female presents with a severe headache.
- Symptoms began last night with 10/10 pain.
- Symptoms partially relieved by sister's pain medication, pain 5/10 today.
- Associated with nausea.
- Notes that frequency of headaches has increased in past year.

Question 1. *What is the differential diagnosis based on this history alone?*

Question 2. *What further questions would you like to ask her to complete her review of symptoms?*

ADDITIONAL HISTORY

- Pain localized to right forehead area.
- Pain is pulsing, throbbing.
- Onset was early evening, partially relieved by pain medication and sleep.
- Feels she needs to lie down in a dark room to feel comfortable.
- No cold symptoms, no fever or chills.
- No visual changes, no numbness tingling in extremities.
- No neck stiffness.
- Two headaches in the past week, probably has had 10 to 15 in the past month. Generally headaches begin in the early evening. Notices she is drowsy and hungry before the headache begins.

Question 3. *What other questions would you like to ask about her medical, family, and social history?*

MORE HISTORY

- Patient denies recent head trauma.
- Drinks occasional glass of wine.
- Drinks 3 or 4 cups of coffee and 3 or 4 diet colas per day.
- Smokes 1 pack per day for 10 years.
- No unusual stress in life.
- Last menstrual period 2 weeks ago, uses OCPs.
- Has been dieting in the past month.
- Mother and sister both have "migraine headaches."

PHYSICAL EXAMINATION

- Alert, well-developed, well-nourished female in moderate distress.
- T = 37.2° C orally; BP = 134/82; P = 80 and regular; RR = 16 and unlabored.
- Skin is warm and dry; no rashes.

HEENT

- No scalp tenderness.
- Face nontender; no pain with percussion of the sinus cavities.
- Tympanic membranes not inflamed; no bulging or retraction.
- Extraocular movements full; visual acuity sharp (20/20 OU with corrective lenses).
- PERRL; + photosensitivity bilaterally; conjunctiva clear; funduscopic demonstrates sharp disks and no hemorrhages.
- Nasal mucosa pink; no drainage.
- Throat not inflamed and without postnasal drainage.

Neck

- Supple with full range of motion.
- No palpable lymphadenopathy in the anterior or posterior chains.
- No bruits heard.

Lungs, Cardiovascular
- Lungs clear to auscultation and percussion.
- Cardiac with RRR without murmurs or gallops.

Abdomen, Extremities
- Abdomen without tenderness or masses.
- Extremities with good pulses, no edema.

Neurologic
- Oriented ×3, memory recent and remote clear.
- No focal motor or sensory deficits.
- Cranial nerves intact.
- Deep tendon reflexes +2 in all groups.
- Negative Kernig and Brudzinski signs.
- Negative Romberg.

Question 4.   *What are the pertinent positive and negative findings on examination?*

Question 5.   *What diagnostic studies are indicated at this time?*

Question 6.   *What is your diagnosis?*

Question 7.   *What should your treatment plan encompass?*

Question 8.   *What further care would you recommend?*

Stroke

DEFINITION

- A stroke (cerebrovascular accident [CVA]) is defined as a focal neurologic disorder developing suddenly because of a pathophysiologic process in cerebral blood vessels. Stroke can be categorized into three major types:
  - Acute brain infarction (ABI).
  - Intracerebral hemorrhage (ICH).
  - Subarachnoid hemorrhage (SAH).

EPIDEMIOLOGY

- In the United States, every 45 seconds someone suffers a stroke such that there are approximately 700,000 strokes per year. Stroke is the third leading cause of death, resulting in 162,000 deaths annually. More women have strokes than men, and blacks have twice the risk compared with whites.
- Stroke is the leading cause of long-term disability in the United States with more than 1 million Americans living with serious functional limitations. According to the National Institutes of Health, of individuals with stroke older than the age of 65, approximately 50% will have persistent hemiparesis, 30% cannot walk without assistance, 19% have aphasia, 35% have depressive symptoms, and 26% require institutional care.
- ABI.
  - 88% of all strokes; 8% to 12% mortality at 1 month, 10% will have a second stroke within one year.
  - Strong association with coronary artery disease; both share many risk factors.
    1. Hypertension (especially systolic) is the most important modifiable risk factor. Individuals with a blood pressure of 120/80 mm Hg have half the risk of stroke than those with hypertension.
    2. Smoking increases risk by two- to threefold. Cessation of smoking returns risk to that of the nonsmoking population after 5 years.
    3. Other factors include age older than 67, diabetes, hyperlipidemia, hyperhomocystinemia, elevated C-reactive protein, male gender or a female after menopause, family history, black race, and recent myocardial infarction.
  - Atrial fibrillation increases the risk of cardioembolic stroke fivefold.
  - Risks related to hypercoagulability include polycythemia, sickle cell disease, oral contraceptives, hormone replacement therapy, pregnancy, inherited thrombotic disorders, migraine.
  - A transient ischemic attack (TIA) is defined as an ischemic focal neurologic deficit lasting less than 24 hours, 5.3% of affected individuals will have an ABI within 2 days and 10.5% within 90 days.

- ICH.
  - 9% of all strokes—mortality is high (37% to 38% at 1 month), especially if there is severe coma upon presentation.
  - Risk factors include hypertension, alcohol abuse, coagulopathies, cocaine or amphetamine abuse, blood dyscrasia, and iatrogenic anticoagulation.
- SAH.
  - 3% of all strokes; 10% die immediately, overall accounts for 25% of stroke deaths.
  - Incidence is higher in young adults and in women.
  - Risk factors include congenital saccular aneurysms, migraine, hypertension, smoking, polycystic kidney, Marfan syndrome, fibromuscular dysplasia, and sickle cell disease.

PATHOPHYSIOLOGY

Genetics

- Multifactorial genetics influence ABI risk including those that are associated with:
  - Genes that contribute to atherosclerosis risk factors (e.g., cholesterol, hypertension, diabetes) and thrombotic disorders (e.g., sickle cell disease, factor V Leiden mutation).
  - Genes that contribute to carotid intimal medial wall thickness such as matrix metalloproteinases (MMP3), inflammation (IL-6), and lipid metabolism (APOE).
  - One gene mapped to chromosome 5 that has been called "the stroke gene" *(STRK1)* and appears to increase the risk of ABI independent of the above-described disorders.
  - The phosphodiesterase 4 D gene and the lipoxygenase gene *ALOX5AP,* but further studies are needed.
- ICH risk is associated with genes that increase the likelihood of hypertension and bleeding. There are also an estimated 50 or more rare monogenic conditions that are associated with ICH including those that cause autosomal dominant amyloid angiopathies (APP, CST3, BRI), cerebral autosomal dominant arteriopathy (NOTCH3), and cavernous hemangiomas (KRIT1).
- SAH risk is associated with polymorphisms of collagen genes *(COL3A1, COL1A2),* polycystic kidney genes *(ADPKD, PKD1, PKD2),* lipoxygenase genes, fibrillin genes *(FBN2),* and α_1-antitrypsin genes.

Cerebral Circulation

- In the normal brain, cerebral blood flow (CBF) is maintained at a relatively constant rate despite changes in cerebral perfusion pressure (mean arterial pressure [MAP] minus intracranial pressure [ICP]). This is accomplished due to the regulation of cerebrovascular resistance (CVR) in a process called **autoregulation**. This relationship can be described by the following formula: CBF = MAP – ICP/CVR. In the injured brain, autoregulation is lost such that small changes in MAP or ICP will affect cerebral blood flow.
- There are many collaterals for cerebral perfusion (circle of Willis) so that the obstruction of a vessel may not lead to infarction of distal tissue, and deficits can be unpredictable.

Tissue Effects

- *Transient ischemic attack (TIA)* describes a sudden loss of neurologic function that resolves within 24 hours (most resolve within 5 minutes).
  - Usually due to atheroemboli from extracranial arteries or cardioemboli.
  - Thrombotic occlusion lyses before infarction can occur.
- ABI.
  - There are four main classifications:
    1. Atherothrombotic occlusion of extracranial (especially at the carotid bifurcation—cause of approximately 30% to 70% of ABI) or intracranial arteries.
    2. Cardioembolic due to atrial fibrillation, recent myocardial infarction with ventricular aneurysm, congestive heart failure, or valvular disease.
    3. Lacunar due to deep cerebral infarcts of the lenticulostriate arteries.
    4. Hemodynamic due to decreased global cerebral perfusion.
  - The neural cellular response to ischemia includes inflammation, release of excitotoxins, cell membrane injury, and both acute and delayed cell death (Figure 19-1).

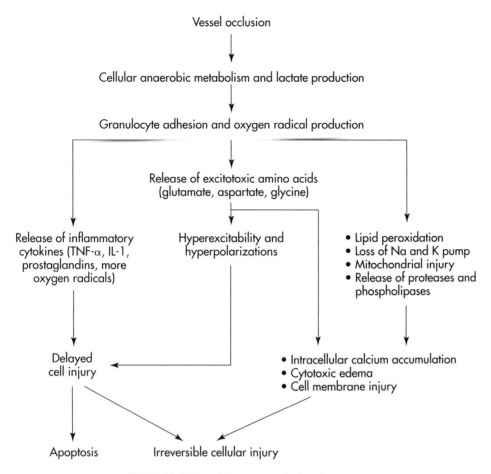

FIGURE **19-1 Neural Response to Ischemia.**

- Patterns of ischemic neuronal injury, sparing and healing.
    1. An area of dense infarction and necrosis forms at the center of ischemic brain tissue.
    2. Spontaneous or therapeutic reperfusion results in the limitation of infarct size, but also contributes to oxygen radical production (reperfusion injury).
    3. Selective neuronal necrosis: Some neurons and glial cells survive, especially if reperfused with 12 hours; sparing may be maximized by rapid reperfusion and neuroprotective therapy.
- Penumbra: Tissue at the periphery of the ischemic zone.
    1. If cerebral blood flow (CBF) falls to approximately 20 mL/100 g/min, neurons remain viable but there is no synaptic function. They may be salvageable if perfusion is restored 90 minutes to several hours after initial event.
    2. Ischemic tissue contains high extracellular potassium causing multiple repetitive depolarizations, leading to ATP depletion and delayed cell death; new therapies are aimed at blocking peri-infarct depolarizations.
- Delayed neuronal death.
    1. Inflammation, excitotoxin release, granulocyte adhesion, oxygen radical production, and cytokine release cause not only acute neuronal damage but also delayed effects, with T lymphocytes and macrophages infiltrating up to 2 weeks after the initial insult.
    2. Cytokines (TNF-α, TGF-β) also induce the activation of cellular endonucleases that cleave neuronal deoxyribonucleic acid (DNA) (apoptosis); this may continue for 2 weeks after infarct.

- Healing and functional recovery.
    1. The brain surrounding the infarct is hypermetabolic; it underscores the need for maximal oxygen and nutrient delivery during the peri-infarction time period.
    2. Polypeptide growth factors (neurotrophins, fibroblast growth factors) result in dendritic sprouting and new axonal growth, and they are protective against delayed neuronal injury. Trials with basic fibroblast growth factor (bFGF) are encouraging.
- Systemic responses to cerebral ischemia.
    1. Arrhythmias (tachy- or bradyarrhythmias), ST-T wave changes, increased creatinine phosphokinase MB (CPK-MB), increased brain natriuretic peptide (BNP), and even myocardial wall motion abnormalities may be seen and are believed to be due to a burst of systemic catecholamines that occurs during cerebral ischemia and infarction.
    2. Neurogenic pulmonary edema (acute respiratory distress syndrome [ARDS]).
    3. Peptic ulcer disease (Cushing ulcer).
    4. Endocrine abnormalities (syndrome of inappropriate antidiuretic hormone [SIADH]).
- ICH.
    - Rupture of artery or arteriole with hematoma formation under arterial pressure.
    - Primary ICH.
        1. Approximately 60% to 75% of ICH results from chronic damage to small perforating vessels of the cerebral arteries due to hypertension. Pathologic vascular changes include atherosclerosis, vasoconstriction, and fragility of the vessel wall.
        2. Cerebral amyloid angiopathy with weakening of vessel walls is a common cause in patients older than age 65 and is associated with pathologic brain changes and dementia similar to Alzheimer disease.
    - Secondary ICH.
        1. Vascular malformations and angiomas cause hemorrhage in children and young adults.
        2. Hemorrhage into intracerebral tumors is an uncommon but important cause of ICH.
        3. Anticoagulant or fibrinolytic use accounts for 10% of all ICH.
    - Mechanisms of brain injury in ICH.
        1. Direct trauma to neurons by ejection of blood into brain tissue.
        2. Mass effect of hematoma and cerebral edema with mechanical compression of surrounding tissues.
            a. Hematoma is surrounded by an ischemic penumbra; ischemic changes of intracellular calcium accumulation, excitotoxic amino acid release, and hyperpolarization will lead to acute and delayed cell death.
            b. Mass effect increases ICP which decreases CBF, and may result in shift of the brain and herniation across the midline or through the foramina.
            c. Expansion of the hematoma occurs in 14% to 26%, usually within 6 hours, with a poor prognosis.
            d. Extravasation of blood into surrounding brain tissue causes vasospasm and worsening ischemia (and causes pain from increased ICP).
- SAH.
    - Rupture of congenital saccular (berry) aneurysms—most common at the junction of the anterior cerebral and anterior communicating arteries; 12% to 31% have multiple aneurysms. Acute presentation may be preceded by one or more promontory bleeds.
    - Mechanism of brain injury in SAH.
        1. Extravasation of blood (oxyhemoglobin) over the brain surface and ventricles.
        2. Results in inflammation, release of excitotoxic amino acids, and toxic oxygen radicals.

 3. Causes cerebrospinal fluid outflow obstruction and hydrocephalus—
   increases ICP.
 4. Delayed vasospasm:
    a. Results from inflammation and decreased nitric oxide.
    b. Occurs in 70% of cases; symptomatic in 36%.
    c. Occurs 3 to 21 days after the initial bleed (peak = days 4 to 12).
    d. Increases overall mortality by threefold and can result in significant
       ischemic neuronal damage.
 5. Rebleeding is common (4% per day acutely, 1% to 2% within the
    first month).
- Hyponatremia.
 1. Common (10% to 34%); linked to a higher rate of secondary cerebral
    infarctions.
 2. May be due to the syndrome of inappropriate antidiuretic hormone
    (SIADH) or cerebral salt-wasting syndrome (mediated by atrial natriuretic
    factor [ANF]).

PATIENT PRESENTATION

- Patient presentation varies widely. Generally, ABI tends to be painless with less change in
  level of consciousness than ICH or SAH. ICH and SAH are characterized by severe headache
  in most cases. However, only 20% to 50% of patients with SAH have the classic "thunderclap
  headache," and only a little more than half have any prodromal headaches at all.

History
Risk factors: history of drug abuse; recent cardiac event; palpitations; recent change in
medications; previous transient painless loss of focal neurologic function (TIA); previous
syncope or seizures; recurrent headaches.

Symptoms
Abrupt painless loss of neurologic function (ABI) or severe headache (ICH) or "thunderclap
headache" (SAH); decreased level of consciousness; focal weakness or numbness; difficulty
speaking; visual changes; difficulty controlling gait; intention tremor; seizures; nausea and
vomiting; nucchal rigidity; photophobia.

Examination
Several studies have determined that three findings are most predictive of stroke: facial
paralysis, arm drift, and abnormal speech.
   Decreased level of consciousness; fever; pupillary asymmetry and decreased reactiveness;
papilledema; cranial nerve palsies, facial droop, meningismus; aphasia or dysarthria; focal
motor or sensory deficit; flaccid or spastic muscle tone; asymmetric deep tendon reflexes;
Babinski reflex; ataxia; other specialized neurologic test abnormalities; ventilatory abnormalities
(e.g., Cheyne-Stokes respirations); tachycardia; premature beats or arrhythmias; carotid bruits;
decreased peripheral pulses or peripheral bruits; evidence of hematologic disease or
coagulopathy (petechiae, ecchymoses).

DIFFERENTIAL DIAGNOSIS

- Primary cardiac event with acute hypotension.
- Primary seizure disorder (especially with Todd paralysis).
- Brain tumor.
- Metabolic or toxic insult (hypoglycemia, drugs).
- Meningitis.
- Trauma (intracranial bleeding [epidural, subdural], concussion).
- Migraine.

KEYS TO ASSESSMENT

- Monitor vital signs and obtain arterial blood gases.
- Careful neurologic examination is imperative. The National Institutes of Health Stroke Scale (NIHSS) uses level of consciousness, gaze, visual fields, facial palsy, arm motor, leg motor, ataxia, sensory, language, dysarthria, and extinction/inattention to assess the amount of neurologic deficit and to provide a baseline examination for continued monitoring.
- Repetitive examinations: Monitor for stroke in evolution with worsening deficits.
- Electrocardiogram (ECG) and cardiovascular assessment; continuous blood pressure monitoring.
- Serum laboratory studies: Arterial blood gases, glucose, electrolytes, coagulation studies, complete blood count (CBC), toxicology screen.
- Computed tomography (CT) scan or magnetic resonance imaging (MRI). CT scan is faster and has 98% sensitivity for ICH and SAH, however CT is less sensitive for acute ABI, and high-speed diffusion-weighted MRI is better for identification of infarction acutely.
- Consider lumbar puncture for suspected SAH: Expect xanthochromia (yellow tinge) and red blood cells; some centers measure CSF bilirubin.
- Vascular studies.
    - Angiography or MRI or CT angiography is indicated urgently in SAH.
    - Noninvasive vascular studies to evaluate cerebral and carotid circulations include:
        1. Carotid duplex ultrasonography.
        2. Quantitative oculopneumoplethysmography.
        3. Transcranial Doppler sonography.
        4. MRI or spiral CT angiography.
    - Echocardiography: Standard or transesophageal to evaluate for cardiac source of emboli.

KEYS TO MANAGEMENT

Acute

- General management.
    - Oxygen: Intubation and mechanical ventilation if hypoxic and/or hypercapnic (some recommend intubation for anyone with Glasgow Coma Scale of 8 or less).
    - Control blood pressure.
        1. Fluid resuscitation increases blood flow and vascular volume in patient with hypotension.
        2. Hypertension should be treated carefully, no more than a decrease of 20% in MAP over 1 hour—IV nitroprusside or labetalol.
    - Monitor and control ICP.
        1. Consider ICP bolt placement.
        2. Consider osmotherapy (mannitol).
        3. Consider hyperventilation: Use only with caution and watch out for decreased CBF.
    - Monitor and manage electrolyte disturbances.
    - Hyperglycemia is associated with worse prognosis and should be treated with insulin.
    - Treat fever with antipyretics; monitor for infectious complications such as pneumonia.
    - Rapid seizure intervention.
    - Attention to nutrition should be begun early (malnutrition results in poorer outcomes).
    - Curling ulcer prophylaxis (sucralfate vs. H_2 blockers).
- ABI.
    - Reperfusion.
        1. Recombinant tissue plasminogen activator (rt-Pa, alteplase) has its greatest efficacy with lowest risk of hemorrhagic conversion if given less than 3 hours after stroke onset. Patient outcomes significantly improved at 3 months. There are numerous contraindications (most relating to bleeding risks) and hemorrhagic conversion of the stroke occurs in approximately 5% of cases.
        2. Intra-arterial prourokinase can be given within 6 hours of onset of symptoms in patients with middle cerebral artery occlusion, with improved outcomes

at 3 months—not as effective as rt-Pa in the first 3 hours after symptom onset.
3. Ultrasound-augmented thrombolysis is used in several prominent stroke centers with improved vessel recannulation.
4. Recent studies combining IV and intra-arterial thrombolysis or intra-arterial thrombolysis plus antiplatelet $GPII_BIII_A$ receptor blockers are promising.
5. Interventional devices such as the Merci retriever are approved for clot removal in selected individuals who are not eligible for thrombolysis.
6. Intravenous desmoteplase (derived from the vampire bat) can be used up to 9 hours after stroke onset—results from recent studies are very promising.
7. Intravenous ancrod (derived from pit viper venom) has also improved stroke outcomes if given within 3 hours of stroke onset; confers a risk of intracranial hemorrhage similar to that of rt-Pa.
8. Heparin is still used occasionally in conjunction with thrombolytic therapy; however, its use is no longer generally recommended.
- Neuroprotection—studies are ongoing.
  1. Candesartan (angiotensin II receptor blocker) in acute stroke decreased 12-month mortality rate in 2 major trials.
  2. Glycerol given within the first days after stroke onset increased short-term survival in a recent meta-analysis of 11 trials.
  3. Caffeinol (combination of caffeine and ethanol) improved outcomes in a recent trial; other studies suggest it is not effective.
  4. *N*-methyl-D-aspartate (NMDA) receptor/channel antagonists block release of glutamate and aspartate, thus decreasing intracellular calcium influx. Preliminary studies were encouraging and they may be used as adjuncts to thrombolysis, but more recent studies suggest that they are not as effective as was hoped.
  5. Hypothermia has been studied with mixed results; most investigators believe that this will be helpful when more sophisticated methods for cooling are developed.
  6. Recombinant human erythropoietin (rh-EPO) improved clinical outcomes and decreased infarct size in one human study. More trials are pending.
  7. Magnesium sulfate reduces excitotoxin release and has reduced infarct severity in some studies, but overall outcomes are not significantly improved.
  8. Activated protein C was effective in decreasing ischemic injury in animal models; human trials under way.
  9. Many other agents: lubeluzole (inhibits presynaptic release of glutamate), α-amino-3-hydroxy-5-methyl-4-isoxazole (AMPA) channel antagonists, calcium channel blockers, γ-aminobutyric agonists, toxic oxygen radical scavengers (tirilazad, ebselen), monoclonal antibodies against leukocyte adhesion molecules, cytokine inhibitors, nitric oxide donors, methylxanthines (pentoxifylline); however, their effectiveness has not been determined.
- ICH.
  - Bed rest, sedate; consider intubation to control airway, administer oxygen, and ventilate if necessary.
  - If on warfarin (secondary ICH), administer fresh frozen plasma, or vitamin K (recombinant factor VIIa [rFVIIa] may work better [studies ongoing]).
  - Control blood pressure: Use labetalol rather than nitrates because it does not cause cerebral vasodilation; balance with fluid administration.
  - Pressure bolt for ICP monitoring: Osmolar therapy with mannitol if indicated; ventriculostomy may be necessary if there is intraventricular hemorrhage; barbiturates and hypothermia are reserved for refractory ICP elevations.
  - Recombinant factor VIIa (rFVIIa) given IV within 4 hours of hemorrhage resulted in smaller volume hemorrhage and improved functional outcomes in a recent large clinical trial but does increase risk for thromboembolic complications (studies ongoing).
  - Surgical decompression in selected patients; less than 12 hours after event for maximal effect; needle aspiration of hematomas can be successful in selected patients with very large IC hematomas.

- Seizure and stress ulcer prophylaxis for most patients; continuous EEG monitoring is used in many large stroke centers.
- SAH.
  - Monitor for arrhythmias and myocardial ischemia.
  - Darkened room; bed rest with head at 30 degrees.
  - Meperidine or codeine for pain; reassess mental status.
  - Ulcer prophylaxis; stool softeners; seizure prophylaxis controversial.
  - Monitor for adequate cerebral perfusion using transcranial doppler (TCD).
  - Monitor for increased ICP—osmolar therapy; ventriculostomy may be needed.
  - Prevent rebleeding.
    1. Perform surgery if in good condition, operate in 1 to 2 days to clip aneurysm (up to 90% successful).
    2. Intra-arterial coils used to block the aneurysm neck are effective in many patients, especially those who are not candidates for surgery.
    3. Antifibrinolytic drugs such as aminocaproic or tranexamic acid are no longer recommended; however, recombinant VIIa (rFVIIa) has decreased aneurysmal hemorrhage in several studies and continues to be evaluated.
  - Prevent vasospasm.
    1. Monitor for headache, mental status changes, and new deficits.
    2. Hyperperfusion with "triple H" (hypervolemic/hypertensive/hemodilution) can be used in the absence of increased ICP to improve perfusion pressure and reduce viscosity.
    3. Calcium channel blocker—nimodipine—clearly reduces severe neurologic deficits and works more by reducing ischemic intracellular calcium influx than by cerebral vasodilation.
    4. Percutaneous transluminal carotid angioplasty (PTCA) is helpful in some patients with refractory vasospasm.
    5. Monitor with daily transcranial Doppler ultrasound.
    6. Prevent hyperglycemia with sliding scale insulin.

Chronic

- Neurologic rehabilitation techniques are varied and of mixed clear therapeutic benefit but all are superior to neglect. Improvements can be seen many months after the acute event.
- Nutrition is vitally important.
- Monitor for depression, recurrent cerebrovascular disease, and cardiac disease, especially coronary artery disease. Pneumonia is also a significant cause of poststroke mortality.

Prevention

- Hypertension is the single most important modifiable risk factor; more than half of all strokes could be prevented with hypertension control.
- Stopping smoking and decreasing alcohol intake can reduce risk.
- Exercise reduces risk significantly in both men and women and in all racial/ethnic groups.
- Cholesterol management reduces risk, especially using HMG CoA reductase inhibitors (statins).
- Use warfarin therapy for nonvalvular atrial fibrillation (INR 2 to 3); direct thrombin inhibitors such as ximelagatran may be superior to warfarin (studies under way).
- Aspirin (50 to 325 mg/day) for primary prevention; aspirin plus dipyridamole is the most effective antithrombotic regimen for secondary prevention of stroke. Others include clopidogrel and ticlopidine.
- Management of transient ischemic attacks (TIAs).
  - Medical therapy with antiplatelet drugs (aspirin, aspirin + dipyridamole, or clopidogrel if aspirin intolerant) and statins.
  - Use warfarin for atrial fibrillation.
  - Surgical intervention (carotid endarterectomy) is suggested for critical stenoses (>70%). Recent studies suggest percutaneous carotid angioplasty with stenting is safer and more effective than endarterectomy for many patients.

PATHOPHYSIOLOGY $\longrightarrow$	CLINICAL LINK
What is going on in the disease process that influences how the patient presents and how he or she should be managed?	*What should you do now that you understand the underlying pathophysiology?*
Ischemic stroke and coronary artery disease share many risk factors and are most often due to atherosclerosis.	Patients with stroke should be monitored for coronary artery disease and vice versa.
Subarachnoid hemorrhage occurs in young, healthy people with few risk factors; many are preceded by promontory bleeds.	Severe headache, stiff neck, and/or decreased level of consciousness must be thoroughly evaluated, even in a young, healthy person.
Acute brain infarction is characterized by both acute ischemic neural cell death and delayed cell death; both are mediated through excitotoxins, oxygen radicals, and inflammation.	New neuroprotection therapies aimed at reducing excitotoxins, oxygen radicals, and inflammation are being studied to see if they can reduce infarct size and improve delayed outcomes.
Intracranial hemorrhage is associated with rapid brain injury, increased intracranial pressure, and poor prognosis.	Rapid and accurate diagnosis and management of ICH are vital to patient survival.
Subarachnoid hemorrhage is characterized by a high likelihood of severe vasospasm that can result in significant ischemic injury.	Patients with SAH must be monitored closely for up to 3 weeks after bleeding and should be treated aggressively to prevent rebleeding and vasospasm.
Brain ischemia and infarction result in relatively little stimulation of meningeal and intracerebral pain receptors, whereas blood in and around the brain stimulates pain receptors widely in meninges and vascular tissue.	ABI tends to present with painless loss of neurologic function, whereas ICH and SAH are most commonly associated with severe headache.
ABI, ICH, and SAH are very different in their pathophysiology, complications, and management.	Rapid evaluation, including CT or MRI, is vital to delivering appropriate care.
Risk of stroke is related to several potentially reversible factors, and a correction of these is associated with a significant decrease in risk.	Management of hypertension, dyslipidemia, smoking, and atherosclerosis is vital to stroke prevention.

SUGGESTED READINGS

Al Mubarak, N. & Iyer, S. S. (2005). Carotid artery stenting for the high surgical risk patients. *Journal of Cardiovascular Surgery*, 46, 1-8.

Amarenco, P., Lavallee, P., & Touboul, P. J. (2004). Statins and stroke prevention. *Cerebrovascular Diseases*, 17(suppl 1), 81-88.

Amarenco, P., Lavallee, P., & Touboul, P. J. (2004). Stroke prevention, blood cholesterol, and statins. *Lancet Neurology*, 3, 271-278.

Anderson, C. S., Hackett, M. L., & House, A. O. (2004). Interventions for preventing depression after stroke. *Cochrane Database of Systematic Reviews*, CD003689.

Andrews, P. J. (2004). Critical care management of acute ischemic stroke. *Current Opinion in Critical Care*, 10, 110-115.

Arboix, A. & Marti-Vilalta, J. L. (2004). New concepts in lacunar stroke etiology: the constellation of small-vessel arterial disease. *Cerebrovascular Diseases*, 17(suppl 1), 58-62.

Aronow, W. S. & Frishman, W. H. (2004). Treatment of hypertension and prevention of ischemic stroke. *Current Cardiology Reports*, 6, 124-129.

Arundine, M. & Tymianski, M. (2004). Molecular mechanisms of glutamate-dependent neurodegeneration in ischemia and traumatic brain injury. *Cellular & Molecular Life Sciences*, 61, 657-668.

Banerji, M. A. (2005). Statins and the prevention of stroke in diabetes. *Current Diabetes Reports*, 5, 1-3.

Bassetti, C. L. (2005). Sleep and stroke. *Seminars in Neurology*, 25, 19-32.

Bath, P. M. & Gray, L. J. (2005). Association between hormone replacement therapy and subsequent stroke: a meta-analysis. *British Medical Journal*, 330, 342.

Benatar, M. (2005). Heparin use in acute ischaemic stroke: does evidence change practice? *QJM*, 98, 147-152.

Bonita, R., Mendis, S., Truelsen, T., Bogousslavsky, J., Toole, J., & Yatsu, F. (2004). The global stroke initiative. *Lancet Neurology*, 3, 391-393.

Broderick, J. P. (2004). Intravenous thrombolysis for acute stroke. *Cleveland Clinic Journal of Medicine*, 71(suppl 1), S28-S30.

Broderick, J. P. (2005). Advances in the treatment of hemorrhagic stroke: a possible new treatment. *Cleveland Clinic Journal of Medicine*, 72, 341-344.

Carley, S. & Harrison, M. (2005). Best evidence topic report. Timing of lumbar puncture in suspected subarachnoid haemorrhage. *Emergency Medicine Journal*, 22, 121-122.

Carley, S. & Sen, A. (2005). Best evidence topic report. Antifibrinolytics for the initial management of sub arachnoid haemorrhage. *Emergency Medicine Journal*, 22, 274-275.

Chamorro, A. (2004). Role of inflammation in stroke and atherothrombosis. *Cerebrovascular Diseases*, 17(suppl 3), 1-5.

Choi, J. H. & Mohr, J. P. (2005). Brain arteriovenous malformations in adults. *Lancet Neurology*, 4, 299-308.

Claassen, J., Mayer, S. A., & Hirsch, L. J. (2005). Continuous EEG monitoring in patients with subarachnoid hemorrhage. *Journal of Clinical Neurophysiology*, 22, 92-98.

Coward, L. J., Featherstone, R. L., & Brown, M. M. (2004). Percutaneous transluminal angioplasty and stenting for carotid artery stenosis. *Cochrane Database of Systematic Reviews*, CD000515.

Cramer, S. C. (2005). Patent foramen ovale and its relationship to stroke. *Cardiology Clinics*, 23, 7-11.

Czlonkowska, A., Ciesielska, A., Gromadzka, G., & Kurkowska-Jastrzebska, I. (2005). Estrogen and cytokines production—the possible cause of gender differences in neurological diseases. *Current Pharmaceutical Design*, 11, 1017-1030.

Davis, S. M. & Donnan, G. A. (2004). Advances in penumbra imaging with MR. *Cerebrovascular Diseases*, 17(suppl 3), 23-27.

Diez-Tejedor, E. & Fuentes, B. (2004). Acute care in stroke: the importance of early intervention to achieve better brain protection. *Cerebrovascular Diseases*, 17(suppl 1), 130-137.

Dobkin, B. H. (2005). Clinical practice. Rehabilitation after stroke. *New England Journal of Medicine*, 352, 1677-1684.

Dodick, D. W., Meissner, I., Meyer, F. B., & Cloft, H. J. (2004). Evaluation and management of asymptomatic carotid artery stenosis. *Mayo Clinic Proceedings*, 79, 937-944.

Doggrell, S. A. (2004). Candesartan for the prevention and treatment of stroke—results of the SCOPE and ACCESS trials. *Expert Opinion on Pharmacotherapy*, 5, 687-690.

Donnan, G. A. (2004). Stroke: prediction, prevention, and outcome. *Lancet Neurology*, 3, 9.

Economides, M. C. & Singh, B. N. (2004). Antithrombotic therapies for stroke prevention in atrial fibrillation. *Minerva Cardioangiologica*, 52, 125-139.

Engelter, S. & Lyrer, P. (2004). Antiplatelet therapy for preventing stroke and other vascular events after carotid endarterectomy. *Stroke*, 35, 1227-1228.

Etminan, M., Takkouche, B., Isorna, F. C., & Samii, A. (2005). Risk of ischaemic stroke in people with migraine: systematic review and meta-analysis of observational studies. *British Medical Journal*, 330, 63.

Fagan, S. C., Hess, D. C., Machado, L. S., Hohnadel, E. J., Pollock, D. M., & Ergul, A. (2005). Tactics for vascular protection after acute ischemic stroke. *Pharmacotherapy*, 25, 387-395.

Fisher, M. (2004). The ischemic penumbra: identification, evolution and treatment concepts. *Cerebrovascular Diseases*, 17(suppl 1), 1-6.

Fleck, J. D. (2005). Antiplatelet medications in the secondary prevention of ischemic stroke. *Current Neurology & Neuroscience Reports*, 5, 1-3.

Frey, J. L. (2005). Recombinant tissue plasminogen activator (rtPA) for stroke. The perspective at 8 years. *Neurologist*, 11, 123-133.

Furlan, A. (2004). Intra-arterial thrombolysis for acute stroke. *Cleveland Clinic Journal of Medicine*, 71(suppl 1), S31-S38.

Gleason, C. E., Cholerton, B., Carlsson, C. M., Johnson, S. C., & Asthana, S. (2005). Neuroprotective effects of female sex steroids in humans: current controversies and future directions. *Cellular & Molecular Life Sciences*, 62, 299-312.

Goldstein, L. B. & Simel, D. L. (2005). Is this patient having a stroke? *Journal of the American Medical Association*, 293, 2391-2402.

Gordon, N. F., Gulanick, M., Costa, F., Fletcher, G., Franklin, B. A., Roth, E. J., Shephard, T., American Heart Association Council on Clinical Cardiology, S. o. E. C. R. a. P., the Council on Cardiovascular Nursing, the Council on Nutrition, P. A. a. M., & and the Stroke Council. (2004). Physical activity and exercise recommendations for stroke survivors: an American Heart Association scientific statement from the Council on Clinical Cardiology, Subcommittee on Exercise, Cardiac Rehabilitation, and Prevention; the Council on Cardiovascular Nursing; the Council on Nutrition, Physical Activity, and Metabolism; and the Stroke Council. *Stroke*, 35, 1230-1240.

Griffin, J. H., Fernandez, J. A., Liu, D., Cheng, T., Guo, H., & Zlokovic, B. V. (2004). Activated protein C and ischemic stroke. *Critical Care Medicine*, 32, S247-S253.

Guadagno, J. V., Donnan, G. A., Markus, R., Gillard, J. H., & Baron, J. C. (2004). Imaging the ischaemic penumbra. *Current Opinion in Neurology*, 17, 61-67.

Hall, C. E. & Grotta, J. C. (2005). New era for management of primary hypertensive intracerebral hemorrhage. *Current Neurology & Neuroscience Reports*, 5, 29-35.

Hanel, R. A., Lopes, D. K., Wehman, J. C., Sauvageau, E., Levy, E. I., Guterman, L. R., & Hopkins, L. N. (2000). Endovascular treatment of intracranial aneurysms and vasospasm after aneurysmal subarachnoid hemorrhage. *Neurosurgery Clinics of North America, 16*, 317-353.

Hankey, G. J. (2004). Ongoing and planned trials of antiplatelet therapy in the acute and long-term management of patients with ischaemic brain syndromes: setting a new standard of care. *Cerebrovascular Diseases, 17*(suppl 3), 11-16.

Harrigan, M. R. & Guterman, L. R. (2005). Endovascular treatment of acute stroke. *Neurosurgery Clinics of North America, 16*, 433-444.

Hopwood, V. & Lewith, G. T. (2005). Does acupuncture help stroke patients become more independent? *Journal of Alternative & Complementary Medicine, 11*, 175-177.

Horiuchi, T., Tanaka, Y., & Hongo, K. (2005). Surgical treatment for aneurysmal subarachnoid hemorrhage in the 8th and 9th decades of life. *Neurosurgery, 56*, 469-475.

Humphries, S. E. & Morgan, L. (2004). Genetic risk factors for stroke and carotid atherosclerosis: insights into pathophysiology from candidate gene approaches. *Lancet Neurology, 3*, 227-235.

Ionita, C. C., Xavier, A. R., Kirmani, J. F., Dash, S., Divani, A. A., & Qureshi, A. I. (2005). What proportion of stroke is not explained by classic risk factors? *Preventive Cardiology, 8*, 41-46.

Jackson, D. M. & Sammut, I. A. (2004). Oxygen free radical traps for the treatment of ischemia-associated organ injury. *Current Opinion in Investigational Drugs, 5*, 50-54.

Janardhan, V. & Qureshi, A. I. (2004). Mechanisms of ischemic brain injury. *Cardiology Reports, 6*, 117-123.

Jensen, M. B. & St Louis, E. K. (2005). Management of acute cerebellar stroke. *Archives of Neurology, 62*, 537-544.

Johnston, D. C. & Hill, M. D. (2004). The patient with transient cerebral ischemia: a golden opportunity for stroke prevention. *CMAJ: Canadian Medical Association Journal, 170*, 1134-1137.

Kappelle, L. J. & Van Der Worp, H. B. (2004). Treatment or prevention of complications of acute ischemic stroke. *Current Neurology & Neuroscience Reports, 4*, 36-41.

Kastin, A. J. & Pan, W. (2005). Targeting neurite growth inhibitors to induce CNS regeneration. *Current Pharmaceutical Design, 11*, 1247-1253.

Kumar, K. (2005). Overview: use of biomarkers for early diagnosis of ischemic stroke. *Current Opinion in Investigational Drugs, 6*, 21-24.

Laurent, S. & Boutouyrie, P. (2005). Arterial stiffness and stroke in hypertension: therapeutic implications for stroke prevention. *CNS Drugs, 19*, 1-11.

Lawes, C. M., Bennett, D. A., Feigin, V. L., & Rodgers, A. (2004). Blood pressure and stroke: an overview of published reviews. *Stroke, 35*, 776-785.

Lawton, M. T., Quinones-Hinojosa, A., Chang, E. F., & Yu, T. (2005). Thrombotic intracranial aneurysms: classification scheme and management strategies in 68 patients. *Neurosurgery, 56*, 441-454.

Lindley, R. I., Wardlaw, J. M., & Sandercock, P. A. (2005). Alteplase and ischaemic stroke: have new reviews of old data helped? *Lancet Neurology, 4*, 249-253.

Mancia, G. (2004). Prevention and treatment of stroke in hypertension. *Clinical Therapeutics, 26*, 631-648.

Manno, E. M., Atkinson, J. L., Fulgham, J. R., & Wijdicks, E. F. (2005). Emerging medical and surgical management strategies in the evaluation and treatment of intracerebral hemorrhage. *Mayo Clinic Proceedings, 80*, 420-433.

Markus, H. S. (2004). Cerebral perfusion and stroke. *Journal of Neurology, Neurosurgery & Psychiatry, 75*, 353-361.

McCullough, P. A., Dorrell, K. A., Sandberg, K. R., & Yerkey, M. W. (2004). Ximelagatran: a novel oral direct thrombin inhibitor for long-term anticoagulation. *Reviews in Cardiovascular Medicine, 5*, 99-103.

Meschia, J. F., Brott, T. G., & Brown, R. D., Jr. (2005). Genetics of cerebrovascular disorders. *Mayo Clinic Proceedings, 80*, 122-132.

Nguyen-Huynh, M. N. & Johnston, S. C. (2005). Transient ischemic attack: a neurologic emergency. *Current Neurology & Neuroscience Reports, 5*, 13-20.

O'Rourke, F., Dean, N., Akhtar, N., & Shuaib, A. (2004). Current and future concepts in stroke prevention. *CMAJ: Canadian Medical Association Journal, 170*, 1123-1133.

Palagummi, P., Saltzman, H., & Ezekowitz, M. (2005). Direct thrombin inhibitors: stroke prevention in atrial fibrillation and potential anti-inflammatory properties. *American Heart Journal, 149*, S32-S35.

Petersen, P. (2005). Ximelagatran—a promising new drug in thromboembolic disorders. *Current Pharmaceutical Design, 11*, 527-538.

Peterson, D. A. (2004). Umbilical cord blood cells and brain stroke injury: bringing in fresh blood to address an old problem. *Journal of Clinical Investigation, 114*, 312-314.

Pitkanen, A. & Kubova, H. (2004). Antiepileptic drugs in neuroprotection. *Expert Opinion on Pharmacotherapy, 5*, 777-798.

Pluta, R. M. (2005). Delayed cerebral vasospasm and nitric oxide: review, new hypothesis, and proposed treatment. *Pharmacology & Therapeutics, 105*, 23-56.

Rajendra, W., Armugam, A., & Jeyaseelan, K. (2004). Neuroprotection and peptide toxins. *Brain Research—Brain Research Reviews, 45*, 125-141.

Rasquin, S. M., Lodder, J., & Verhey, F. R. (2005). Predictors of reversible mild cognitive impairment after stroke: a 2-year follow-up study. *Journal of the Neurological Sciences, 229-230*, 21-25.

Read, S. J. & Barone, F. C. (2005). Introduction to stroke genomics. *Methods in Molecular Medicine, 104*, 3-16.

Righetti, E., Celani, M. G., Cantisani, T., Sterzi, R., Boysen, G., & Ricci, S. (2004). Glycerol for acute stroke. *Cochrane Database of Systematic Reviews*, CD000096.

Rimmer, J. H. & Wang, E. (2005). Aerobic exercise training in stroke survivors. *Topics in Stroke Rehabilitation, 12*, 17-30.

Ringleb, P. A., Schellinger, P. D., & Schwark, C. (2004). Clopidogrel in the management of cerebrovascular events. *International Journal of Clinical Practice, 58*, 402-410.

Rinkel, G. J., Feigin, V. L., Algra, A., van den Bergh, W. M., Vermeulen, M., & van Gijn, J. (2005). Calcium antagonists for aneurysmal subarachnoid haemorrhage. *Cochrane Database of Systematic Reviews*, CD000277.

Rodi, D., Couture, R., Ongali, B., & Simonato, M. (2005). Targeting kinin receptors for the treatment of neurological diseases. *Current Pharmaceutical Design, 11*, 1313-1326.

Rubattu, S., Gigante, B., Stanzione, R., De Paolis, P., Tarasi, D., & Volpe, M. (2004). In the search for stroke genes: a long and winding road. *American Journal of Hypertension, 17*, 197-202.

Ruigrok, Y. M., Rinkel, G. J., & Wijmenga, C. (2005). Genetics of intracranial aneurysms. *Lancet Neurology, 4*, 179-189.

Sacco, R. L. (2004). Risk factors for TIA and TIA as a risk factor for stroke. *Neurology, 62*, S7-11.

Saxena, R. & Koudstaal, P. J. (2004). Anticoagulants for preventing stroke in patients with nonrheumatic atrial fibrillation and a history of stroke or transient ischaemic attack. *Cochrane Database of Systematic Reviews*, CD000185.

Schaller, B. & Graf, R. (2004). Cerebral ischemia and reperfusion: the pathophysiologic concept as a basis for clinical therapy. *Journal of Cerebral Blood Flow & Metabolism, 24*, 351-371.

Schellinger, P. D. & Hacke, W. (2005). Stroke: advances in therapy. *Lancet Neurology, 4*, 2.

Schellinger, P. D., Kaste, M., & Hacke, W. (2004). An update on thrombolytic therapy for acute stroke. *Current Opinion in Neurology, 17,* 69-77.

Schmidtke, K. & Hull, M. (2005). Cerebral small vessel disease: how does it progress? *Journal of the Neurological Sciences, 229-230,* 13-20.

Sherman, D. G. (2004). Antithrombotic and hypofibrinogenetic therapy in acute ischemic stroke: what is the next step? *Cerebrovascular Diseases, 1*(suppl 1), 138-143.

Sila, C. A. (2004). Antiplatelet therapy for acute stroke: aspirin and beyond. *Cleveland Clinic Journal of Medicine, 71*(suppl 1), S57-S59.

Slevin, M., Krupinski, J., Kumar, P., Gaffney, J., & Kumar, S. (2005). Gene activation and protein expression following ischaemic stroke: strategies towards neuroprotection. *Journal of Cellular & Molecular Medicine, 9,* 85-102.

Solenski, N. J. (2004). Transient ischemic attacks: Part I. Diagnosis and evaluation. *American Family Physician, 69,* 1665-1674.

Solenski, N. J. (2004). Transient ischemic attacks: Part II. Treatment. *American Family Physician, 69,* 1681-1688.

Sterzi, R. & Vidale, S. (2004). Treatment of intracerebral hemorrhage: the clinical evidences. *Neurological Sciences, 25*(suppl 1), S12.

Stone, T. W. (2005). Adenosine, neurodegeneration and neuroprotection. *Neurological Research, 27,* 161-168.

Sun, F. Y. & Guo, X. (2005). Molecular and cellular mechanisms of neuroprotection by vascular endothelial growth factor. *Journal of Neuroscience Research, 79,* 180-184.

Sztriha, L. K., Sas, K., & Vecsei, L. (2005). Aspirin resistance in stroke: 2004. *Journal of the Neurological Sciences, 229-230,* 163-169.

Trubelja, N., Vaughan, C., & Coplan, N. L. (2005). The role of statins in preventing stroke. *Preventive Cardiology, 8,* 98-101.

van Gijn, J. (2004). The future of stroke neurology. *Journal of Neurology, 251,* 235-239.

Vespa, P. (2005). Continuous EEG monitoring for the detection of seizures in traumatic brain injury, infarction, and intracerebral hemorrhage: "to detect and protect." *Journal of Clinical Neurophysiology, 22,* 99-106.

Wahlgren, N. G. & Ahmed, N. (2004). Neuroprotection in cerebral ischaemia: facts and fancies—the need for new approaches. *Cerebrovascular Diseases, 17*(suppl 1), 153-166.

Wardlaw, J. M. & Mielke, O. (2005). Early signs of brain infarction at CT: observer reliability and outcome after thrombolytic treatment—systematic review. *Radiology, 235,* 444-453.

Wechsler, L. R. (2004). Stem cell transplantation for stroke. *Cleveland Clinic Journal of Medicine, 71*(suppl 1), S40-S41.

Weinberger, J. (2005). Adverse effects and drug interactions of antithrombotic agents used in prevention of ischaemic stroke. *Drugs, 65,* 461-471.

Weir, N. U., Demchuk, A. M., Buchan, A. M., & Hill, M. D. (2005). Stroke prevention. MATCHing therapy to the patient with TIA. *Postgraduate Medicine, 117,* 26-30.

Wijdicks, E. F., Kallmes, D. F., Manno, E. M., Fulgham, J. R., & Piepgras, D. G. (2005). Subarachnoid hemorrhage: neurointensive care and aneurysm repair. *Mayo Clinic Proceedings, 80,* 550-559.

Wilson, S. R., Hirsch, N. P., & Appleby, I. (2005). Management of subarachnoid haemorrhage in a non-neurosurgical centre. *Anaesthesia, 60,* 470-485.

Stroke

INITIAL HISTORY

- 76-year-old man, slightly confused.
- Wife describes symptoms starting 30 minutes ago.
- Sudden onset of difficulty getting his mouth to form words, speech is slurred.
- Face and mouth numb; tongue felt "thick."
- Unable to hold his coffee cup in his right hand.
- Right leg weak, needed to hold on to the table to stand.

Question 1.   *What is your differential diagnosis based on the information you have now?*

Question 2.   *What other questions would you like to ask?*

☐ **Gail L. Kongable, MSN, FNP, MPH contributed this case study.**

ADDITIONAL HISTORY

- History of essential hypertension, uncontrolled.
- Has not been taking his thiazide diuretic because it makes him feel "bad."
- Was told he has high cholesterol, but has not returned to see his primary care provider.
- Has experienced several brief spells of right-sided weakness that resolved in a few minutes—thought this was his arm falling asleep.
- No head trauma or recent infections.
- Family history: mother died of stroke, father died of acute myocardial infarction (AMI).
- Smokes 1 pack per day for past 30 years.
- Sedentary life-style.

Question 3.   *Now what do you think?*

PHYSICAL EXAMINATION

- Alert and anxious white male.
- Slurred speech, uses appropriate words.
- T = 37° C, orally; RR = 16 and regular; HR = 86 and irregular; BP = 190/120 mm Hg (reclining).

HEENT
- Conjunctivae are clear without exudate or lesions.
- Fundi are without lesions, nicking, or cotton tufts.
- Nasal mucosa is pink without drainage.
- Oral mucous membranes are moist, no lesions, poor dentition.
- Pharynx is pink without lesions or exudate.

Skin, Neck
- Pale with senile lentigines, no lesions or bruises.
- No lesions or bruises, no tenting; dry and flaky.
- Supple, no lymphadenopathy or thyromegaly.
- Bruit auscultated over left carotid artery.

Lungs
- Chest expansion is symmetric and full.
- Diaphragmatic excursion is equal at 4 cm.
- Lung sounds are clear to auscultation.

Cardiac
- Heart sounds: irregular rate and rhythm.
- No murmurs, gallops, or clicks.

Abdomen
- Nondistended; bowel sounds are present and not hyperactive.
- Liver percusses 2 cm below right costal margin but overall 12 cm in size.
- No tenderness or masses; no bruits.

Extremities
- Cool but good capillary refill at 3 seconds.
- 1+ pitting edema of bilateral ankles.
- Radial artery pulses full and equal; anterior pedal pulses diminished but equal.
- No clubbing.

Neurologic
- Alert and oriented.
- Facial droop on right, with loss of nasolabial fold.
- Diminished gag reflex.
- Strength 3/5 in the right upper extremity and 4/5 in the right lower extremity; 5/5 in the left upper and lower extremities.
- Deep tendon reflexes (DTRs) 1+ on right, 2+ on left.
- Sensory intact to touch, no neglect.

Question 4.   *What studies would you initiate now while preparing your interventions?*

Question 5.   *What therapies would you initiate immediately while awaiting results of the laboratory studies?*

LABORATORY RESULTS

- ECG; atrial fibrillation.
- Serum glucose = 130 mg/dL.
- PT = 12.5 seconds; PTT = 28 seconds.
- Platelet count = 220,000/mm^3.
- Head CT scan without contrast media did not reveal evidence of bleeding.

EMERGENCY DEPARTMENT COURSE

- Risks and benefits of thrombolytic therapy are explained to patient and family.
- Patient does not improve neurologically.
- BP improves with labetalol.

PHYSICAL EXAMINATION UPDATE

- Vital signs.
  - BP = 170/86; HR = 100, irregular.
- Neurologic examination.
  - Alert and oriented.
  - Follows commands.
  - Right hemiparesis worsening; strength is now 2/5 in both the upper and lower extremities on the right, still 5/5 on the left.
  - Moderate dysarthria.
  - Decreased sensation on right.

Question 6. *What do you think is happening? Why is the hemiparesis worsening? What does his CT scan mean? Should you continue to treat his hypertension to bring it down to normal?*

Question 7. *What interventions should be initiated now?*

Question 8. *Now what should be done and what can the patient expect?*

HOSPITAL COURSE

- Patient does well with digoxin 0.125 mg po daily for atrial fibrillation. He converts to normal sinus rhythm; P = 82, regular.
- Total cholesterol = 270; HDL = 25, ratio 6:6.
- Antihypertensive therapy with an ACE inhibitor is initiated.
- Antiplatelet therapy; aspirin 325 mg po daily.
- HbA_{1c} = 6.8%.
- He has not smoked while hospitalized.
- Cardiac echo was normal (no mural thrombus); carotid Doppler showed <40% stenosis on right and <50% stenosis on the left with no hemodynamic changes (not a candidate for carotid endarterectomy at this point).

Question 9. *What instructions and medication should this patient go home with?*

Question 10. *What steps can he take to prevent future attacks?*

Alzheimer Disease

DEFINITION

- Alzheimer disease (AD) is defined as a gradual onset and continuing decline of cognitive function from a previously higher level, resulting in impairment of social and occupational function.
- Impairment of recent memory occurs and at least one of the following:
  - Language disturbances (aphasia).
  - Word-finding difficulties.
  - Disturbances of praxis.
  - Visual agnosia.
  - Constructional disturbances.
  - Disturbances of executive function, including abstract reasoning and concentration.
- Cognitive deficits are not due to other psychiatric, neurologic, or systemic diseases.
- Cognitive deficits do not exclusively occur in the setting of delirium.

EPIDEMIOLOGY

- Most common dementia of older adults; more than 4.5 million people in the United States have AD.
- Older than age 65, 5% to 10% of the U.S. population is affected; older than age 80, 20% to 40% of the population is affected.
- Time from AD diagnosis to death averages 8 to 10 years.
- Risk factors.
  - Increasing age.
  - Family history.
    1. Increased risk in siblings and even greater risk in identical twins.
    2. Autosomal dominant inheritance of presenilin genes (see following) with early-onset familial AD.
  - Female gender.
  - Use of hormone replacement therapy with conjugated equine estrogen and medroxyprogesterone acetate.
  - Down syndrome (nearly everyone with trisomy 21 will develop AD by age 40).
  - Head trauma with a loss of consciousness results in a threefold increase in risk; the latest studies suggest this is only true if epsilon-4 allele on the *apolipoprotein E* gene (*APOE$_4$*) is also present (see below).

- Other associated risk factors include alcohol abuse, depression, and sleep disturbance.
- Possible infection with *Chlamydia pneumoniae* or herpes simplex virus (controversial).
- Possible increased serum levels of copper, iron, or aluminum (controversial).

PATHOPHYSIOLOGY

Genetics

Four genes have been clearly identified so far.

- Familial AD.
    - *Presenilin 1 (PS1)* gene on chromosome 14 (leads to increased β-secretase activity and β-amyloid synthesis, also contributes to apoptosis of neurons); associated with early onset dementia in particular families.
    - *Presenilin 2 (PS2)* gene on chromosome 1 (leads to increased β-secretase activity and β-amyloid synthesis, also contributes to apoptosis of neurons); associated with early onset dementia in particular families.
- Sporadic AD.
    - A β-*amyloid precursor protein (APP)* gene on chromosome 21 (β-amyloid found in structural lesions commonly seen in AD brain tissue) (Figure 20-1).

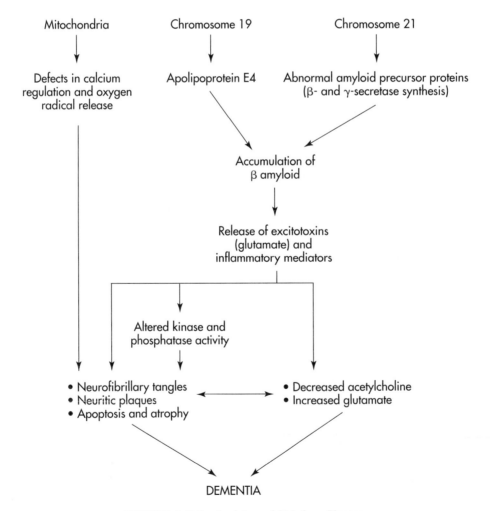

FIGURE **20-1 Pathophysiology of Alzheimer Disease.**

- Epsilon-4 allele on the *apolipoprotein E* gene *(APOE$_4$)* on chromosome 19.
    1. APOE is required for normal cholesterol transport, which is necessary for removal of β-amyloid protein from the central nervous system.
    2. APOE$_4$ results in accumulation of β-amyloid protein.
    3. It may also contribute to AD pathology by causing abnormal binding of APOE protein to τ protein of neurofibrillary tangles and to β-amyloid proteins of senile plaques (see Figure 20-1).
    4. Heterozygous APOE$_4$ doubles the risk of AD and occurs in 34% to 65% of people with AD, but also occurs in 24% to 31% of people without AD; homozygous mutation increases risk fivefold.
- Probable mutations in glutathione-S transferase (GST01) and insulin-degrading enzyme (IDE) genes.
- The primary genetic defect for sporadic AD may be located in the mitochondrial deoxyribonucleic acid (DNA) with defects in intracellular calcium regulation, oxygen radical production, and cell death.

Tissue Effects (see Figure 20-1)

- Amyloid precursor protein (APP) is cleaved by β- and γ-secretase enzymes to β-amyloid protein. Mutations in APP result in overproduction of abnormal β-amyloid.
- The APOE$_4$ isoform results in decreased transport of β-amyloid out of the central nervous system.
- β-amyloid protein accumulates in neurons and results in increased release of glutamate, which is an excitotoxin.
    - Increased glutamate contributes to intracellular calcium influx, cellular edema, and necrosis and apoptosis of neurons.
    - In normal memory and learning functions, glutamate is transiently released at the synapse in high concentrations and displaces magnesium binding to the *N*-methyl-D-aspartate (NMDA) receptor, thus providing a neuronal signal. In AD, chronically increased glutamate release causes low-level signaling that creates "background noise," making the physiologic signals necessary for learning and memory undetectable.
- There is a 40% to 90% decrease in choline acetyltransferase with decreased levels of acetylcholine (ACH) occurring even in the first year of dementia symptoms.
- Inflammatory mediators are also released that contribute to alterations in kinase and phosphatase activity resulting in structural defects and neuronal cell death. Toxic oxygen radicals generated from inflammation and mitochondrial injury further contribute to structural defects and cell death.
- There is some evidence for an autoimmune contribution to the disease process (increased T lymphocytes) but this is not fully understood.
- Several structural abnormalities are common to AD brain tissue.
    - Neuritic plaques: Clusters of degenerating nerve-terminals with β-amyloid protein fragments that occur in greatest numbers in the parietotemporal region and hippocampus (memory).
    - Neurofibrillary tangles: Bundles of filamentous τ proteins in the cytoplasm of neurons.
    - Atrophy and apoptosis necrosis of neurons.

PATIENT PRESENTATION

History

Often obtained from family; patient may be unaware of changes; family history; history of head trauma; absence of other causes such as heavy alcohol abuse, nutritional deficits, and drug use (illicit or prescribed); seizures; other neurologic complaints (focal weakness or numbness; cerebral or meningeal infections; syphilis; thyroid disease.

Symptoms

Insidious and gradually progressive loss of memory with apraxias, aphasias, and visual and cognitive disturbances; clear consciousness with absence of hallucinations and delusions until late in the disease course; absence of asterixis or tremor.

Examination

Cognitive memory deficits without focal neurologic findings or evidence of delirium or systemic disease as the cause of mental status changes.

DIFFERENTIAL DIAGNOSIS

Other forms of idiopathic dementia such as dementia-associated with Lewy bodies (DLB).
- Depression.
- Vascular dementia.
    - Alcohol and/or drug use.
    - Pernicious anemia.
    - Mass lesions.
    - Thyroid disorders.
    - Huntington chorea, Creutzfeldt-Jakob disease.
    - Chronic infection (syphilis, viral [HIV], fungal).
    - Toxins (lead).
    - Chronic subdural hematoma.
    - Normal pressure hydrocephalus.
    - Parkinson disease.
    - Anoxic brain injury.

KEYS TO ASSESSMENT

- Begin evaluation by questioning the patient about instrumental activities of daily living: driving, managing money, shopping, doing the laundry, medications, etc.
- Establish dementia using the DSM IV criteria: use established mental-status tests such as: Information-Orientation-Concentration Test, Mini-Mental State Examination (MMSE), Dementia Rating Scale, Geriatric Depression Scale, AD Assessment Scale, etc.
- Rule out treatable causes of dementia.
    - Review current medications and inquire about substance abuse.
    - Obtain complete blood count, serum electrolytes, blood urea nitrogen (BUN), and creatinine (Cr) levels, liver function tests (LFTs).
    - Obtain serum B_{12} and thyroid studies.
    - Evaluate for depression (pseudodementia).
    - Obtain brain magnetic resonance imaging (MRI).
    - Other studies to be considered in selected patients.
        1. Electroencephalogram (EEG).
        2. Toxin screens (heavy metals).
        3. Syphilis and human immunodeficiency virus (HIV) serology.
        4. Evaluation for cerebrovascular disease (see Chapter 19).
        5. Positron emission tomography (PET)—clinical role still being defined.
        6. Lumbar puncture to measure cerebrospinal fluid (CSF) β-amyloid and τ proteins is possible but is not routinely indicated and these biomarkers have not yet been adequately validated for screening.
- Differentiate from delirium, which has a sudden onset, fluctuating course, reduced consciousness, globally oriented attention, visual hallucinations, fleeting delusions, complete disorientation, reduced or greatly exaggerated activity, incoherent speech, and asterixis or tremor.
- The family is an important source of information about the underlying disease process and for identifying the key issues in patient management.

- Establish the stage of AD progression.
  - Mild: Forget where things are placed, get lost, forget appointments (both recent and remote memory); depression and anxiety.
  - Moderate: Language trouble, spatial disorientation, poor problem solving, confusion, denial.
  - Severe: Aimlessness, hallucinations, agitation, aphasia.

KEYS TO MANAGEMENT

- Prevention and early intervention.
  - Although nothing has been proven to prevent Alzheimer disease, controlling hypertension, preventing and treating cerebrovascular disease, and active participation in cognitive activities such as reading have been associated with a decreased risk for dementia.
  - There is increasing evidence that HMG CoA reductase inhibitors (statins) may decrease the risk for AD independent of serum cholesterol levels.
  - Antioxidants such as vitamin E, and nonsteroidal anti-inflammatory drugs (NSAIDs) may also decrease risk; studies are ongoing.
- Nonpharmacologic methods.
  - Involve the family early and assess the "caregiver burden" to decide on the need for alternative living options and for monitoring changes in the patient with therapy.
  - Obtain patient participation in drafting advance directives and power of attorney while the patient is still competent.
  - Maintain the socialization of the patient. Walking daily with a care provider has been shown to improve the AD patient's cognitive abilities.
  - Prevent injury, especially in later stages when disorientation worsens.
  - Maintain good nutrition and exercise.
  - Refer families to support organizations.
- Pharmacologic agents.
  - Treating primary cognitive deficits.
    1. Donepezil, rivastigmine, and galantamine are cholinesterase inhibitors that increase acetylcholine; they provide some improvements in memory, orientation, and ability to care for self, but it is not clear how well these improvements are maintained. The drugs are associated with fatigue, insomnia, and significant gastrointestinal distress, including nausea and diarrhea.
    2. Memantine is an *N*-methyl-D-asparate (NMDA) receptor antagonist that has been approved for AD and has been documented to result in a decrease in clinical deterioration and increase in functioning in moderate to severe AD. It acts by blocking low-level glutamate stimulation of the synapse, while allowing for adequate signal transduction during memory and learning.
    3. Ginkgo biloba (high-purity extract [EGb 761]) improves cognitive function and global clinical state over 6 months.
  - Slowing disease progression.
    1. Blockers of β-secretase are being developed and show promise in early studies.
    2. APP vaccines are under investigation.
    3. Anti-APP monoclonal antibodies have some effect but toxicities are high and most trials have been halted.
    4. Probucol and statins are being evaluated in established AD.
    5. Selegiline (an antiparkinsonian drug) may slow the rate of functional decline in some patients with AD, but is of yet unproved benefit.
    6. Propentofylline inhibits glutamate release and increases cerebral blood flow; studies have demonstrated cognitive improvements; awaiting approval for use in the United States.
    7. NSAIDs have not been shown to affect the progression of AD.
    8. Antioxidants such as vitamin E (α-tocopherol) have shown some promise in slowing functional decline in AD but study results are inconsistent.

9. Newer estrogen-based compounds are being tested (estrogen promotes neuronal function and cerebral blood flow, but has not been effective in treating AD).
10. Nerve growth factors prevent cholinergic cell loss and are being intensively studied.

- Controlling behavior and agitation.
    1. Selective serotonin reuptake inhibitors (SSRIs) trazodone and nefazodone can reduce anxiety and improve depressive symptoms, but patients should be monitored carefully.
    2. Short-acting anxiolytics may help with anxiety and insomnia but often result in confusion and ataxia.
    3. Atypical antipsychotics such as risperdal may be needed in severe AD.

PATHOPHYSIOLOGY →	CLINICAL LINK
What is going on in the disease process that influences how the patient presents and how he or she should be managed?	*What should you do now that you understand the underlying pathophysiology?*
The genetics of AD are very complicated and polygenic (except in the case of early-onset familial inheritance), and more genetic links are still being defined.	Population screening for AD is not possible or desirable at this time; a family history of early-onset AD (50s or younger) should be investigated.
Two protein gene products, β-amyloid protein and $APOE_4$, have been identified as being key components of the structural abnormalities characteristic of AD.	Further understanding of these processes, and identification of others, may lead to more specific AD prevention options and therapies such as β-secretase inhibitors and vaccination.
The clinical manifestations of AD, especially in the late stages, can be easily confused with delirium, which is an acute state that requires rapid intervention.	Evaluation for the rapidity of onset of symptoms, amount of agitation, and severity or disorientation and reduced consciousness must be done quickly and carefully to rule out a treatable and potentially life-threatening cause of delirium.
Numerous other causes for dementia include vascular disease, depression, chronic infection, endocrine or metabolic disease, and drugs.	The diagnosis of AD is one of exclusion; careful examination and lab analysis are necessary to rule out treatable causes of dementia.
Decreased acetylcholine is a primary feature of AD pathophysiology.	Donepezil, rivastigmine, and galantamine improve cognition by increasing ACH, but more effective drugs with fewer side effects are needed.
Continuous glutamate overexcitation at the synapse (excitotoxin) is a key feature of AD pathophysiology and results in an inability of the neurons to send adequate memory and learning signals.	Memantine, a new drug approved for AD, blocks low-level glutamate at the receptor but allows for signal transduction.
AD occurs in older adults, who are particularly susceptible to the side effects of medications.	Although caregiver burden is very significant in AD, treatment with neuroleptics, anxiolytics, or antidepressants is associated with considerable toxicity.

SUGGESTED READINGS

Areosa, S. A., McShane, R., & Sherriff, F. (2004). Memantine for dementia. *Cochrane Database of Systematic Reviews*, CD003154.

Beal, M. F. (2004). Mitochondrial dysfunction and oxidative damage in Alzheimer's and Parkinson's diseases and coenzyme Q10 as a potential treatment. *Journal of Bioenergetics & Biomembranes*, 36, 381-386.

Berman, K. & Brodaty, H. (2004). Tocopherol (vitamin E) in Alzheimer's disease and other neurodegenerative disorders. *CNS Drugs*, 18, 807-825.

Bertram, L. & Tanzi, R. E. (2004). The current status of Alzheimer's disease genetics: what do we tell the patients? *Pharmacological Research*, 50, 385-396.

Binder, L. I., Guillozet-Bongaarts, A. L., Garcia-Sierra, F., & Berry, R. W. (2005). Tau, tangles, and Alzheimer's disease. *Biochimica et Biophysica Acta*, 1739, 216-223.

Bishop, G. M. & Robinson, S. R. (2004). Physiological roles of amyloid-beta and implications for its removal in Alzheimer's disease. *Drugs & Aging*, 21, 621-630.

Braak, H. & Del Tredici, K. (2004). Alzheimer's disease: intraneuronal alterations precede insoluble amyloid-beta formation. *Neurobiology of Aging*, 25, 713-718.

Bullock, R. (2004). Future directions in the treatment of Alzheimer's disease. *Expert Opinion on Investigational Drugs*, 13, 303-314.

Caballero, J. & Nahata, M. (2004). Do statins slow down Alzheimer's disease? A review. *Journal of Clinical Pharmacy & Therapeutics*, 29, 209-213.

Cacquevel, M., Lebeurrier, N., Cheenne, S., & Vivien, D. (2004). Cytokines in neuroinflammation and Alzheimer's disease. *Current Drug Targets*, 5, 529-534.

Carro, E. & Torres-Aleman, I. (2004). The role of insulin and insulin-like growth factor I in the molecular and cellular mechanisms underlying the pathology of Alzheimer's disease. *European Journal of Pharmacology*, 490, 127-133.

Carter, D. B. (2005). The interaction of amyloid-beta with ApoE. *Sub-Cellular Biochemistry*, 38, 255-272.

Casserly, I. & Topol, E. (2004). Convergence of atherosclerosis and Alzheimer's disease: inflammation, cholesterol, and misfolded proteins. *Lancet*, 363, 1139-1146.

Chang, C. Y. & Silverman, D. H. (2004). Accuracy of early diagnosis and its impact on the management and course of Alzheimer's disease. *Expert Review of Molecular Diagnostics*, 4, 63-69.

Citron, M. (2004). Beta-secretase inhibition for the treatment of Alzheimer's disease—promise and challenge. *Trends in Pharmacological Sciences*, 25, 92-97.

Citron, M. (2004). Strategies for disease modification in Alzheimer's disease. *Nature Reviews Neuroscience*, 5, 677-685.

Coleman, P., Federoff, H., & Kurlan, R. (2004). A focus on the synapse for neuroprotection in Alzheimer disease and other dementias. *Neurology*, 63, 1155-1162.

Counts, S. E. & Mufson, E. J. (2005). The role of nerve growth factor receptors in cholinergic basal forebrain degeneration in prodromal Alzheimer disease. *Journal of Neuropathology & Experimental Neurology*, 64, 263-272.

Cummings, J. L. (2004). Alzheimer's disease. *New England Journal of Medicine*, 351, 56-67.

Dougall, N. J., Bruggink, S., & Ebmeier, K. P. (2004). Systematic review of the diagnostic accuracy of 99mTc-HMPAO-SPECT in dementia. *American Journal of Geriatric Psychiatry*, 12, 554-570.

Eikelenboom, P. & van Gool, W. A. (2004). Neuroinflammatory perspectives on the two faces of Alzheimer's disease. *Journal of Neural Transmission*, 111, 281-294.

Fillit, H. (2004). Intravenous immunoglobulins for Alzheimer's disease. *Lancet Neurology*, 3, 704.

Fratiglioni, L., Paillard-Borg, S., & Winblad, B. (2004). An active and socially integrated lifestyle in late life might protect against dementia. *Lancet Neurology*, 3, 343-353.

Fuentealba, R. A., Farias, G., Scheu, J., Bronfman, M., Marzolo, M. P., & Inestrosa, N. C. (2004). Signal transduction during amyloid-beta-peptide neurotoxicity: role in Alzheimer disease. *Brain Research—Brain Research Reviews*, 47, 275-289.

Gasparini, L., Ongini, E., & Wenk, G. (2004). Non-steroidal anti-inflammatory drugs (NSAIDs) in Alzheimer's disease: old and new mechanisms of action. *Journal of Neurochemistry*, 91, 521-536.

Gelinas, D. S., DaSilva, K., Fenili, D., George-Hyslop, P., & McLaurin, J. (2004). Immunotherapy for Alzheimer's disease. *Proceedings of the National Academy of Sciences of the United States of America*, 101(suppl 2), 14657-14662.

Gibson, G. E. & Huang, H. M. (2005). Oxidative stress in Alzheimer's disease. *Neurobiology of Aging*, 26, 575-578.

Golde, T. E. (2005). The abeta hypothesis: leading us to rationally designed therapeutic strategies for the treatment or prevention of Alzheimer disease. *Brain Pathology*, 15, 84-87.

Goni, F. & Sigurdsson, E. M. (2005). New directions towards safer and effective vaccines for Alzheimer's disease. *Current Opinion in Molecular Therapeutics*, 7, 17-23.

Gupta, V. B., Anitha, S., Hegde, M. L., Zecca, L., Garruto, R. M., Ravid, R., Shankar, S. K., Stein, R., Shanmugavelu, P., & Jagannatha Rao, K. S. (2005). Aluminium in Alzheimer's disease: are we still at a crossroad? *Cellular & Molecular Life Sciences*, 62, 143-158.

Hardy, J. (2004). Toward Alzheimer therapies based on genetic knowledge. *Annual Review of Medicine*, 55, 15-25.

Hartman, T. (2005). Cholesterol and Alzheimer's disease: statins, cholesterol depletion in APP processing and Abeta generation. *Sub-Cellular Biochemistry*, 38, 365-380.

Huang, X., Moir, R. D., Tanzi, R. E., Bush, A. I., & Rogers, J. T. (2004). Redox-active metals, oxidative stress, and Alzheimer's disease pathology. *Annals of the New York Academy of Sciences*, 1012, 153-163.

Hynd, M. R., Scott, H. L., & Dodd, P. R. (2004). Glutamate-mediated excitotoxicity and neurodegeneration in Alzheimer's disease. *Neurochemistry International*, 45, 583-595.

Iqbal, K., Alonso, A. C., Chen, S., Chohan, M. O., El Akkad, E., Gong, C. X., Khatoon, S., Li, B., Liu, F., Rahman, A., Tanimukai, H., & Grundke-Iqbal, I. (2005). Tau pathology in Alzheimer disease and other tauopathies. *Biochimica et Biophysica Acta*, 1739, 198-210.

Itzhaki, R. F., Wozniak, M. A., Appelt, D. M., & Balin, B. J. (2004). Infiltration of the brain by pathogens causes Alzheimer's disease. *Neurobiology of Aging*, 25, 619-627.

Kamboh, M. I. (2004). Molecular genetics of late-onset Alzheimer's disease. *Annals of Human Genetics*, 68, 381-404.

Kar, S., Slowikowski, S. P., Westaway, D., & Mount, H. T. (2004). Interactions between beta-amyloid and central cholinergic neurons: implications for Alzheimer's disease. *Journal of Psychiatry & Neuroscience*, 29, 427-441.

Kerr, M. L. & Small, D. H. (2005). Cytoplasmic domain of the beta-amyloid protein precursor of Alzheimer's disease: function, regulation of proteolysis, and implications for drug development. *Journal of Neuroscience Research*, 80, 151-159.

Lee, H. G., Moreira, P. I., Zhu, X., Smith, M. A., & Perry, G. (2004). Staying connected: synapses in Alzheimer disease. *American Journal of Pathology*, 165, 1461-1464.

Letenneur, L. (2004). Risk of dementia and alcohol and wine consumption: a review of recent results. *Biological Research*, 37, 189-193.

LeVine, H., III (2004). The amyloid hypothesis and the clearance and degradation of Alzheimer's beta-peptide. *Journal of Alzheimer's Disease*, 6, 303-314.

Liu, H., Wang, H., Shenvi, S., Hagen, T. M., & Liu, R. M. (2004). Glutathione metabolism during aging and in Alzheimer disease. *Annals of the New York Academy of Sciences,* 1019, 346-349.

Lott, I. T. & Head, E. (2005). Alzheimer disease and Down syndrome: factors in pathogenesis. *Neurobiology of Aging,* 26, 383-389.

Loy, C. & Schneider, L. (2004). Galantamine for Alzheimer's disease. *Cochrane Database of Systematic Reviews* CD001747.

Luchsinger, J. A. & Mayeux, R. (2004). Dietary factors and Alzheimer's disease. *Lancet Neurology,* 3, 579-587.

Lyketsos, C. G. & Lee, H. B. (2004). Diagnosis and treatment of depression in Alzheimer's disease. A practical update for the clinician. *Dementia & Geriatric Cognitive Disorders,* 17, 55-64.

Mattson, M. P. (2004). Pathways towards and away from Alzheimer's disease. *Nature,* 430, 631-639.

Moreira, P. I., Smith, M. A., Zhu, X., Honda, K., Lee, H. G., Aliev, G., & Perry, G. (2005). Oxidative damage and Alzheimer's disease: are antioxidant therapies useful? *Drug News & Perspectives,* 18, 13-19.

Nestor, P. J., Scheltens, P., & Hodges, J. R. (2004). Advances in the early detection of Alzheimer's disease. *Nature Medicine,* 10(suppl), S34-S41.

Nitsch, R. M. (2004). Immunotherapy of Alzheimer disease. *Alzheimer Disease & Associated Disorders,* 18, 185-189.

Pinkerton, J. V. & Henderson, V. W. (2005). Estrogen and cognition, with a focus on Alzheimer's disease. *Seminars in Reproductive Medicine,* 23, 172-179.

Plosker, G. L. & Lyseng-Williamson, K. A. (2005). Memantine: a pharmacoeconomic review of its use in moderate-to-severe Alzheimer's disease. *Pharmacoeconomics,* 23, 193-206.

Poirier, J. (2005). Apolipoprotein E, cholesterol transport and synthesis in sporadic Alzheimer's disease. *Neurobiology of Aging,* 26, 355-361.

Polidori, M. C. (2004). Oxidative stress and risk factors for Alzheimer's disease: clues to prevention and therapy. *Journal of Alzheimer's Disease,* 6, 185-191.

Pollack, S. J. & Lewis, H. (2005). Secretase inhibitors for Alzheimer's disease: challenges of a promiscuous protease. *Current Opinion in Investigational Drugs,* 6, 35-47.

Popescu, B. O. & Ankarcrona, M. (2004). Mechanisms of cell death in Alzheimer's disease: role of presenilins. *Journal of Alzheimer's Disease,* 6, 123-128.

Rachakonda, V., Pan, T. H., & LE, W. D. (2004). Biomarkers of neurodegenerative disorders: how good are they? *Cell Research,* 14, 347-358.

Refolo, L. M. & Fillit, H. M. (2004). Apolipoprotein E4 as a target for developing new therapeutics for Alzheimer's disease. *Journal of Molecular Neuroscience,* 23, 151-155.

Rossner, S., Lange-Dohna, C., Zeitschel, U., & Perez-Polo, J. R. (2005). Alzheimer's disease beta-secretase BACE1 is not a neuron-specific enzyme. *Journal of Neurochemistry,* 92, 226-234.

Schenk, D., Hagen, M., & Seubert, P. (2004). Current progress in beta-amyloid immunotherapy. *Current Opinion in Immunology,* 16, 599-606.

Selkoe, D. J. (2005). Defining molecular targets to prevent Alzheimer disease. *Archives of Neurology,* 62, 192-195.

Shen, Z. X. (2004). Brain cholinesterases: II. The molecular and cellular basis of Alzheimer's disease. *Medical Hypotheses,* 63, 308-321.

Silverman, D. H. & Alavi, A. (2000). PET imaging in the assessment of normal and impaired cognitive function. *Radiologic Clinics of North America,* 43, 67-77.

Sonkusare, S. K., Kaul, C. L., & Ramarao, P. (2005). Dementia of Alzheimer's disease and other neurodegenerative disorders—memantine, a new hope. *Pharmacological Research,* 51, 1-17.

Spires, T. L. & Hyman, B. T. (2004). Neuronal structure is altered by amyloid plaques. *Reviews in the Neurosciences,* 15, 267-278.

Standridge, J. B. (2004). Pharmacotherapeutic approaches to the prevention of Alzheimer's disease. *American Journal Geriatric Pharmacotherapy,* 2, 119-132.

Standridge, J. B. (2004). Pharmacotherapeutic approaches to the treatment of Alzheimer's disease. *Clinical Therapeutics,* 26, 615-630.

Stojakovic, T., Scharnagl, H., & Marz, W. (2004). ApoE: crossroads between Alzheimer's disease and atherosclerosis. *Seminars in Vascular Medicine,* 4, 279-285.

Stutzmann, G. E. (2005). Calcium dysregulation, IP3 signaling, and Alzheimer's disease. *Neuroscientist,* 11, 110-115.

Szekely, C. A., Thorne, J. E., Zandi, P. P., Ek, M., Messias, E., Breitner, J. C., & Goodman, S. N. (2004). Nonsteroidal anti-inflammatory drugs for the prevention of Alzheimer's disease: a systematic review. *Neuroepidemiology,* 23, 159-169.

Tanzi, R. E. & Bertram, L. (2005). Twenty years of the Alzheimer's disease amyloid hypothesis: a genetic perspective. *Cell,* 120, 545-555.

Thal, L. J. (2004). The Alzheimer's Disease Cooperative Study in 2004. *Alzheimer Disease & Associated Disorders,* 18, 183-185.

Tomita, T. & Iwatsubo, T. (2004). The inhibition of gamma-secretase as a therapeutic approach to Alzheimer's disease. *Drug News & Perspectives,* 17, 321-325.

Tsai, V. W., Scott, H. L., Lewis, R. J., & Dodd, P. R. (2005). The role of group I metabotropic glutamate receptors in neuronal excitotoxicity in Alzheimer's disease. *Neurotoxicity Research,* 7, 125-141.

Tuppo, E. E. & Arias, H. R. (2005). The role of inflammation in Alzheimer's disease. *International Journal of Biochemistry & Cell Biology,* 37, 289-305.

Vassar, R. (2004). BACE1: the beta-secretase enzyme in Alzheimer's disease. *Journal of Molecular Neuroscience,* 23, 105-114.

Vassar, R. (2005). beta-Secretase, APP and Abeta in Alzheimer's disease. *Sub-Cellular Biochemistry,* 38, 79-103.

Verdier, Y., Zarandi, M., & Penke, B. (2004). Amyloid beta-peptide interactions with neuronal and glial cell plasma membrane: binding sites and implications for Alzheimer's disease. *Journal of Peptide Science,* 10, 229-248.

Verdile, G., Fuller, S., Atwood, C. S., Laws, S. M., Gandy, S. E., & Martins, R. N. (2004). The role of beta amyloid in Alzheimer's disease: still a cause of everything or the only one who got caught? *Pharmacological Research,* 50, 397-409.

Walker, L. C., Ibegbu, C. C., Todd, C. W., Robinson, H. L., Jucker, M., LeVine, H., III, & Gandy, S. (2005). Emerging prospects for the disease-modifying treatment of Alzheimer's disease. *Biochemical Pharmacology,* 69, 1001-1008.

Walsh, D. M. & Selkoe, D. J. (2004). Deciphering the molecular basis of memory failure in Alzheimer's disease. *Neuron,* 44, 181-193.

Whitehead, A., Perdomo, C., Pratt, R. D., Birks, J., Wilcock, G. K., & Evans, J. G. (2004). Donepezil for the symptomatic treatment of patients with mild to moderate Alzheimer's disease: a meta-analysis of individual patient data from randomised controlled trials. *International Journal of Geriatric Psychiatry,* 19, 624-633.

Winblad, B. & Jelic, V. (2004). Long-term treatment of Alzheimer disease: efficacy and safety of acetylcholinesterase inhibitors. *Alzheimer Disease & Associated Disorders,* 18(suppl 1), S2-S8.

Wisniewski, T. & Frangione, B. (2005). Immunological and anti-chaperone therapeutic approaches for Alzheimer disease. *Brain Pathology,* 15, 72-77.

Zamrini, E., De Santi, S., & Tolar, M. (2004). Imaging is superior to cognitive testing for early diagnosis of Alzheimer's disease. *Neurobiology of Aging,* 25, 685-691.

Zhu, X., Raina, A. K., Perry, G., & Smith, M. A. (2004). Alzheimer's disease: the two-hit hypothesis. *Lancet Neurology,* 3, 219-226.

Zhu, X., Smith, M. A., Perry, G., & Aliev, G. (2004). Mitochondrial failures in Alzheimer's disease. *American Journal of Alzheimer's Disease & Other Dementias,* 19, 345-352.

Zlokovic, B. V. (2005). Neurovascular mechanisms of Alzheimer's neurodegeneration. *Trends in Neurosciences,* 28, 202-208.

Alzheimer Disease

INITIAL HISTORY

- 76-year-old woman.
- More socially withdrawn lately, told daughter she had not been feeling well.
- While shopping for groceries with daughter, patient became separated in the aisles. She became anxious, confused, and angry when store employees and others tried to assist her.
- Presented 30 minutes later.

Question 1.   *What is your differential diagnosis based on the information you now have?*

Question 2.   *What other questions would you like to ask now? (These questions should be asked of the patient first and then of a reliable historian separately.)*

ADDITIONAL HISTORY

- The daughter has noticed increased anxiety and confusion in her mother on several occasions.
- No personal or family history of psychologic illness.
- Daughter describes language problems such as trouble finding words.
- Problems with abstract thinking.
- Poor or decreased judgment.
- Disorientation in place and time.
- Changes in mood and behavior.
- Changes in personality.

□ **Gail L. Kongable, MSN, FNP, MPH contributed this case study.**

FURTHER HISTORY

- No history of trauma or recent infection.
- Family history: father and brother died from stroke and heart disease; mother had Alzheimer disease.
- Current medications: aspirin, 325 mg daily; hydrochlorothiazide, 25 mg bid.
- No other medical history.
- No known allergies.

Question 3.   *Now what do you think about her history?*

PHYSICAL EXAMINATION

- Alert elderly woman in no acute distress, anxious.
- T = 37° C orally; P = 85 and regular; RR = 15 and unlabored; BP 158/88 right arm (sitting).

HEENT, Skin, Neck

- Pupils are small and react to light sluggishly.
- Ocular fundus is pale; vessels are narrow and attenuated.
- Dentures present; buccal and pharyngeal membranes are moist without lesions or exudate.
- Skin is pale, dry with senile lentigines.
- Skin is transparent with decreased turgor.
- Multiple minor ecchymosis noted on forearms and dorsum of hands.
- No other lesions or abrasions.
- No lymphadenopathy, no thyromegaly.
- Trachea is midline.
- Carotid pulses full and equal bilaterally without bruit.
- No jugular venous distention.

Lungs

- Increased anterior/posterior diameter, with mild kyphosis.
- No shortness of breath.
- Lungs clear to auscultation throughout, bilaterally.

Cardiac

- Apical pulse at fifth ICS, L MCL.
- Regular rate and rhythm.
- Normal S_1, S_2; no murmurs, clicks, or rubs.

Abdomen, Extremities, Neurologic

- Round, symmetric with no apparent masses or hernias.
- No scars or lesions.
- Bowel sounds present; no bruits.
- Tympany to percussion in all quadrants; no masses or organomegaly.
- No redness, cyanosis, skin lesions.
- Symmetric with no swelling or atrophy.
- Warm bilaterally.
- All pulses present and equal bilaterally.
- No lymphadenopathy.
- Orientation to person, time, and place inconsistent—does not know the day or date.
- Pinprick, light touch, vibration intact; able to identify a key.
- Motor: No atrophy, weakness, or tremor; rapid alternating movements smooth.
- DTRs all 2+.
- No Babinski.

Musculoskeletal
- Gait slightly wide based; unable to tandem walk.
- No Romberg.
- Joints and muscles symmetric; no swelling, masses, deformities, tenderness.
- Mild kyphosis of the spine.
- Joints: Full, smooth range of motion; no crepitation, tenderness.
- Extremities: Able to maintain flexion and extension against resistance without tenderness.

Question 4.   *What studies would you initiate now while preparing your interventions?*

Question 5.   *What therapies would you initiate immediately while awaiting the results of the laboratory studies?*

LABORATORY RESULTS

- Head CT scan showed one small capsular infarction, no mass lesion or edema, no hydrocephalus.
- No significant abnormal results of chemistry, hematology, and metabolism screens.
- MMSE findings of impairment of memory and three other cognitive areas.
- Geriatric Depression Scale (GDS) is positive for memory difficulty, disrupted sleep-wake cycle, apathy, increased dependence (classic for Alzheimer disease).

Question 6.   *What does Alzheimer dementia look like on CT scan?*

EMERGENCY DEPARTMENT COURSE

- Patient is cooperative, in no apparent distress.
- Becomes less confused with repeated explanation of circumstances.
- Physical examination unchanged.
- Repeat laboratory studies: None.

Question 7.   *What do you think is happening?*

Question 8. *Now what should be done and what can the patient expect?*

HOSPITAL COURSE

- Response to therapy: Stable condition.
- Discharged to home in the care of daughter after 24 hours.
- Referral to neurologist for further evaluation of cognitive deficits and treatment.

Question 9. *What instructions and medications should this patient go home with?*

Question 10. *What steps can she take to prevent future problems?*

21

Epilepsy

DEFINITION

- Epilepsy, as defined by the Commission on Epidemiology and Prognosis of Epilepsy, is the occurrence of at least two unprovoked seizures with at least a 24-hour separation between them.
- Neither seizure nor epilepsy is a diagnosis or disease entity itself; it is a symptom of other processes that affect the brain in a variety of ways but have seizures as their final common clinical expression.
- Seizures are the cardinal manifestation of epilepsy, though not all patients with seizures have epilepsy.
- A seizure is an excessive or abnormal sudden, high-frequency discharge of the brain's neurons.
- Status epilepticus is defined as continuous or repeating seizures that occur so rapidly that the patient does not recover consciousness between them.

CLASSIFICATION

- The diagnosis, treatment, and prognosis of seizure disorders depend on the correct identification of types of seizures and epilepsy. There are two currently accepted classification schemes: the International Classification of Epileptic Seizures [ICES] and the International Classification of Epilepsies and Epileptic Syndromes [ICEES].
- **Overview of ICES.**
  - **Partial seizures:** Begin in a focal or restricted part of the cortex. They may evolve into secondarily generalized seizures.
    1. Simple partial seizures: Consciousness is not impaired. They are further subdivided into various categories based on signs and symptoms produced by the seizure.
    2. Complex partial seizures: Consciousness is impaired. Complex partial seizures can arise from any cortical area, yet they are frequently considered equivalent to temporal lobe seizures and are frequently preceded by an aura.
  - **Generalized seizures:** Begin with epileptiform activity over the entire cortex. There are two major types of generalized seizures (and many other less common types).
    1. Absence seizures are brief generalized seizures without prominent motor manifestations and are typically associated with a generalized 3-Hz spike-and-wave pattern on an electroencephalogram (EEG).
    2. Tonic-clonic seizures often evolve from tonic to clonic movements. The tonic phase causes sudden, sustained tone, and is frequently manifested as flexor or extensor posturing. This may be accompanied by a guttural cry as air is forced out

□ Lucy R. Paskus, RN, MSN, CPNP coauthored this chapter.

of closed vocal cords. The clonic phase results in a relatively symmetric, bilateral, synchronous, and semirhythmic jerking of the upper and lower extremities, increasing in amplitude and decreasing in frequency as the seizure progresses.

- Unclassified epileptic seizures: In practice, seizures may not always fall clearly into one category, although it is important to remember that a single patient may present with several different seizure types.
- Overview of ICEES.
  - Like ICES, ICEES divides seizure types into partial, generalized, and undetermined. Whereas ICES categorizes seizure type, ICEES expands this classification scheme to include more information about the cause and clinical manifestations of the seizure. Subcategories of the epilepsies and epileptic syndromes include the following:
    1. Idiopathic: Most common; no obvious underlying cause or pathologic alteration other than a presumed genetic predisposition.
    2. Symptomatic: Occur as a result of a defined cerebral disorder.
    3. Cryptogenic: Suspected to be symptomatic despite absence of definitive proof of the underlying cause.
- Both the ICES and ICEES are useful but they also they have their limitations. Both are so detailed as to be impractical for most nonneurologists; new classification schemes are being proposed.

EPIDEMIOLOGY

- Epilepsy is one of the most common chronic neurologic disorders in the United States, with a prevalence of approximately 0.5%.
- The cumulative lifetime risk of having a seizure is 8%.
- Half the lifetime risk of developing epilepsy occurs during childhood or adolescence.
- During childhood, rates are highest during the first year of life and then drop sharply; rates drop off again during adolescence; older than age 50, the rate of epilepsy begins to increase again, secondary to cerebrovascular disease and cerebral vascular accidents.
- The mortality rate of a patient with epilepsy is two to four times that of the nonepileptic population, with the mortality being highest in the 10 years after diagnosis.
- 10% of deaths in patients with epilepsy are directly related to a seizure or status epilepticus, whereas 5% of deaths are secondary to a fatal accident during a seizure.
- The suicide risk in people with epilepsy is 25 times that of the general population.

PATHOPHYSIOLOGY

Genetics

- A few of the familial epilepsies have been found to have a genetic basis, with mutations in the ion channels that modulate neuronal firing. However, for the vast majority of the epilepsies, a genetic link has yet to be discovered.
- Mutations in *SCN1B*, which encodes a voltage-gated sodium-channel subunit, are associated with generalized epilepsy, and mutations in *KCNQ2* and *KCNQ3*, which both encode potassium channels, are associated with benign familial neonatal convulsions.

Tissue Effects

- One or more of the following mechanisms are postulated to be involved in the genesis and spread of epileptic discharges.
  - Disturbance in the excitation/inhibition balance in the hypothalamus is thought to be a major factor in the etiology of epilepsy.
    1. Excitatory amino acids (EAAs) are in a physiologic balance with the inhibitory neurotransmitters. Glutamate, an EAA, is the primary excitatory neurotransmitter in the central nervous system and acts primarily through activation of the *N*-methyl-D-aspartate (NMDA) receptors.

2. Gamma-aminobutyric acid (GABA) is the primary inhibitory neurotransmitter, and decreases in GABA activity are common in epileptic conditions.

3. Both decreased GABAergic inhibition and increased glutamatergic excitation are thought to be critically involved in the cellular mechanisms underlying the initiation and spread of epileptic seizures and the processes that lead to epileptogenesis and, as a consequence, chronic epilepsy.

4. Many new antiepileptic drugs (AEDs) are targeted at enhancing GABA activity. Decreasing glutamatergic activity is more difficult because available NMDA antagonists are excessively neurotoxic. Studies are ongoing to evaluate newer drugs aimed at inhibiting glutamate activity.

- Changes in voltage-regulated ion channels in neuronal membranes lead to excessive depolarization or excessive action potential firing. Potential ion channel defects include those involving the voltage-sensitive calcium, potassium, or sodium channels, and sodium/hydrogen exchangers.

- Changes in gap junctions result in altered interneuronal communication and changes in neural synchrony. These gap junctions are influenced by serum pH (alkalosis tends to stimulate epileptogenic communication, whereas acidosis inhibits it), but there are no current pharmacologic therapies that target the gap junction. A ketogenic diet may affect the gap junction via changes in pH.

- Hippocampal sclerosis with aberrant neuronal connections due to sprouting of dentate granule cells may lead to hyperexcitability and has been implicated in partial seizure pathogenesis.

- Cortical malformations are also implicated in epileptogenesis. These malformations include localized cellular dysplasias or more global abnormalities, and can be classified as disorders of neuronal proliferation, neuronal migration, or cortical organization.

PATIENT PRESENTATION

History

Positive family history of seizures; febrile seizures as a child; head injury; central nervous system (CNS) infection; stroke; heart disease; reported lapses of consciousness; episodes of incontinence; seizure activity witnessed by others; history of motor vehicle accidents or other unexplained injuries; alcohol or drug abuse or toxicity.

Symptoms

Localized seizure-like movements on one part of the body; episodic loss of consciousness; focal neurologic deficits; visual changes; headache; confusion; incontinence, tongue-biting; fatigue; tearfulness; incontinence; symptoms from injuries.

Examination

Between seizures, the examination may be completely normal; witnessed seizures allow for confirmation of the diagnosis; focal neurologic findings; evidence of injury; evidence of drug or alcohol abuse.

DIFFERENTIAL DIAGNOSIS

- Not seizures.
  - Syncope: Cardiogenic (arrhythmias), orthostatic changes, cerebral, neurocardiogenic (e.g., vasovagal).
  - Psychogenic "seizures"; parasomnias; somatoform disorder; malingering; factitious disorder (e.g., Munchausen syndrome).
  - Migraines.
- Seizures.
  - Metabolic: Fat embolism, porphyria.
  - Vascular pathology (transient ischemic attacks, stroke), hypertensive encephalopathy, eclampsia.

- Neoplastic: Tumor, lymphoma, leukemia, metastatic cancer.
- Drug induced: Antipsychotics, theophylline, tricyclic antidepressants, meperidine, cyclosporin, cisplatin, and β-lactam antibiotics can cause seizures at therapeutic doses.
- Drug withdrawal: Anticonvulsants, benzodiazepines, barbiturates, baclofen, alcohol and illicit drug abuse/withdrawal.
- Endocrine: Hypoglycemia, hypo-/hypernatremia, hypo-/hypercalcemia.
- Anoxia: Cardiac arrest, carbon monoxide poisoning, asphyxiation.
- Fever: More common in young children.
- Infections: Cerebral abscess, meningitis/encephalitis, cerebral malaria.
- Cranial trauma: Especially penetrating.
- Immune: Acute demyelination, cerebral vasculitis.

KEYS TO ASSESSMENT

- Goals of evaluation are as follows:
    - Verify that a seizure has occurred.
        1. Post-event confusion and lateral tongue-biting are strong indicators that a seizure has occurred.
        2. Epilepsy is essentially a clinical diagnosis, and more than one witnessed classical generalized tonic-clonic or absence seizures can be diagnostic of epilepsy.
        3. Obtain a detailed patient interview and, if possible, an interview of those who witnessed the seizure; these subjective accounts can assist in differential diagnosis, as well as establishing seizure type.
    - Rapidly identify potential life-threatening causes (trauma, myocardial infarction, stroke, metabolic disarray, drug toxicity).
        1. When a seizure occurs within well-defined circumstances, such as a stroke or head injury, the focus should be on treating the underlying cause and preventing recurrence of the seizure.
        2. An urgent metabolic and toxic screening is necessary for every patient presenting with a first generalized seizure, with particular attention paid to natremia and glycemia.
    - When the patient is known to have epilepsy and is under treatment, a seizure should not be managed in the atmosphere of an emergency; priority should be placed on understanding what triggered the seizure (e.g., improper medication use, alcohol, skipped meals, sleep deprivation, stress, fever, menstrual period, strong emotions, intense exercise, flashing lights, loud music).
    - Patient history.
        1. Medication history: To rule out iatrogenic seizures.
        2. Medical history: Head injury, stroke, Alzheimer disease, intracranial infection, drug or alcohol abuse.
        3. Family history: Family history of seizures, in particular absence and myoclonic seizures may be inherited.
    - Physical examination should include a thorough neurologic examination to look for focal deficits.
        1. When the neurologic examination is abnormal, magnetic resonance imaging (MRI) becomes urgent.
        2. Following a normal neurologic examination, patients should have an EEG and MRI on an outpatient basis; the MRI should be scheduled as soon as possible if the EEG shows abnormal activity.
        3. In addition to the neurologic examination, a cardiovascular examination that includes heart auscultation and orthostatic blood pressure should be undertaken.
    - EEG.
        1. EEG is essential for the use of the ICES and ICEES to appropriately categorize and manage epilepsy.
        2. EEG can support but never exclude the diagnosis of epilepsy.

3. In an isolated first seizure, EEG findings may be of little value in predicting risk of recurrence, but may be used in deciding when to initiate treatment with AEDs.
4. Incidence of epileptiform activity in people without seizures is 0% to 3.8%.
5. Many patients with epilepsy have a normal EEG on one or more occasions.
6. Repetition of EEGs and the use of different activations (hyperventilation, photic stimulation, sleep deprivation) increase the chances of finding paroxysmal activity in epileptic patients.
7. The interictal EEG recording is an important localizing and prognostic tool in epilepsy surgery evaluation.

- MRI.
    1. Demonstrates structural lesions (cortical dysplasias, infarcts, or tumors), though not necessarily epileptogenic focus.
    2. Crucial in presurgical evaluation.
    3. Experimental: Functional MRI (fMRI) and MR spectroscopic imaging (MRSI).
- ECG.
    1. Recommended in older adults.
    2. May be useful if seizure or syncope occurred with exertion.
- Lumbar puncture (LP): Indicated if an acute infectious process is suspected, after neuroimaging studies have ruled out intracranial hypertension.
- Positron emission tomography (PET): May identify the foci of epileptogenesis as areas of interictal hypometabolism.
- Single photon emission computed tomography (SPECT): Measures distribution of blood flow; can be applied during seizures because tracers can be mixed at the bedside.

KEYS TO MANAGEMENT

- Goals of management.
    - To control seizures.
    - Avoid side effects of treatment.
    - Maintain or restore quality of life.
- Initiating treatment.
    - Not all patients with seizures require a referral to a neurologist; however, those who present with focal neurologic findings (by history, examination, or EEG) should be referred.
    - The optimal treatment plan is derived following an accurate diagnosis of the patient's seizure type(s), an objective measure of the intensity and frequency of seizures, awareness of medication side effects, and an evaluation of disease-related psychosocial issues.
- Pharmacologic agents.
    - In a patient with one seizure and without risk factors for recurrence (prior neurologic injury or lesions, history of epilepsy in a sibling, or an EEG with generalized epileptiform discharges), it is reasonable to withhold AEDs if the patient is willing and informed.
    - After a second seizure, the risk for recurrence is 80% to 90%, and the patient should be treated with AEDs. Risks for recurrence include history of serious brain injury, brain lesion on CT or MRI, focal neurologic examination, mental retardation, abnormal EEG, and that the first seizure was a partial seizure.
    - AEDs: The common link among older and new AEDs is their ability to moderate excitatory and inhibitory neurotransmission by affecting several different sites such as ion channels, neurotransmitter receptors, and neurotransmitter metabolism.
        1. Drugs that block voltage-dependent sodium channels: Carbamazepine, phenytoin, lamotrigine, oxcarbazepine, zonisamide.
        2. Drugs that affect calcium channels: Ethosuximide.
        3. Drugs that affect GABA metabolism: Phenobarbital, tiagabine, vigabatrin, benzodiazepines.

4. Drugs with multiple mechanisms of action: Valproate, felbamate, topiramate, pregabalin (under U.S. Food and Drug Administration [FDA] review).
5. Drugs with unknown mechanism of action: Gabapentin, levetiracetam.

- Generally the "newer" AEDs have lower side effect rates, little or no need for serum monitoring, once or twice daily dosing for some, and fewer drug interactions. However, the newer AEDs are expensive and may pose a significant financial burden on many patients. The more commonly used "older" and "newer" AEDs are listed below.

"Older" AEDs	"Newer" AEDs
Phenytoin	Felbamate
Carbamazepine	Gabapentin
Phenobarbital	Lamotrigine
Valproic acid	Tiagabine
Benzodiazepines	Topiramate
	Vigabatin
	Zonisamide
	Oxcarbazepine
	Ethosuximide
	Levetiracetam

- A working knowledge of available AEDs including their mechanism of action, pharmacokinetics, drug-drug interactions, and adverse effects is essential.
- The goal for pharmacologic therapy in epilepsy is monotherapy. Monotherapy is often equally or more effective than combination therapy and better tolerated; it has fewer drug interactions, better compliance, lower cost, and improved quality of life.
- The nature of the seizure that the patient is experiencing, as well as the specific epileptic syndrome, may influence the choice of AED.
- Approximately 70% of patients can achieve seizure control with AEDs.
- Dosing of medications.
    1. A very low dose is given for the first few days, then dosage is gradually increased.
    2. Generalized tonic-clonic seizures typically require a lower dose than partial seizures.
    3. With an increase in dosage level comes increased adverse drug reactions.
    4. The final decision about which dosage level is appropriate will take into account the individual characteristics of the patient and a complete and detailed medical and social history is helpful in choosing the appropriate AED dosage level.
- The best AED is the one that controls seizures without causing unacceptable side effects.
- Patients should be urged to not start any other prescription, over-the-counter medication, or herbal remedies without first contacting the primary care provider because these might affect the serum concentration of their AED.
- Combination or polytherapy in drug-resistant epilepsy.
    1. Combination therapy is generally used after failure of successive monotherapy (at least two adequate sequential trials of single agents).
    2. Combine drugs with different mechanisms of action.
    3. Avoid drugs with similar adverse effects.
- The role of plasma drug concentrations.
    1. Routine drug monitoring is not recommended at this time; however, measurement of drug levels may provide important references in adjusting dosages, ruling out noncompliance, and toxicity.
    2. Many of the new AEDs demonstrate marked inter- and intraindividual pharmacodynamic variability, and the role of therapeutic drug monitoring is being explored.
- Deciding when to stop drug therapy in the seizure-free patient.
    1. A patient on monotherapy who has been seizure free more than 2 years may be a candidate for drug withdrawal.

2. An abnormal EEG offers a poor prognosis of successful medication withdrawal.
3. Implications of drug withdrawal should be discussed with the patient, especially the probability of relapse.
4. If withdrawal is indicated and agreed upon, it should take place gradually over no less than 2 to 6 months.
5. For patients on combination therapy, taper one drug at a time.

- Surgical management.
  - Surgery is typically reserved for those patients who fail medical management, but it is probably underused in the management of refractory epilepsy.
  - There must be a well-localized epileptogenic focus, and the focus must be located such that the surgery would not result in severe speech or memory deficits.
  - The prototype of surgically remediable epilepsy syndromes is temporal lobe epilepsy, one of the most common forms of epilepsy and also one of the most refractory.
  - Surgical options include anterior corpus callostomy, functional hemispherectomy, resective surgery, multiple subpial resections, gamma-knife surgery, vagus nerve stimulation, and deep brain stimulation.
  - Only complete resection of the epileptogenic brain region offers the possibility of cure. Other surgical options are palliative.
  - Pediatric epilepsy surgery is increasing secondary to the delineation of certain catastrophic epileptic disorders of infants and young children and the greater understanding of the plasticity of the developing brain.
- Treatment of epilepsy in women.
  1. There are increasing concerns about the interaction of AEDs and endocrine function that can affect ovarian function, induce polycystic ovary–like syndrome, and threaten fertility.
  2. Sex hormone fluctuations during maturation may exacerbate seizures at particular points during the life cycle for women, including menarche, menses, pregnancy, and perimenopausal years. Seizures may become less predictable with menopause due to the abrupt decline of estrogen and progesterone.
  3. There is the potential for catamenial epilepsy (seizures associated with menstrual cycle) related to relative lack of progesterone during the luteal phase of the cycle (estrogen is proconvulsant, and progesterone is anticonvulsant).
  4. Complex partial seizures usually arise from the medial temporal lobe structures, and epileptic activity may propagate to the hypothalamus, altering normal pituitary gonadotropic hormone release, which in turn alters sex steroid release, resulting in anovulatory cycles, infertility, and irregular menses.
  5. Seizure frequency may be increased during pregnancy, with serum levels of AEDs gradually decreasing as pregnancy progresses.
  6. In children born to women with epilepsy, there is an increased risk for infant mortality, congenital malformation, low birthweight, developmental delays, and neonatal hemorrhage (important to supplement with vitamin K during the last month of pregnancy in women taking AEDs).
  7. Use of AEDs may reduce folate levels; higher maintenance doses of 0.4 to 5 mg/day are often used to decrease the risk of fetal neural tube defects in patients with epilepsy who have childbearing potential.
  8. Enzyme-inducing AEDs (EIAEDs) may substantially reduce circulating estrogen levels, reducing the effectiveness of some oral contraceptive pills (OCPs); therefore OCPs containing 50 mcg of ethinyl estradiol are recommended for all women taking EIAEDs. OCPs with progesterone (anticonvulsant) may actually result in seizure modification.
  9. Osteopathies are being reported with increasing frequency; metabolic bone disease is a recognized consequence of using hepatic EIAEDs, due to interference with calcium absorption and vitamin D metabolism. Early measures of bone health should be considered, and all patients who have been taking AEDs for

more than 5 years should be evaluated. Vitamin D and calcium should be supplemented as indicated.

10. The choice of AED should be based on the stage of the woman's reproductive age, including efficacy for her type of epilepsy and potential for adverse events, interaction with contraception, and teratogenicity.

- Special issues in the elderly.
    1. The occurrence of new-onset seizures rises sharply in older adults; cerebrovascular accidents account for as much as 40% to 50% of new-onset symptomatic epilepsy.
    2. New-onset seizures in older adults are typically cryptogenic or symptomatic partial seizures that require long-term treatment.
    3. These seizures have a high risk for recurrence because of their identified or suspected focal pathology; even with nonspecific or unrevealing MRI and EEG findings it is appropriate to begin AED treatment following the first seizure.
    4. AED treatment for these seizures should be presumed to be lifelong, and selection of an AED should consider tolerability, side effects, and pharmacokinetics as much as efficacy.
    5. New-onset epileptic seizures in the older adult are often controlled with relatively modest dosages; titrate the drug slowly with a low target dose to reduce side effects.
    6. Take into consideration that even healthy older adult patients have age-dependent decreases in renal and hepatic function, as well as decreased volume of distribution and degree of protein binding.

- Social issues.
    1. Patients newly diagnosed with epilepsy may suffer a number of losses including loss of independence, employment, insurance, ability to drive, and self-esteem. Driving is legally restricted in most states following a new diagnosis of epilepsy.
    2. Long-term effects include social stigma and possible cognitive decline.
    3. Awareness of comorbid conditions such as depression and adverse medication effects is important.
    4. There is the potential for adverse cosmetic effects of treatment such as coarsening of facial features, excessive hair growth, gingival hyperplasia, weight gain, and tremor, which for some patients may be worse than the original condition.

PATHOPHYSIOLOGY $\longrightarrow$	CLINICAL LINK
What is going on in the disease process that influences how the patient presents and how he or she should be managed?	*What should you do now that you understand the underlying pathophysiology?*
Seizures are categorized by their clinical appearance and EEG pattern; these categories are correlated with prognosis and response to medication.	A careful history of a seizure from observers, as well as an EEG, is essential to the appropriate identification of the seizure type and selection of the proper drug.
Seizures are most likely the result of an imbalance of excitatory (glutamate) and inhibitory (GABA) neurotransmitters and/or abnormal ionic exchange at the neuronal membrane.	The older AEDs work primarily by stabilizing neuronal membrane ionic activity; the newer drugs are aimed at modulating glutamate and/or GABA activity.
Seizures can result from many causes, including anoxia, space-occupying lesions, infarctions, toxins, metabolic disarray, trauma, and infections.	A thorough evaluation with special emphasis on the neurologic examination and laboratories is essential in the new-onset seizure patient, and an MRI should be done quickly if there is any evidence of localized neurologic disease.
An EEG can be abnormal in people without epilepsy and can be normal in patients with epilepsy.	The EEG is most useful in the evaluation of new-onset seizures if it can be correlated by observed epileptic activity; thus activators, such as sleep deprivation, hyperventilation, and photic stimulation with observation of the patient, may be indicated to confirm the diagnosis.
The efficacy and side effects of the AEDs vary significantly among individual patients.	The selection of appropriate pharmacologic management must also be based on psychosocial information obtained from the patient and family.
Hormone changes in women throughout the menstrual cycle, with the use of oral contraceptives, and with pregnancy are associated with an increased risk of seizures. In addition, epilepsy and the use of AEDs during pregnancy is associated with many potential complications for the infant.	Women with epilepsy require a high level of vigilance for potential complications, and expert management especially during pregnancy.

SUGGESTED READINGS

Arunkumar, G. & Morris H. (1998). Epilepsy update: new medical and surgical treatment options. *Cleveland Clinic Journal of Medicine*, 65(10), 527-532, 534-537.

Beaumont, A. & Whittle, I. R. (2000). The pathogenesis of tumour associated epilepsy. *Acta Neurochirurgica*, 142(1), 1-15.

Bergey, G. (2004). Initial treatment of epilepsy: special issues in treating the elderly. *Neurology*, 63(10 suppl 4), S40-S48.

Bernard, C., Cossart, R., Hirsch, J. C., Esclapez, M., & Ben Ari, Y. (2000). What is GABAergic inhibition? How is it modified in epilepsy? *Epilepsia*, 41(suppl 6), S90-S95.

Binnie, C. D. (2000). Vagus nerve stimulation for epilepsy: a review. *Seizure*, 9(3), 161-169.

Bowman, E. S. & Coons, P. M. (2000). The differential diagnosis of epilepsy, pseudoseizures, dissociative identity disorder, and dissociative disorder not otherwise specified. *Bulletin of the Menninger Clinic*, 64(2), 164-180.

Burgess, D. L. & Noebels, J .L. (2000). Calcium channel defects in models of inherited generalized epilepsy. *Epilepsia*, 41(8), 1074-1075.

Carlen, P. L., Skinner, F., Zhang, L., Naus, C., Kushnir, M., & Perez Velazquez, I. J. (2000). The role of gap junctions in seizures. *Brain Research—Brain Research Reviews*, 32(1), 235-241.

Chapman, A. G. (2000). Glutamate and epilepsy. *Journal of Nutrition*, 130(4S), 1043S-1045S.

Cramer, J. A., Fisher, R., Ben Menachem, E., French, J., & Mattson, R. H. (1999). New antiepileptic drugs: comparison of key clinical trials. *Epilepsia*, 40(5), 590-600.

Devinsky, O. (1999). Patients with refractory seizures. *New England Journal of Medicine*, 340(20), 1565-1570.

Dubeau, F. & McLachlan, R. S. (2000). Invasive electrographic recording techniques in temporal lobe epilepsy. *Canadian Journal of Neurological Sciences*, 27(Suppl), 34.

Engel, J., Jr. (1999). The timing of surgical intervention for mesial temporal lobe epilepsy: a plan for a randomized clinical trial. *Archives of Neurology*, 56(11), 1338-1341.

Ensom, M. H. (2000). Gender-based differences and menstrual cycle-related changes in specific diseases: implications for pharmacotherapy. *Pharmacotherapy*, 20(5), 523-539.

Feely, M. (1999). Fortnightly review: drug treatment of epilepsy. *British Medical Journal*, 318(7176), 106-109.

Fowle, A. J. & Binnie, C. D. (2000). Uses and abuses of the EEG in epilepsy. *Epilepsia*, 41(suppl 3), S10-S18.

Gilliam, F., Carter, J., & Vahle, V. (2004). Tolerability of antiseizure medications: implications for health outcomes. *Neurology*, 63(10 suppl 4), S9-S12.

Gordon, N. (2000). Cognitive functions and epileptic activity. *Seizure*, 9(3), 184-188.

Greenwood, R. S. (2000). Adverse effects of antiepileptic drugs. *Epilepsia*, 41(suppl 2), S42-S52.

Greenwood, R. S. & Tennison, M. B. (1999). When to start and stop anticonvulsant therapy in children. *Archives of Neurology*, 56(9), 1073-1077.

Harden, C. (2003). Menopause and bone density issues for women with epilepsy. *Neurology*, 61(6 suppl 2), S16-S22.

Hirose, S., Okada, M., Kaneko, S., & Mitsudome, A. (2000). Are some idiopathic epilepsies disorders of ion channels? A working hypothesis. *Epilepsy Research*, 41(3), 191-204.

Jones, M. W. & Anderman, F. (2000). Temporal lobe epilepsy surgery: definition of candidacy. *Canadian Journal of Neurological Sciences*, 27(suppl 1), S11-S13.

Juhasz, C., Chugani, D. C., Muzik, O., Watson, C., Shah, J., Shah, A., & Chugani, H. T. (2000). Relationship between EEG and positron emission tomography abnormalities in clinical epilepsy. *Journal of Clinical Neurophysiology*, 17(1), 29-42.

Krumholz, A. (1999). Nonepileptic seizures: diagnosis and management. *Neurology*, 53(5 suppl 2), S76-S83.

Lester, H. A. & Karschin, A. (2000). Gain of function mutants: ion channels and G protein-coupled receptors. *Annual Review of Neuroscience*, 23, 89-125.

Liporace, J. & D'Abreu, A. (2003). Epilepsy and women's health: family planning, bone health, menopause, and menstrual related seizures. *Mayo Clinic Proceedings*, 78(4), 497-506.

Logsdon-Pokorny, V. K. (2000). Epilepsy in adolescents: hormonal considerations. *Journal of Pediatric & Adolescent Gynecology*, 13(1), 9-13.

Loscher, W. (1998). Pharmacology of glutamate receptor antagonists in the kindling model of epilepsy. *Progress in Neurobiology*, 54(6), 721-741.

Mattson, R.H. (1998). Medical management of epilepsy in adults. *Neurology*, 51(5 suppl 4), S15-S20.

McAbee, G. N. & Wark, J. E. (2000). A practical approach to uncomplicated seizures in children. *American Family Physician*, 62(5), 1109-1116.

Morrell, M. J. (1999). Epilepsy in women: the science of why it is special. *Neurology*, 53(4 suppl 1), S42-S48.

Moshe, S. L. (2000). Mechanisms of action of anticonvulsant agents. *Neurology*, 55(5 suppl 1), S32-S40.

Nguyen, D. & Spencer, S. (2003). Recent advances in the treatment of epilepsy. *Archives of Neurology*, 60(7), 929-935.

Nsour, W. M., Lau, C. B. S., & Wong, I. C. (2000). Review on phytotherapy in epilepsy. *Seizure*, 9(2), 96-107.

Pachlatko, C. (1999). The relevance of health economics to epilepsy care. *Epilepsia*, 40(suppl 7).

Parrent, A. G. & Lozano, A. M. (2000). Stereotactic surgery for temporal lobe epilepsy. *Canadian Journal of Neurological Sciences*, 27(suppl 1), S79-S84.

Pellock, J. M. (1999). Managing pediatric epilepsy syndromes with new antiepileptic drugs. *Pediatrics*, 104(5:Pt 1), 1106-1116.

Perucca, E. (2000). Is there a role for therapeutic drug monitoring of new anticonvulsants? *Clinical Pharmacokinetics*, 38(3), 191-204.

Pimentel, J. (2000). Current issues on epileptic women. *Current Pharmaceutical Design*, 6(8), 865-872.

Prasad, A. N., Prasad, C., & Stafstrom, C. E. (1999). Recent advances in the genetics of epilepsy: insights from human and animal studies. *Epilepsia*, 40(10), 1329-1352.

Rho, J. M. & Sankar, R. (1999). The pharmacologic basis of antiepileptic drug action. *Epilepsia*, 40(11), 1471-1483.

Rogawski, M. A. (2000). KCNQ2/KCNQ3 K+ channels and the molecular pathogenesis of epilepsy: implications for therapy. *Trends in Neurosciences*, 23(9), 393-398.

Schachter, S. (2005). Evaluation of the first seizure in adults. *UpToDate* online 13.2. www.uptodate.com [literature review for version 13.2 is current through April 2005, topic last changed on May 10, 2005].

Schachter, S. (2005). Overview of the management of epilepsy in adults. *UpToDate* online 13.2. www.uptodate.com [literature review for version 13.2 is current through April 2005, topic last changed on May 5, 2005].

Schachter, S. (2005). Pharmacology of antiepileptic drugs. *UpToDate* online 13.2. www.uptodate.com [literature review for version 13.2 is current through April 2005, topic last changed on May 6, 2005].

Silfvenius, H. (1999). Cost and cost-effectiveness of epilepsy surgery. *Epilepsia*, 40(suppl 8), 32-39.

Sloviter, R. S. (1999). Status epilepticus-induced neuronal injury and network reorganization. *Epilepsia*, 40(suppl 1), S34-S39.

So, E. L. (2000). Integration of EEG, MRI, and SPECT in localizing the seizure focus for epilepsy surgery. *Epilepsia*, 41(suppl 3), S48-S54.

So, E. L., O'Brien, T. J., Brinkmann, B. H., & Mullan, B. P. (2000). The EEG evaluation of single photon emission computed tomography abnormalities in epilepsy. *Journal of Clinical Neurophysiology*, 17(1), 10-28.

Smith, P. & Cossburn, M. (2004). Seizures: assessment and management in the emergency unit. *Clinical Medicine*, 4(2), 118-122.

Stephen, L. J. & Brodie, M. J. (2000). Epilepsy in elderly people. *Lancet*, 355(9213), 1441-1446.

Swann, J. W., Lee, C. L., Smith, K. L., & Hrachovy, R. A. (2000). Developmental neuroplasticity and epilepsy. *Epilepsia*, 41(8), 1078-1079.

Tatum, W., Liporace, J., Benbadis, S., & Kaplan, P. (2004). Updates on the treatment of epilepsy in women. *Archives of Internal Medicine*, 164(2), 137-145.

Tomson, T. (2000). Mortality in epilepsy. *Journal of Neurology*, 247(1), 15-21.

Tomson, T. & Johannessen, S. I. (2000). Therapeutic monitoring of the new antiepileptic drugs. *European Journal of Clinical Pharmacology*, 55(10), 697-705.

Tuxhorn, I., Moch, A., & Holthausen, H. (2000). Pediatric epilepsy surgery: state of the art, recent developments and future perspectives. *Epileptic Disorders*, 2(1), 53-55.

Vazquez, B. (2004). Monotherapy in epilepsy: role of the newer antiepileptic drugs. *Archives of Neurology*, 61(9), 1361-1365.

Waagepetersen, H. S., Sonnewald, U., & Schousboe, A. (1999). The GABA paradox: multiple roles as metabolite, neurotransmitter, and neurodifferentiative agent. *Journal of Neurochemistry*, 73(4), 1335-1342.

Wiebe, S. (2000). Epidemiology of temporal lobe epilepsy. *Canadian Journal of Neurological Sciences*, 27(suppl 1), S6-S10.

Willmore, L. J. (1998). Epilepsy emergencies: the first seizure and status epilepticus. *Neurology*, 51(5 suppl 4), S34-S38.

Yerby, M. S. (2000). Quality of life, epilepsy advances, and the evolving role of anticonvulsants in women with epilepsy. *Neurology*, 55(5 suppl 1), S54-S58.

Epilepsy

INITIAL HISTORY

- 15-year-old boy.
- Playing touch football when symptoms developed.
- Became unreasonably angry at his friend.
- Fell to the ground with sudden onset of unconsciousness.
- His body stiffened with arms and legs extended.
- He did not breathe for about 10 seconds.
- He then began violent, rhythmic, muscular contractions accompanied by strenuous hyperventilation that lasted 2 to 3 minutes.
- Incontinent of urine.
- He then lay limp, breathing rapidly, and woke up confused.
- Presented 1 hour later in the emergency department.

Question 1. *What is your differential diagnosis based on the information you now have?*

Question 2. *What other questions would you like to ask now?*

ADDITIONAL HISTORY

- No memory of the event; first memory was of finding himself on the ground.
- No history of seizures.
- Denies taking any drugs or alcohol.
- No recent upper respiratory or other infections of ears or sinuses.
- History of minor head injury as a child with loss of consciousness.
- Had complained of headache to his mother earlier in the day.

□ **Gail L. Kongable, MSN, FNP, MPH contributed this case study.**

- No nausea or vomiting.
- Had been having a stressful time in school; 4 to 5 hours of sleep nightly.
- Older sister had a seizure with high fever at age 3; none since.

Question 3. *What do you think about his history?*

PHYSICAL EXAMINATION

- Alert but tired teenager in no apparent distress.
- T = 37° C orally; P = 72, regular; RR = 14, regular and unlabored; BP = 115/72 mm Hg, (sitting).

Skin, HEENT
- Skin pink, warm, dry; no lesions or abrasions.
- Conjunctivae pink, moist.
- Visual acuity 20/20 without glasses.
- Fundi without lesions or hemorrhages.
- Nasal mucosa pink, moist without lesions, no exudate.
- Bite wound left lateral tongue; no bleeding, no exudate.
- Pharynx pink without exudate.

Neck
- Supple.
- No adenopathy, no thyromegaly.
- No bruits.

Lungs
- Chest expansion full, symmetric.
- Normal diaphragmatic position and excursion.
- Lung sounds clear to auscultation throughout all lobes bilaterally.

Cardiac
- Apical pulse palpated at fourth intercostal space, midclavicular line.
- Heart rate and rhythm regular.
- No murmurs, clicks, gallops, extra systoles.

Abdomen, Extremities
- Nondistended.
- Bowel sounds present and not hyperactive.
- Liver percusses 2 cm below right costal margin (RCM); overall size is 8 cm.
- No tenderness, masses, organomegaly; no bruit.
- Brisk capillary refill at 3 seconds; no edema, no clubbing.

Neurologic
- Alert, oriented, somewhat sleepy.
- Cranial nerves II through XII intact, face symmetric.
- Strength 5/5 throughout.
- DTRs 2+ and symmetric.
- Sensory intact to touch.
- No Romberg.
- Able to perform rapid alternating movements (RAM) smoothly without error.

Question 4. *What studies would you initiate now while preparing your interventions?*

Question 5. *What therapies would you initiate immediately while awaiting results of the laboratory studies?*

LABORATORY RESULTS

- CBC, chemistries, liver function studies, and urinalysis are all within normal ranges.
- Head CT and MRI are normal.

EMERGENCY DEPARTMENT COURSE

- Patient becomes increasingly irritable and anxious.
- He experiences a second seizure with loss of consciousness; generalized tonic convulsion is closely followed by alternating clonic convulsions.
- The event lasts about 2 minutes.
- The patient appears to sleep for about 5 minutes (postictal).
- The patient awakens confused.

PATIENT UPDATE

- P = 110, regular; RR = 20; BP = 130/76.
- Lungs are clear to auscultation, no aspiration.
- Skin diaphoretic, warm.
- Patient sleepy, oriented to name only.
- Neurologic examination remains normal.

Question 6. *What interventions should be initiated now?*

RESPONSE TO THERAPY

- No further seizure activity over the next 4 hours.
- Patient is drowsy and oriented when awakened from sleep.
- RR = 12.

Question 7. *Now what should be done and what can the patient expect?*

HOSPITAL COURSE

- The patient does well with no further seizures.
- He continues to be tired, but has no other adverse effects.
- EEG shows no epileptiform activity with and without hyperventilation.
- He is treated with phenobarbital 30 mg/day and phenytoin 100 mg at bedtime.
- He is discharged home on the second day.

Question 8. *What instructions and medications should the patient go home with?*

Chapter 22

Acute Bacterial Meningitis

DEFINITION

- Infection of the meninges by bacteria, usually with an underlying encephalitis.

EPIDEMIOLOGY

- Two to five cases of bacterial meningitis per 100,000 people are diagnosed annually in the United States; median age is 25 years. It is one of the top 10 causes of infection-related death worldwide and causes significant neurologic sequelae in nearly half of those who survive.
- The risk factors for bacterial meningitis include extremes of age, splenectomy, sickle cell disease, alcoholism, liver disease, otitis media, sinusitis, pneumonia, diabetes mellitus, immunodeficiency (inherited or acquired), ventricular shunt, cerebrospinal fluid (CSF) leak, and recent neurosurgical procedures.
- Since the use of the *Haemophilus influenzae* vaccine became widespread, the incidence of bacterial meningitis has declined and there has been a shift in the most likely etiologic organisms.
- The most common cause of bacterial meningitis in children and adults is *Streptococcus pneumoniae* (pneumococcus). Mortality rates for adults with pneumococcal meningitis in the United States are 21% to 28% even with treatment. Of survivors, up to 30% have long-term sequelae such as hearing loss and neurologic deficits. Penicillin resistance of streptococcal infections is now estimated at 25% to 35% (40% to 90% in children older than 6 years of age), and resistance to cefotaxime is 15%.
- *Neisseria meningitidis* (meningococcus) is common in ages 2 to 18 years. Fatality rates with treatment are approximately 10%.
- *Staphylococcus* and gram-negative organisms are more common in older patients and in infections due to trauma and nosocomial exposure.
- *Listeria monocytogenes* causes up to 10% of infections, especially in immunocompromised adults.
- Likely pathogens based on age and predisposing factors are listed in Table 22-1.
- Overall, acute bacterial meningitis is nearly always fatal without treatment; there is a 10% mortality even with therapy.

PATHOPHYSIOLOGY

Genetics

- Genetic polymorphisms associated with increased host susceptibility to bacterial meningitis include those affecting Toll-like receptor genes, lipopolysaccharide (LPS)-binding protein gene, angiotensin-converting enzyme genes, complement genes, properdin genes, leukocyte receptor genes, inflammatory cytokine genes (tumor necrosis factor-α [TNF-α], interleukins) and coagulation genes (tissue plasminogen activator factor V Leiden, protein C).

TABLE **22-1** IDSA Practice Guidelines for Empirical Antimicrobial Therapy for Purulent Meningitis, Based on Patient Age and Specific Predisposing Condition (2004)

Predisposing Factor	Common Bacterial Pathogens	Antimicrobial Therapy
Age		
<1 month	*Streptococcus agalactiae, Escherichia coli, Listeria monocytogenes, Klebsiella* spp.	Ampicillin plus cefotaxime or ampicillin plus an aminoglycoside
1-23 months	*Streptococcus pneumoniae, Neisseria meningitidis, S. agalactiae, Haemophilus influenzae, E. coli*	Vancomycin plus a third-generation cephalosporin
2-50 years	*N. meningitidis, S. pneumoniae*	Vancomycin plus a third-generation cephalosporin
>50 years	*S. pneumoniae, N. meningitidis, L. monocytogenes,* aerobic gram-negative bacilli	Vancomycin plus ampicillin plus a third-generation cephalosporin
Head Trauma		
Basilar skull fracture	*S. pneumoniae, H. influenzae,* group A β-hemolytic streptococci	Vancomycin plus a third-generation cephalosporin
Penetrating trauma	*Staphylococcus aureus,* coagulase-negative staphylococci (especially *Staphylococcus epidermidis*), aerobic gram-negative bacilli (including *Pseudomonas aeruginosa*)	Vancomycin plus cefepime, vancomycin plus ceftazidime, or vancomycin plus meropenem
Postneurosurgery	Aerobic gram-negative bacilli (including *P. aeruginosa*), *S. aureus,* coagulase-negative staphylococci (especially *S. epidermidis*)	Vancomycin plus cefepime, vancomycin plus ceftazidime, or vancomycin plus meropenem
CSF Shunt	Coagulase-negative staphylococci (especially *S. epidermidis*), *S. aureus,* aerobic gram-negative bacilli (including *P. aeruginosa*), *Propionibacterium acnes*	Vancomycin plus cefepime, vancomycin plus ceftazidime, or vancomycin plus meropenem

From Tunkel, A. R., Hartman, B. J., Kaplan, S. L., Kaufman, B. A., Roos, K. L., Scheld, W. M., & Whitley, R. J. (2004). Practice guidelines for bacterial meningitis. *Clinical Infectious Disease*, 39, 1267-1284; © 2004 by The Infectious Disease Society of America.

Tissue Effects

- Bacteria invade the central nervous system (CNS) due to infection by an aggressive organism, host immunosuppression and/or direct or repetitive seeding of the subarachnoid space.
- Bacteria invade the CNS via one of three pathways (Figure 22-1). Of these, the hematogenous route is the most common.
    - Hematogenous: Mucosal colonization of the nasopharynx, or infections of the lung and skin result in seeding of the blood and transport to the meninges.
    - Contiguous: Spreads directly to the meninges from otitis media or sinusitis.
    - Direct entry: Trauma, lumbar puncture, or surgery can lead to direct inoculation of the CSF.
- Encapsulated organisms are the most common pathogens (pneumococcus, meningococcus). They are usually from a respiratory or cranial source and they multiply rapidly in the CSF.
- Once in the CSF, bacterial products (especially LPS and peptidoglycan) stimulate the production of inflammatory cytokines from macrophages (through stimulation of Toll-like receptors [TLR2, TLR4]), endothelial cells, and astrocytes. Inflammatory and injurious mediators released in meningitis include TNF-α, interleukin (IL)-1, IL-6 IL-8, nitrous oxide (NO), matrix metalloproteinases, caspases, excitotoxins (glutamate), and vascular endothelial growth factor (VEGF).
- Cytokines chemotactic for neutrophils and lymphocytes are also released and adhesion molecules are expressed, resulting in the adhesion of the leukocytes to the endothelium, endothelial injury, and disruption of the blood-brain barrier, leading to protein and cellular accumulation in the CSF.
- Endothelial injury also causes initiation of the coagulation cascade with microthrombosis and vasogenic edema.
- Increased intracranial pressure (ICP) due to cerebral edema and CSF outflow obstruction causes reduced cerebral blood flow (CBF), leading to brain ischemia and eventually death.

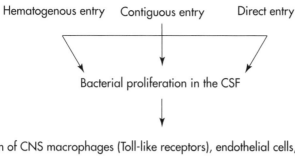

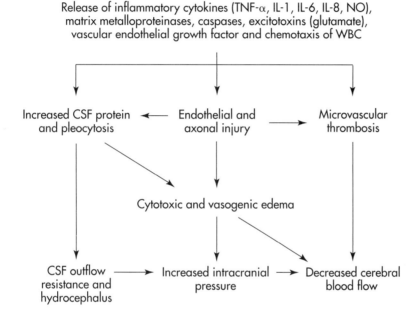

FIGURE **22-1 Pathogenesis of Bacterial Meningitis.**

- There is concern that the use of bacteriolytic antibiotics that cleave the cell membranes may lead to release of bacterial toxins (e.g., pneumolysin from pneumococci), which can worsen inflammation. The administration of corticosteroids with antibiotics is now recommended.

PATIENT PRESENTATION

There are two types of onset:
  - Rapid (25%): hospitalized within 24 hours of the onset of symptoms; high mortality rate.
  - Slow (75%): days to weeks of preceding prodromal symptoms.

History

Recent upper respiratory symptoms; exposure to other ill individuals; sinusitis or otitis media; recent neurosurgery; immunosuppression; sickle cell disease.

Symptoms

Headache; fever; stiff neck; rash; somnolence or irritability; photophobia; vomiting; seizures; blurred vision; diplopia; numbness; or weakness.

Examination

Fever; decreased level of consciousness; nuchal rigidity; Brudzinski and Kernig signs; cranial nerve palsies; disconjugate gaze; focal neurologic deficits; rashes.

DIFFERENTIAL DIAGNOSIS

- Viral meningitis.
- Subarachnoid hemorrhage.
- Encephalitis.
- Migraine.
- Influenza.
- Carcinomatous meningitis.
- Parameningeal foci of infection.

KEYS TO ASSESSMENT

- Lumbar puncture should not be delayed for radiologic testing unless the patient is immunocompromised, has a history of CNS disease, has a new-onset seizure, or there is evidence of papilledema, abnormal level of consciousness, or focal neurologic signs (see below).
- CSF findings consistent with bacterial meningitis include:
  - Pressure: Increased (mean pressure = 30 cm H_2O).
  - Protein: Increased (>150 mg/dL).
  - Leukocytes: Presence of any polymorphonuclear neutrophils (PMNs) in the CSF is suggestive of bacterial meningitis (however lymphocytosis may occur in *Listeria* infections).
  - Glucose: Decreased (<40 mg/dL); lactate: increased.
  - C-reactive protein: Increased and distinguishes bacterial from viral causes with high negative predictive value.
  - Lactic dehydrogenase (LDH): Increased.
  - Gram stain: 60% to 80% sensitive, >90% specific.
  - Culture: 70% to 85% sensitive.
  - Rapid antigen test for CSF pneumococcal antigens (Binax Now).
  - India ink: Look for cryptococcus.
  - Counter-immunoelectrophoresis (CIE), latex agglutination, and polymerase chain reaction (PCR) provide 70% to 100% sensitivity for the presence of *S. pneumoniae, N. meningitidis, H. influenzae, Streptococcus agalactiae,* herpes simplex virus (HSV), enterovirus, and *Listeria.*
- Other CSF studies.
  - CSF procalcitonin is highly specific for bacterial meningitis but not highly sensitive; its clinical utility continues to be investigated.
  - CSF TNF-α, IL-1, IL-6, IL-8 complement, and endothelins are all being evaluated.
- Serum reveals increased white blood cells (WBCs) and possible electrolyte disturbances, (e.g., hyponatremia from the syndrome of inappropriate antidiuretic hormone (SIADH) or cerebral salt-wasting syndrome).
- Computed tomography (CT) or magnetic resonance imaging (MRI) should be obtained if there is evidence of increased intracranial pressure, an immunocompromised patient, focal neurologic findings on the physical examination, or equivocal CSF results (see above).

KEYS TO MANAGEMENT

- Early recognition, early identification, and rapid initiation of therapy are crucial to patient survival.
- Isolation of the patient is indicated until the organism has been identified.
- Antibiotics should not be delayed while obtaining a CSF specimen; CSF cultures will not be decreased in diagnostic sensitivity if antibiotics are begun 1 to 2 hours before lumbar puncture.

- Antibiotics: Empiric indicated until a specific organism can be identified.
  - They should cover likely organisms including antibiotic-resistant strains.
  - They must penetrate the blood-brain barrier and be bactericidal (leukocyte phagocytosis is inefficient in CSF due to deficiency of complement and specific antibodies).
  - Currently recommended antibiotics according to the Practice Guidelines published by the Infectious Disease Society of America are listed in Table 22-1.
- Recent guidelines support the use of adjunctive corticosteroids in all adults with bacterial meningitis, especially for pneumococcal meningitis, correlated with increased survival and decreased sequelae. Most studies recommend 10 mg of dexamethasone IV with or just before the first dose of antibiotics and continued every 6 hours for 4 days.
- Experimental efforts are directed at limiting endothelial and neuronal damage including oxygen radical scavengers, protease inhibitors, and caspase inhibitors.
- Monitoring and managing sequelae.
  - ICP pressure bolt and management of increased ICP.
  - Anticonvulsants for recurrent seizures.
  - Support for sepsis.
  - Shunt for refractory hydrocephalus.
  - Support for disseminated intravascular coagulation (DIC), SIADH, or cerebral salt-wasting syndrome.
- Reassess for long-term sequelae: Up to 25% have prolonged complications such as deafness, mental retardation, seizure disorder, spasticity, or paresis.
- Prevention.
  - Vaccination.
    1. *H. influenzae:* Vaccinate all children older than 2 months of age.
    2. *N. meningitidis:* Recommendations recently updated to include all adolescents ages 11 and 12 as well as individuals who are asplenic or immunocompromised, travelers to endemic areas, all individuals exposed to community and college outbreaks, and household contacts of infected individuals. Most universities recommend vaccination for all incoming students.
    3. *S. pneumoniae:* Vaccinate adults older than 65 years of age; those with chronic cardiovascular, pulmonary, hepatic, renal disease; diabetes; alcoholism; CSF leak; asplenia; lymphoma; HIV; nephrotic syndrome; or multiple myeloma; and those who are immunocompromised.
  - Chemoprophylaxis medications that are indicated for those who are in close contact with individuals who have meningococcal infection may include rifampin, ciprofloxacin, ceftriaxone, minocycline, or spiramycin.

PATHOPHYSIOLOGY →	CLINICAL LINK
What is going on in the disease process that influences how the patient presents and how he or she should be managed?	*What should you do now that you understand the underlying pathophysiology?*
Encapsulated organisms are common pathogens in bacterial meningitis, and the immune defenses in the CSF are relatively weak, so these organisms can multiply quickly.	Meningitis can progress rapidly to significant neurologic injury and must be treated with empiric antibiotics as soon as possible.
The first step in host response to CSF bacterial invasion is via the production of inflammatory cytokines from endothelial cells and astrocytes (TNF-α, IL-1, NO).	Meningitis is characterized by intense inflammation of the meninges and underlying brain tissue; steroids should be administered along with antibiotics.
Increased intracranial pressure is the most ominous sequela of meningitis and can result in decreased cerebral blood flow, brain ischemia, and herniation.	Patients must be monitored for deteriorating mental status, changes in vital signs, and papilledema; ICP monitoring and treatment with osmotic agents may be necessary.
Meningitis and subarachnoid hemorrhage can occur in otherwise young and healthy people, and both present with headache, change in mental status, meningismus, and focal neurologic deficits, particularly cranial nerve palsies.	Subarachnoid hemorrhage must be ruled out in a patient who does not describe the usual infectious prodromal symptoms and who has clinical evidence of increased intracranial pressure with MRI or CT scanning.
Bacteria in the CSF cause changes in the blood-brain barrier that allow cells (usually neutrophils) and protein into the CSF, use up the glucose, and produce lactate with their metabolism, and can often be seen on Gram stain or can be cultured and tested for with polymerase chain reaction (PCR).	Diagnosis of meningitis is usually made by lumbar puncture with CSF analysis indicating increased protein, neutrophils, and lactate, decreased glucose, and positive stains, cultures, and PCR testing.
The CSF has limited immunologic protection and organisms can multiply quickly with rapid deterioration of the patient and risk for long-term sequelae and death.	Rapid institution of broad-spectrum empiric antibiotics is crucial to patient outcomes and should not be delayed because of performing diagnostic tests including the lumbar puncture.

SUGGESTED READINGS

Bottcher, T., Ren, H., Goiny, M., Gerber, J., Lykkesfeldt, J., Kuhnt, U., Lotz, M., Bunkowski, S., Werner, C., Schau, I., Spreer, A., Christen, S., & Nau, R. (2004). Clindamycin is neuroprotective in experimental *Streptococcus pneumoniae* meningitis compared with ceftriaxone. *Journal of Neurochemistry, 91,* 1450-1460.

Campos-Outcalt, D. (2005). Meningococcal vaccine: new product, new recommendations. *Journal of Family Practice, 54,* 324-326.

Cardona-Bonet, L. L. & Cortes, A. (2004). Management of perioperative infectious complications in the neurologic patient. *Neurologic Clinics, 22,* 329-345.

Chaudhuri, A. (2004). Adjunctive dexamethasone treatment in acute bacterial meningitis. *Lancet Neurology, 3,* 54-62.

Coenjaerts, F. E., van der Flier, M., Mwinzi, P. N., Brouwer, A. E., Scharringa, J., Chaka, W. S., Aarts, M., Rajanuwong, A., van de Vijver, D. A., Harrison, T. S., & Hoepelman, A. I. (2004). Intrathecal production and secretion of vascular endothelial growth factor during cryptococcal meningitis. *Journal of Infectious Diseases, 190,* 1310-1317.

Cottagnoud, P. H. & Tauber, M. G. (2004). New therapies for pneumococcal meningitis. *Expert Opinion on Investigational Drugs, 13,* 393-401.

Ebert, S., Gerber, J., Bader, S., Muhlhauser, F., Brechtel, K., Mitchell, T. J., & Nau, R. (2005). Dose-dependent activation of microglial cells by Toll-like receptor agonists alone and in combination. *Journal of Neuroimmunology, 159,* 87-96.

Emonts, M., Hazelzet, J. A., de Groot, R., & Hermans, P. W. (2003). Host genetic determinants of *Neisseria meningitidis* infections. *The Lancet Infectious Diseases, 3,* 565-577.

Flores-Cordero, J. M., Amaya-Villar, R., Rincon-Ferrari, M. D., Leal-Noval, S. R., Garnacho-Montero, J., Llanos-Rodriguez, A. C., & Murillo-Cabezas, F. (2003). Acute community-acquired bacterial meningitis in adults admitted to the intensive care unit: clinical manifestations, management and prognostic factors. *Intensive Care Medicine, 29,* 1967-1973.

Gendelman, H. E. & Persidsky, Y. (2005). Infections of the nervous system. *Lancet Neurology, 4,* 12-13.

Gerber, J., Lotz, M., Ebert, S., Kiel, S., Huether, G., Kuhnt, U., & Nau, R. (2005). Melatonin is neuroprotective in experimental *Streptococcus pneumoniae* meningitis. *Journal of Infectious Diseases, 191,* 783-790.

Gielchinsky, Y., Cohen, R., Revel, A., & Ezra, Y. (2005). Postpartum maternal group B streptococcal meningitis. *Acta Obstetricia et Gynecologica Scandinavica, 84,* 490-491.

Ginsberg, L. (2004). Difficult and recurrent meningitis. *Journal of Neurology, Neurosurgery & Psychiatry, 75*(suppl 1), i16-i21.

Hasbun, R., Abrahams, J., Jekel, J., & Quagliarello, V. (2001). Computed tomography of the head before lumbar puncture in adults with suspected meningitis. *New England Journal of Medicine, 345,* 1727-1733.

Hirst, R. A., Kadioglu, A., O'Callaghan, C., & Andrew, P. W. (2004). The role of pneumolysin in pneumococcal pneumonia and meningitis. *Clinical & Experimental Immunology, 138,* 195-201.

Iliev, A. I., Stringaris, A. K., Nau, R., & Neumann, H. (2004). Neuronal injury mediated via stimulation of microglial Toll-like receptor-9 (TLR9). *FASEB Journal, 18,* 412-414.

Kaper, J. B., Nataro, J. P., & Mobley, H. L. (2004). Pathogenic *Escherichia coli. Nature Reviews, Microbiology, 2,* 123-140.

Koedel, U., Scheld, W. M., & Pfister, H. W. (2002). Pathogenesis and pathophysiology of pneumococcal meningitis. *The Lancet Infectious Diseases, 2,* 721-736.

Maiden, M. C. (2004). Dynamics of bacterial carriage and disease: lessons from the meningococcus. *Advances in Experimental Medicine & Biology, 549,* 23-29.

McCracken, G. H., Jr. (2004). Current management of bacterial meningitis. *Advances in Experimental Medicine & Biology, 549,* 31-33.

Nathan, B. R. & Scheld, W. M. (2002). The potential roles of C-reactive protein and procalcitonin concentrations in the serum and cerebrospinal fluid in the diagnosis of bacterial meningitis. *Current Clinical Topics in Infectious Diseases, 22,* 155-165.

Nau, R. & Bruck, W. (2002). Neuronal injury in bacterial meningitis: mechanisms and implications for therapy. *Trends in Neurosciences, 25,* 38-45.

Nau, R. & Eiffert, H. (2002). Modulation of release of proinflammatory bacterial compounds by antibacterials: potential impact on course of inflammation and outcome in sepsis and meningitis. *Clinical Microbiology Reviews, 15,* 95-110.

Nau, R., Gerber, J., Bunkowski, S., & Bruck, W. (2004). Axonal injury, a neglected cause of CNS damage in bacterial meningitis. *Neurology, 62,* 509-511.

Oliver, W. J., Shope, T. C., & Kuhns, L. R. (2003). Fatal lumbar puncture: fact versus fiction—an approach to a clinical dilemma. *Pediatrics, 112,* e174-e176.

Patel, M. & Lee, C. K. (2005). Polysaccharide vaccines for preventing serogroup A meningococcal meningitis. *Cochrane Database of Systematic Reviews,* CD001093.

Pathan, N., Faust, S. N., & Levin, M. (2003). Pathophysiology of meningococcal meningitis and septicaemia. *Archives of Disease in Childhood, 88,* 601-607.

Pathan, N., Hemingway, C. A., Alizadeh, A. A., Stephens, A. C., Boldrick, J. C., Oragui, E. E., McCabe, C., Welch, S. B., Whitney, A., O'Gara, P., Nadel, S., Relman, D. A., Harding, S. E., & Levin, M. (2004). Role of interleukin 6 in myocardial dysfunction of meningococcal septic shock. *Lancet, 363,* 203-209.

Pathan, N., Sandiford, C., Harding, S. E., & Levin, M. (2002). Characterization of a myocardial depressant factor in meningococcal septicemia. *Critical Care Medicine, 30,* 2191-2198.

Pile, J. C. & Longworth, D. L. (2005). Should adults with suspected acute bacterial meningitis get adjunctive corticosteroids? *Cleveland Clinic Journal of Medicine, 72,* 67-70.

Pomar, V., Martinez, S., Paredes, R., & Domingo, P. (2004). Advances in adjuvant therapy against acute bacterial meningitis. *Current Drug Targets—Infectious Disorders, 4,* 303-309.

Pracht, D., Elm, C., Gerber, J., Bergmann, S., Rohde, M., Seiler, M., Kim, K. S., Jenkinson, H. F., Nau, R., & Hammerschmidt, S. (2005). PavA of *Streptococcus pneumoniae* modulates adherence, invasion, and meningeal inflammation. *Infection & Immunity, 73,* 2680-2689.

Prasad, K., Singhal, T., Jain, N., & Gupta, P. K. (2004). Third generation cephalosporins versus conventional antibiotics for treating acute bacterial meningitis. *Cochrane Database of Systematic Reviews,* CD001832.

Rosa, D. D., Pasqualotto, A. C., de Quadros, M., & Prezzi, S. H. (2004). Deficiency of the eighth component of complement associated with recurrent meningococcal meningitis—case report and literature review. *Brazilian Journal of Infectious Diseases, 8,* 328-330.

Scheld, W. M., Koedel, U., Nathan, B., & Pfister, H. W. (2002). Pathophysiology of bacterial meningitis: mechanism(s) of neuronal injury. *Journal of Infectious Diseases, 186*(suppl 2), S225-S233.

Schneider, J. I. (2004). Rapid infectious killers. *Emergency Medicine Clinics of North America, 22,* 1099-1115.

Sinner, S. W. & Tunkel, A. R. (2000). Antimicrobial agents in the treatment of bacterial meningitis. *Infectious Disease Clinics of North America, 18,* 581-602.

Snape, M. D. & Pollard, A. J. (2005). Meningococcal polysaccharide-protein conjugate vaccines. *The Lancet Infectious Diseases, 5,* 21-30.

Spreer, A., Kerstan, H., Bottcher, T., Gerber, J., Siemer, A., Zysk, G., Mitchell, T. J., Eiffert, H., & Nau, R. (2003). Reduced release of pneumolysin by *Streptococcus pneumoniae* in vitro and in vivo after treatment with nonbacteriolytic antibiotics in comparison to ceftriaxone. *Antimicrobial Agents & Chemotherapy*, 47, 2649-2654.

Spreer, A., Lis, A., Gerber, J., Reinert, R. R., Eiffert, H., & Nau, R. (2004). Differences in clinical manifestation of *Streptococcus pneumoniae* infection are not correlated with in vitro production and release of the virulence factors pneumolysin and lipoteichoic and teichoic acids. *Journal of Clinical Microbiology*, 42, 3342-3345.

Stringaris, A. K., Geisenhainer, J., Bergmann, F., Balshusemann, C., Lee, U., Zysk, G., Mitchell, T. J., Keller, B. U., Kuhnt, U., Gerber, J., Spreer, A., Bahr, M., Michel, U., & Nau, R. (2002). Neurotoxicity of pneumolysin, a major pneumococcal virulence factor, involves calcium influx and depends on activation of p38 mitogen-activated protein kinase. *Neurobiology of Disease*, 11, 355-368.

Tunkel, A. R., Hartman, B. J., Kaplan, S. L., Kaufman, B. A., Roos, K. L., Scheld, W. M., & Whitley, R. J. (2004). Practice guidelines for bacterial meningitis. *Clinical Infectious Diseases*, 39, 1267-1284.

Tunkel, A. R. & Scheld, W. M. (2002). Corticosteroids for everyone with meningitis. *New England Journal of Medicine*, 347, 1613-1615.

van de Beek, D., de Gans, J., McIntyre, P., & Prasad, K. (2004). Steroids in adults with acute bacterial meningitis: a systematic review. *The Lancet Infectious Diseases*, 4, 139-143.

van der Flier, M., Geelen, S. P., Kimpen, J. L., Hoepelman, I. M., & Tuomanen, E. I. (2003). Reprogramming the host response in bacterial meningitis: how best to improve outcome. *Clinical Microbiology Reviews*, 16, 415-429.

van der Flier, M., Hoppenreijs, S., van Rensburg, A. J., Ruyken, M., Kolk, A. H., Springer, P., Hoepelman, A. I., Geelen, S. P., Kimpen, J. L., & Schoeman, J. F. (2004). Vascular endothelial growth factor and blood-brain barrier disruption in tuberculous meningitis. *Pediatric Infectious Disease Journal*, 23, 608-613.

Xie, Y., Kim, K. J., & Kim, K. S. (2004). Current concepts on *Escherichia coli* K1 translocation of the blood-brain barrier. *FEMS Immunology & Medical Microbiology*, 42, 271-279.

Zysk, G., Bethe, G., Nau, R., Koch, D., Grafin, V. B., V, Heinz, H. P., & Reinert, R. R. (2003). Immune response to capsular polysaccharide and surface proteins of *Streptococcus pneumoniae* in patients with invasive pneumococcal disease. *Journal of Infectious Diseases*, 187, 330-333.

Bacterial Meningitis

INITIAL HISTORY

- 21-year-old male college student, preparing for fall final exams.
- Reports increasingly severe headache, fever for past 24 hours, and extreme light sensitivity.
- Reports nausea but has not vomited.
- Profoundly tired, feels "weak all over."

Question 1. *What other questions about his symptoms would you like to ask this patient?*

ADDITIONAL HISTORY

- Describes headache as throbbing, bitemporal.
- Wearing sunglasses in dim room because the "light hurts my eyes."
- States, "I just got a bad head cold with a sore throat about 2 weeks ago. I hoped I was getting better."
- Denies any history of migraine, tension, or cluster headache.
- Reports neck feels stiff.
- Reports "having trouble concentrating on materials for finals."
- States he is unsure how high his fever has gotten and that he sometimes has chills.
- Denies chest pain or dyspnea.

Question 2. *What questions would you like to ask this patient about his medical and social history?*

MEDICAL HISTORY

- Surgical history: Tonsillectomy, age 9.
- Medical history: Recent URI.
- Currently taking no medications or supplements; no known allergies.
- Denies receiving vaccination for meningitis, otherwise up to date on immunizations.
- Denies history of meningitis, head or back trauma, severe infections, or immunodeficiency.
- Denies history of any serious infection or having to be hospitalized.
- Has never been tested for HIV; no history of cancer/leukemia/lymphoma.

LIFE-STYLE AND SOCIAL HISTORY

- College student, senior.
- Lives in fraternity house with approximately 60 other young men.
- Nonsmoker.
- Drinks alcoholic beverages primarily on weekends, 6 to 8 beers per week.
- Well-balanced diet.
- Exercises 4 or 5 days per week at local gym; running and weightlifting.
- Sexually active in monogamous relationship for 1 year.

PHYSICAL ASSESSMENT

- Well-built, well-nourished male appearing tired but in no acute distress.
- T = 38.5° C tympanic; P = 98 and regular; RR = 20; BP= 102/68 right arm (sitting).

HEENT
- PERRLA, photophobia makes fundal examination difficult, no obvious papilledema.
- Conjunctivae clear.
- Sinus tenderness over maxillary sinuses bilaterally.
- Throat examination reveals postnasal drainage; no lesions or exudate.
- No lymphadenopathy.

Neck
- Stiff and painful with flexion.
- Positive Kernig and Brudzinski signs.

Skin
- No rash or lesions over trunk or extremities.

Chest
- Lungs clear to auscultation.
- Heart sounds S_1, S_2 regular without murmurs, rubs, or gallops.

Abdomen
- Nondistended.
- Bowel sounds positive in all four quadrants.
- Soft, nontender.
- No palpable mass or organomegaly.

Neurologic
- Oriented ×4.
- Mildly lethargic.
- Cranial nerves II through XII intact.
- Strengths 5/5 in bilateral upper and lower extremities.
- DTR 2+ symmetric.
- No gait disturbance; able to perform heel-to-shin test without difficulty.

Question 3.   *What are the pertinent positives and negatives on this examination?*

Question 4.   *What is your differential diagnosis at this time?*

Question 5.   *What laboratory tests and therapeutic interventions would be indicated at this time?*

LABORATORY RESULTS

- Serum chemistries normal.
- CBC.
    - WBCs = 14,000 (90% PMNs).
    - Hgb/Hct = 14/42.
- Platelets 225,000.
    - Rapid strep throat culture = negative.

LUMBAR PUNCTURE

- Opening pressure = 30 cm H_2O.
- Increased protein, decreased glucose, increased lactate.
- 120 WBC/mm^3, all PMNs.
- Gram stain positive for gram-positive diplococci.
- India ink negative for fungi.

Question 6.   *How would you interpret these laboratory findings?*

Question 7.   *What antibiotics/therapeutic interventions would be indicated?*

HOSPITAL COURSE

- Patient is admitted.
- Symptoms gradually improve.

Question 8.   *For what complications should this patient be monitored?*

Chapter 23

Osteoarthritis

DEFINITION

- Osteoarthritis (OA) is defined as a heterogeneous group of conditions that leads to joint symptoms and signs that are associated with defective integrity of articular cartilage in addition to related changes in the underlying bone.
- Primary osteoarthritis is idiopathic and can be generalized or localized.
- Secondary osteoarthritis occurs due to an identifiable risk factor or cause such as joint trauma, anatomic abnormalities, infection, neuropathy, hemophilia, metabolic alterations in cartilage (hemochromatosis), or subchondral bone alteration (acromegaly, Paget disease).

EPIDEMIOLOGY

- OA is the most common form of debilitating joint disease in the world.
- OA affects 60% to 70% of people older than age 65 in the United States.
- There is increasing risk for OA with increasing age; therefore prevalence is rising rapidly as the population ages.
- Other risk factors for primary OA include obesity, repetitive joint overuse, immobilization, and increased bone density (less "shock absorption" [see below]).

PATHOPHYSIOLOGY

Genetics

- Rare forms of familial OA are related to dominant inheritance of mutations of the type II collagen gene, human lymphocyte antigen (HLA) A1 B8 haplotype, familial chondrocalcinosis (crystal deposition in joints), and chondrodysplasias.
- Primary OA has been linked to a large number of genes including genes for collagen types II, IX, XI, COMP, matrilin 3, and frizzled-related protein 3. Other genes that have been linked to OA risk include those for the inflammatory cytokines such as interleukins and prostaglandins.

Tissue Effects

- Cartilage components become disorganized and degraded in OA.
  - Mechanical factors result in the release of enzymes (matrix metalloproteinases, collagenase, and stromelysin), resulting in proteoglycan depletion and type II collagen disordering.
  - Proteolytic cleavage of collagen fibrils contributes to the loss of the cartilage matrix, especially at the medial cartilage surface.
  - Inflammatory cytokines (interleukin [IL]-1, prostaglandin E_2 [PGE_2], tumor necrosis factor [TNF]-α, IL-6, IL-17, and nitric oxide) promote joint inflammation and cartilage degradation. IL-1 is believed to be a crucial stimulator of joint destruction, and PGE_2 causes the pain of OA, so both are primary targets for therapy (see below).

- Chondrocytes become unresponsive to growth factors such as transforming growth factor-β and insulin-like growth factor, and cannot fully compensate for matrix loss. An imbalance of cartilage synthesis and degradation develops with abrasions, pitting, and fissuring of the articular surface.
- Matrix degradation and overhydration of articular cartilage lead to a loss in compressive stiffness and elasticity with transmission of greater mechanical stress to the subchondral bone.
- The subchondral trabecular bone is damaged and loses its normal hydraulic "shock absorption"; bone cysts may form from this excess subchondral bone stress.
- Repair mechanisms at the edge of the articular surface (cartilage-bone interface) result in increased synthesis of cartilage and bone-forming overgrowths called osteophytes.

- Some patients are found to have various forms of calcium crystals concentrated in the damaged articular cartilage. The pathogenesis of this crystal deposition is unclear but is correlated with a more rapid disease progression in these patients.
- Articular cartilage requires physiologic weight loading and motion to allow adequate penetration of nutrients from the synovial fluid into the cartilage; nonphysiologic loads (either in excess or insufficient) result in poor cartilage nutrition.
- Human joints require maximal mobility while avoiding articular tissue injury. One hypothesis is that there is a "protective muscular reflex" that prevents the joint from exceeding its normal range of excursion; it has been postulated that disordered neuromuscular activity may play a role in the pathogenesis of OA.
- Joint instability is correlated with a high risk of OA. Increasing the strength of the "bridging" muscles across a joint can improve joint stability, decrease joint loading, and reduce mechanical stress. Thus exercise can improve symptoms and joint function, even in the absence of radiographic improvement.
- The pain of OA is related to hypersensitivity of periarticular nociceptors caused by PGE_2. These nociceptors are stimulated by abnormal movement from mechanical factors, synovial inflammation, and intraosseous hypertension. Articular cartilage is aneural, so OA joint damage may be significant before pain develops.

PATIENT PRESENTATION

History

Family history of OA; history of joint trauma; weight gain; occupation that includes repetitive movements, especially of the knees (squatting), elbows and back (heavy lifting), and hands (assembly line and mill work).

Symptoms

Nagging pain that has been present for years in one or more joints, and waxes and wanes in intensity according to the weather and exertion; stiffness after prolonged inactivity that "loosens up" with activity (may become permanent in late stages); swelling and deformity, especially of the knees and fingers, with development of "knobby" joints at the distal and proximal interphalangeal joints (DIPs and PIPs); inability to grip with the hands or comb the hair; restricted walking and fatigue.

Examination

Limping gait; Heberden nodes (DIP osteophytes) and Bouchard nodes (PIP osteophytes); flexor and lateral deviations of the distal phalanx; decreased range of motion and crepitus with passive motion; swelling, warmth, and tenderness (inflammation) during "flares."

DIFFERENTIAL DIAGNOSIS

- Secondary osteoarthritis.
- Rheumatoid arthritis.
- Gout.

- Systemic lupus erythematosus.
- Rheumatic fever.
- Septic arthritis.

KEYS TO ASSESSMENT

- Carefully assess all joints for deformity, crepitation, and decreasing range of motion.
- Examine the eyes, skin, and organs for evidence of systemic rheumatic disease.
- In a patient with (1) a classic history for OA; (2) a joint examination revealing Heberden nodes and decreased range of motion without evidence of significant joint deformity or inflammation; and (3) a general physical examination without evidence of systemic disease, consideration should be given for empiric treatment without further diagnostic testing.
- Specific joint involvement is frequently assessed with radiograph (weight bearing for the knee), looking for joint space narrowing, subchondral bone cysts and sclerosis, and osteophytes.
- Serum markers for evidence of articular cartilage destruction are used experimentally as a means of detecting OA before there is radiologic evidence. These include keratan sulfate and cartilage oligomeric matrix protein; these are not yet indicated for routine clinical evaluation.
- Magnetic resonance imaging (MRI) is a sensitive indicator of OA, and its role is expanding as innovative surgical interventions are explored.
- In a patient with severe disease or suspicious aspects to the history and physical, further diagnostic testing is indicated.
  - Chemistries including blood urea nitrogen (BUN) and creatinine (Cr).
  - Erythrocyte sedimentation rate (ESR), C-reactive protein, and rheumatoid factor.
  - Other specific tests for rheumatologic disease such as anti-deoxyribonucleic acid (anti-DNA), HLA-B27, and uric acid.
  - Arthrocentesis with chemistries, cell counts, cultures and stain, and rheumatoid factor.

KEYS TO MANAGEMENT

- The American College of Rheumatology Guidelines for OA Management suggest beginning therapy with nonpharmacologic modalities and then adding acetaminophen (see below) and then proceeding to other medications if symptoms are refractory.
- Nonpharmacologic management.
  - Exercise improves symptoms and quality of life in patients with mild to moderate OA. Muscle-strengthening exercises and walking have been shown to improve symptoms.
  - Physical therapy including passive range-of-motion and water exercises can improve function. Therapists may also recommend joint braces, canes, walkers, and other assist devices for increasing mobility and for joint protection.
  - Occupational therapy can help with assistive devices for activities of daily living.
  - Heat application, transcutaneous electric nerve stimulation (TENS), and acupuncture can be considered.
  - Diet for weight loss if appropriate.
  - Increased intake of vitamin C has been correlated with decreased OA progression and pain.
  - Ultrasound (diathermy) facilitates tendon extensibility, relaxes muscles, and decreases pain.
- Pharmacologic therapies.
  - Acetaminophen has been shown in many studies to be as effective as nonsteroidal anti-inflammatory drugs (NSAIDs) in reducing pain for mild to moderate OA. It has been recommended by the American College of Rheumatology as the first-line drug for treatment of OA. Acetaminophen may act by blocking cyclooxygenase 3 enzyme (COX-3) and can be given in doses as high as 1 g four times per day. Hepatic toxicity is the primary serious potential complication of this form of therapy.
  - Use of capsaicin as a topical analgesic (decreases neuronal substance P, which is a neurotransmitter implicated in arthritis pain) can reduce symptoms, as can topical methylsalicylate creams. These are usually considered adjunctive to acetaminophen therapy.

- Although OA is now known to have an inflammatory component, NSAID use is associated with some risk, and these drugs should be used only when simple analgesics such as acetaminophen fail to control symptoms.
    1. The primary side effects of NSAIDs (upper gastrointestinal ulceration and bleeding) are of particular risk in older adults. There is also increasing evidence that NSAIDs may increase the risk for cardiovascular events.
    2. Some patients will have greater analgesia with NSAIDs than with acetaminophen; these individuals should be started at low doses to reduce the risk of side effects.
    3. Cyclooxygenase 2 enzyme (COX-2) inhibitors reduce the risk of gastrointestinal ulceration when compared with nonselective NSAIDs, but the risk is not reduced to zero. Furthermore, rofecoxib was taken off the market in September 2004 because of increased cardiovascular risks. Other COX-2 inhibitors are also undergoing safety analyses. Although many patients derive great relief with these medications, meta-analyses of comparative studies show no consistent differences in response rates to COX-2 inhibitors when compared with other forms of analgesia in patients with OA.
    4. Drugs that block several of the inflammatory pathways simultaneously (COX-1, COX-2, and lipoxygenase-5 [LOX-5]) (e.g., licofelone) are in development.
- Chondroprotective drugs undergoing extensive research include glucosamine polysulfate, chondroitin sulfate, sodium pentosan polysulfate, and glycosaminoglycan peptide complex orally. These have been found to improve symptoms in many patients, with few side effects.
- Intra-articular injection of steroids during acute inflammatory "flares" can provide rapid symptom relief; frequency of steroid injections greater than three or four times a year may be associated with decreased cartilage repair.
- Viscosupplementation via joint injection of low-molecular-weight hyaluronic acid can provide sustained pain relief (weeks to months) in many individuals, but onset of benefit is slow and can take up to 12 weeks to develop.
- Opioid analgesic drugs should be used only when other methods fail, or as an adjunct during episodes of extreme pain.
- Surgical management.
  - Orthopedic surgery (including arthroscopic procedures) such as joint debridement, abrasion arthroplasty, chondral shaving, bone "scaffolding," and joint replacement, can be used with selected patients, often with dramatic improvements in mobility and pain.
- Experimental therapies.
  - Autologous chondrocyte implantation for severe disease; studies are positive.
  - Cytokine blockers are used in rheumatoid arthritis; studies pending in OA.
  - Gene therapy.
    1. IL-1 receptor antagonist delivery via adeno-associated viral vector.
    2. Introduction of chondroprotective genes into chondrocytes.
    3. Growth factor gene introduction into periarticular tissues.
  - Stem cell growth of chondrocytes and cartilage.

PATHOPHYSIOLOGY	→	CLINICAL LINK
What is going on in the disease process that influences how the patient presents and how he or she should be managed?		*What should you do now that you understand the underlying pathophysiology?*
Mechanical factors contribute to enzyme release that can cause articular cartilage degradation, and joint instability is correlated with a high risk of OA.	→	Overuse and trauma to joints are risk factors for OA.
The articular cartilage requires some joint "loading" to receive maximal supply of synovial fluid nutrients; exercise that improves muscle strength can improve joint function.	→	Exercise is beneficial to the health and healing of the articular cartilage.
Inflammatory cytokines have been found to play a significant role in the pathophysiology of OA, but their inhibition with anti-inflammatory drugs has not resulted in an improvement in disease progression.	→	OA is no longer considered a purely noninflammatory joint disease, but the role of anti-inflammatory medications in the long-term management of OA is highly controversial.
Unresponsiveness of chondrocytes to growth factors and the loss of "chondroprotection" have been implicated in the pathogenesis of OA.	→	New treatments for OA include chondroprotective drugs that may prevent cartilage degradation and improve healing.
Bone is laid down at the perimeter of the articular cartilage, forming growth of bone called osteophytes.	→	OA is characterized by bony protuberances in the joints, especially at the distal interphalangeal joints (Heberden nodes) and at the vertebral disk spaces that can limit range of motion.
OA is a complex interaction of inflammation and articular cartilage destruction for which simple analgesia may not be sufficient therapy.	→	Cytokine blockers, gene therapy, and stem cell introduction are all potentially effective approaches to the management of OA.

SUGGESTED READINGS

Aggarwal, A. & Sempowski, I. P. (2004). Hyaluronic acid injections for knee osteoarthritis. Systematic review of the literature. *Canadian Family Physician*, 50, 249-256.

Aigner, T., Kim, H. A., & Roach, H. I. (2004). Apoptosis in osteoarthritis. *Rheumatic Diseases Clinics of North America*, 30, 639-653.

Akarca, U. S. (2005). Gastrointestinal effects of selective and non-selective non-steroidal anti-inflammatory drugs. *Current Pharmaceutical Design*, 11, 1779-1793.

Altman, R. D. (2004). Pain relief in osteoarthritis: the rationale for combination therapy. *Journal of Rheumatology*, 31, 5-7.

Alvaro-Gracia, J. M. (2004). Licofelone—clinical update on a novel LOX/COX inhibitor for the treatment of osteoarthritis. *Rheumatology*, 43(suppl 1), i21-i25.

American College of Obstetricians and Gynecologists Women's Health Care Physicians. (2004). Osteoarthritis. *Obstetrics & Gynecology*, 104, 62S-65S.

Anderson, J. W., Nicolosi, R. J., & Borzelleca, J. F. (2005). Glucosamine effects in humans: a review of effects on glucose metabolism, side effects, safety considerations and efficacy. *Food & Chemical Toxicology*, 43, 187-201.

Ashworth, N. L., Chad, K. E., Harrison, E. L., Reeder, B. A., & Marshall, S. C. (2005). Home versus center based physical activity programs in older adults. *Cochrane Database of Systematic Reviews*, CD004017.

Avci, D. & Bachmann, G. A. (2004). Osteoarthritis and osteoporosis in postmenopausal women: clinical similarities and differences. *Menopause*, 11, 615-621.

Bailey, A. J., Mansell, J. P., Sims, T. J., & Banse, X. (2004). Biochemical and mechanical properties of subchondral bone in osteoarthritis. *Biorheology*, 41, 349-358.

Balazs, E. A. (2004). Viscosupplementation for treatment of osteoarthritis: from initial discovery to current status and results. *Surgical Technologies International*, 12, 278-289.

Berenbaum, F. (2004). Signaling transduction: target in osteoarthritis. *Current Opinion in Rheumatology*, 16, 616-622.

Biggee, B. A. & McAlindon, T. (2004). Glucosamine for osteoarthritis: part II, biologic and metabolic controversies. *Medicine & Health, Rhode Island*, 87, 180-181.

Bjordal, J. M., Ljunggren, A. E., Klovning, A., & Slordal, L. (2004). Non-steroidal anti-inflammatory drugs, including cyclo-oxygenase-2 inhibitors, in osteoarthritic knee pain: meta-analysis of randomised placebo controlled trials. *British Medical Journal*, 329, 1317.

Bonnet, C. S. & Walsh, D. A. (2005). Osteoarthritis, angiogenesis and inflammation. *Rheumatology*, 44, 7-16.

Borzi, R. M., Mazzetti, I., Marcu, K. B., & Facchini, A. (2004). Chemokines in cartilage degradation. *Clinical Orthopaedics & Related Research*, Oct(427 Suppl), S53-S61.

Bradley, L. A. (2004). Recent approaches to understanding osteoarthritis pain. *Journal of Rheumatology—Supplement*, 70, 54-60.

Brouwer, R. W., Jakma, T. S., Bierma-Zeinstra, S. M., Verhagen, A. P., & Verhaar, J. (2005). Osteotomy for treating knee osteoarthritis. *Cochrane Database of Systematic Reviews* CD004019.

Brouwer, R. W., Jakma, T. S., Verhagen, A. P., Verhaar, J. A., & Bierma-Zeinstra, S. M. (2005). Braces and orthoses for treating osteoarthritis of the knee. *Cochrane Database of Systematic Reviews*, CD004020.

Brune, K. (2004). Safety of anti-inflammatory treatment—new ways of thinking. *Rheumatology*, 43(suppl 1), i16-i20.

Buckwalter, J. A. & Brown, T. D. (2004). Joint injury, repair, and remodeling: roles in post-traumatic osteoarthritis. *Clinical Orthopaedics & Related Research*, Jun(423), 7-16.

Buckwalter, J. A. & Martin, J. A. (2004). Sports and osteoarthritis. *Current Opinion in Rheumatology*, 16, 634-639.

Buescher, J. S., Meadows, S., & Saseen, J. (2004). Clinical inquiries. Does acetaminophen and NSAID combined relieve osteoarthritis pain better than either alone? *Journal of Family Practice*, 53, 501-503.

Burr, D. B. (2004). The importance of subchondral bone in the progression of osteoarthritis. *Journal of Rheumatology—Supplement*, 70, 77-80.

Carter, D. R., Beaupre, G. S., Wong, M., Smith, R. L., Andriacchi, T. P., & Schurman, D. J. (2004). The mechanobiology of articular cartilage development and degeneration. *Clinical Orthopaedics & Related Research*, Oct(127 Suppl), S69-S77.

Chadderdon, R. C., Shimer, A. L., Gilbertson, L. G., & Kang, J. D. (2004). Advances in gene therapy for intervertebral disc degeneration. *Spine Journal: Official Journal of the North American Spine Society*, 4, 341S-347S.

Cook, S. D., Barrack, R. L., Patron, L. P., & Salkeld, S. L. (2004). Osteogenic protein-1 in knee arthritis and arthroplasty. *Clinical Orthopaedics & Related Research*, Nov(428), 140-145.

Dieppe, P. A. (2004). Relationship between symptoms and structural change in osteoarthritis: what are the important targets for osteoarthritis therapy? *Journal of Rheumatology—Supplement*, 70, 50-53.

Dieppe, P. A. & Lohmander, L. S. (2005). Pathogenesis and management of pain in osteoarthritis. *Lancet*, 365, 965-973.

Doherty, M. (2004). How important are genetic factors in osteoarthritis? *Journal of Rheumatology—Supplement*, 70, 22-27.

Dougados, M. (2004). Monitoring osteoarthritis progression and therapy. *Osteoarthritis & Cartilage*, 12(suppl A), S55-S60.

Dougados, M. (2004). Outcome measures for clinical trials of disease modifying osteoarthritis drugs in patients with hip osteoarthritis. *Journal of Rheumatology—Supplement*, 70, 66-69.

Edwards, J. E., McQuay, H. J., & Moore, R. A. (2004). Efficacy and safety of valdecoxib for treatment of osteoarthritis and rheumatoid arthritis: systematic review of randomised controlled trials. *Pain*, 111, 286-296.

Evans, C. H. (2004). Gene therapies for osteoarthritis. *Current Rheumatology Reports*, 6, 31-40.

Evans, C. H. (2005). Gene therapy: what have we accomplished and where do we go from here? *Journal of Rheumatology—Supplement*, 72, 17-20.

Evans, C. H., Gouze, J. N., Gouze, E., Robbins, P. D., & Ghivizzani, S. C. (2004). Osteoarthritis gene therapy. *Gene Therapy*, 11, 379-389.

Felson, D. T. (2004). Risk factors for osteoarthritis: understanding joint vulnerability. *Clinical Orthopaedics & Related Research*, S16-S21.

Fenton, C., Keating, G. M., & Wagstaff, A. J. (2004). Valdecoxib: a review of its use in the management of osteoarthritis, rheumatoid arthritis, dysmenorrhoea and acute pain. [Review] [93 refs]. *Drugs*, 64, 1231-1261.

Garner, S. E., Fidan, D. D., Frankish, R., & Maxwell, L. (2005). Rofecoxib for osteoarthritis. *Cochrane Database of Systematic Reviews*, CD005115.

Gidwani, S. & Fairbank, A. (2004). The orthopaedic approach to managing osteoarthritis of the knee. *British Medical Journal*, 329, 1220-1224.

Gokhale, J. A., Frenkel, S. R., & Dicesare, P. E. (2004). Estrogen and osteoarthritis. *American Journal of Orthopedics*, 33, 71-80.

Goldring, S. R. & Goldring, M. B. (2004). The role of cytokines in cartilage matrix degeneration in osteoarthritis. *Clinical Orthopaedics & Related Research*, S27-S36.

Gossec, L. & Dougados, M. (2004). Intra-articular treatments in osteoarthritis: from the symptomatic to the structure modifying. *Annals of the Rheumatic Diseases*, 63, 478-482.

Gouttenoire, J., Valcourt, U., Ronziere, M. C., Aubert-Foucher, E., Mallein-Gerin, F., & Herbage, D. (2004). Modulation of collagen synthesis in normal and osteoarthritic cartilage. *Biorheology*, 41, 535-542.

Grubb, B. D. (2004). Activation of sensory neurons in the arthritic joint. *Novartis Foundation Symposium, 260,* 28-36.

Guilak, F., Fermor, B., Keefe, F. J., Kraus, V. B., Olson, S. A., Pisetsky, D. S., Setton, L. A., & Weinberg, J. B. (2004). The role of biomechanics and inflammation in cartilage injury and repair. *Clinical Orthopaedics & Related Research,* Jun(423), 17-26.

Gupta, K. B., Duryea, J., & Weissman, B. N. (2004). Radiographic evaluation of osteoarthritis. *Radiologic Clinics of North America, 42,* 11-41

Hanna, F. S., Wluka, A. E., Bell, R. J., Davis, S. R., & Cicuttini, F. M. (2004). Osteoarthritis and the post-menopausal woman: epidemiological, magnetic resonance imaging, and radiological findings. *Seminars in Arthritis & Rheumatism, 34,* 631-636.

Herzog, W., Clark, A., & Longino, D. (2004). Joint mechanics in osteoarthritis. *Novartis Foundation Symposium, 260,* 79-95.

Hinz, B. & Brune, K. (2004). Pain and osteoarthritis: new drugs and mechanisms. *Current Opinion in Rheumatology, 16,* 628-633.

Jawad, A. S. (2005). Analgesics and osteoarthritis: are treatment guidelines reflected in clinical practice? *American Journal of Therapeutics, 12,* 98-103.

Jordan, J. M. (2004). Cartilage oligomeric matrix protein as a marker of osteoarthritis. *Journal of Rheumatology—Supplement, 70,* 45-49.

Jordan, J. M., Kraus, V. B., & Hochberg, M. C. (2004). Genetics of osteoarthritis. *Current Rheumatology Reports, 6,* 7-13.

Kelly, M. A., Kurzweil, P. R., & Moskowitz, R. W. (2004). Intra-articular hyaluronans in knee osteoarthritis: rationale and practical considerations. *American Journal of Orthopedics, 33,* 15-22.

Kelly, M. A., Moskowitz, R. W., & Lieberman, J. R. (2004). Hyaluronan therapy: looking toward the future. *American Journal of Orthopedics, 33,* 23-28.

Kidd, B. L., Photiou, A., & Inglis, J. J. (2004). The role of inflammatory mediators on nociception and pain in arthritis. *Novartis Foundation Symposium, 260,* 122-133.

Kuettner, K. E. & Cole, A. A. (2005). Cartilage degeneration in different human joints. *Osteoarthritis & Cartilage, 13,* 93-103.

Lohmander, L. S. (2004). Markers of altered metabolism in osteoarthritis. *Journal of Rheumatology—Supplement, 70,* 28-35.

Malemud, C. J. (2004). Cytokines as therapeutic targets for osteoarthritis. *Biodrugs, 18,* 23-35.

Malemud, C. J. (2004). Protein kinases in chondrocyte signaling and osteoarthritis. *Clinical Orthopaedics & Related Research,* Oct(427 Suppl), S145-S151.

Martel-Pelletier, J. (2004). Pathophysiology of osteoarthritis. *Osteoarthritis & Cartilage,* 12(suppl A), S31-S33.

Moskowitz, R. W., Kelly, M. A., Lewallen, D. G., & Vangsness, C. T., Jr. (2004). Nonsurgical approaches to pain management for osteoarthritis of the knee. *American Journal of Orthopedics, 33,* 10-14.

Owens, S., Wagner, P., & Vangsness, C. T., Jr. (2004). Recent advances in glucosamine and chondroitin supplementation. *The Journal of Knee Surgery, 17,* 185-193.

Palacios, L. C., Jones, W. Y., Mayo, H. G., & Malaty, W. (2004). Clinical inquiries. Do steroid injections help with osteoarthritis of the knee? *Journal of Family Practice, 53,* 921-922.

Radin, E. L. (2004). Who gets osteoarthritis and why? *Journal of Rheumatology—Supplement, 70,* 10-15.

Roddy, E., Zhang, W., & Doherty, M. (2005). Aerobic walking or strengthening exercise for osteoarthritis of the knee? A systematic review. *Annals of the Rheumatic Diseases, 64,* 544-548.

Roddy, E., Zhang, W., Doherty, M., Arden, N. K., Barlow, J., Birrell, F., Carr, A., Chakravarty, K., Dickson, J., Hay, E., Hosie, G., Hurley, M., Jordan, K. M., McCarthy, C.,

McMurdo, M., Mockett, S., O'Reilly, S., Peat, G., Pendleton, A., & Richards, S. (2005). Evidence-based recommendations for the role of exercise in the management of osteoarthritis of the hip or knee—the MOVE consensus. *Rheumatology, 44,* 67-73.

Schurman, D. J., & Smith, R. L. (2004). Osteoarthritis: current treatment and future prospects for surgical, medical, and biologic intervention. *Clinical Orthopaedics & Related Research,* Oct(427 Suppl), S183-S189.

Sharma, L. (2004). The role of proprioceptive deficits, ligamentous laxity, and malalignment in development and progression of knee osteoarthritis. *Journal of Rheumatology—Supplement, 70,* 87-92.

Spector, T. D. & MacGregor, A. J. (2004). Risk factors for osteoarthritis: genetics. *Osteoarthritis & Cartilage,* 12(suppl A), S39-S44.

Steinmeyer, J. (2004). Cytokines in osteoarthritis-current status on the pharmacological intervention. *Frontiers in Bioscience, 9,* 575-580.

Tesche, F. & Miosge, N. (2005). New aspects of the pathogenesis of osteoarthritis: the role of fibroblast-like chondrocytes in late stages of the disease. *Histology & Histopathology, 20,* 329-337.

Trippel, S. B. (2004). Growth factor inhibition: potential role in the etiopathogenesis of osteoarthritis. *Clinical Orthopaedics & Related Research,* Oct(427 Suppl), S47-S52.

Verstraete, K. L., Almqvist, F., Verdonk, P., Vanderschueren, G., Huysse, W., Verdonk, R., & Verbrugge, G. (2004). Magnetic resonance imaging of cartilage and cartilage repair. *Clinical Radiology, 59,* 674-689.

Volpi, N. (2004). The pathobiology of osteoarthritis and the rationale for using the chondroitin sulfate for its treatment. *Current Drug Targets—Immune Endocrine & Metabolic Disorders, 4,* 119-127.

Walsh, D. A. (2004). Angiogenesis in osteoarthritis and spondylosis: successful repair with undesirable outcomes. *Current Opinion in Rheumatology, 16,* 609-615.

Wegman, A., van der Windt, D., van Tulder, M., Stalman, W., & de Vries, T. (2004). Nonsteroidal antiinflammatory drugs or acetaminophen for osteoarthritis of the hip or knee? A systematic review of evidence and guidelines. *Journal of Rheumatology, 31,* 344-354.

Wieland, H. A., Michaelis, M., Kirschbaum, B. J., & Rudolphi, K. A. (2005). Osteoarthritis—an untreatable disease? *Nature Reviews, Drug Discovery, 4,* 331-344.

Zerkak, D. & Dougados, M. (2004). The use of glucosamine therapy in osteoarthritis. *Current Pain & Headache Reports, 8,* 507-511.

Zerkak, D. & Dougados, M. (2004). The use of glucosamine therapy in osteoarthritis. *Current Rheumatology Reports, 6,* 41-45.

Zhang, W., Doherty, M., Arden, N., Bannwarth, B., Bijlsma, J., Gunther, K. P., Hauselmann, H. J., Herrero-Beaumont, G., Jordan, K., Kaklamanis, P., Leeb, B., Lequesne, M., Lohmander, S., Mazieres, B., Martin-Mola, E., Pavelka, K., Pendleton, A., Punzi, L., Swoboda, B., Varatojo, R., Verbruggen, G., Zimmermann-Gorska, I., Dougados, M., & EULAR Standing Committee for International Clinical Studies Including Therapeutics. (2005). EULAR evidence based recommendations for the management of hip osteoarthritis: report of a task force of the EULAR Standing Committee for International Clinical Studies Including Therapeutics (ESCISIT). *Annals of the Rheumatic Diseases, 64,* 669-681.

Zhang, W., Jones, A., & Doherty, M. (2004). Does paracetamol (acetaminophen) reduce the pain of osteoarthritis? A meta-analysis of randomised controlled trials. *Annals of the Rheumatic Diseases, 63,* 901-907.

Menopausal Osteoporosis

DEFINITION

- Menopausal osteoporosis refers to the type of osteoporosis that occurs in women after menopause (type I).
- The World Health Organization (WHO) defines osteoporosis as a value of bone mineral density 2.5 standard deviations or more below the young adult mean. The National Institutes of Health defines osteoporosis as a skeletal disorder characterized by compromised bone strength predisposing to an increased risk of fracture. Bone strength reflects the integration of two main features: bone density and bone quality.
- The disease is characterized by low bone mass and microarchitectural deterioration of bone tissue, leading to enhanced bone fragility and a consequent increase in fracture risk.

EPIDEMIOLOGY

- Affects more than 5 million U.S. women; another 15 million are at risk due to low bone mass.
- One in every two white women will suffer an osteoporotic fracture in her lifetime; 90% of hip fractures in white women are attributable to osteoporosis. One year after hip fracture mortality is 20%, and 40% of women are still unable to walk independently.
- After vertebral fracture, 80% to 90% of women still have pain at 1 year.
- An estimated 15% of young adults in the United States have osteopenia.
- Risk factors.
  - Age older than 65.
  - History of fracture as an adult.
  - Family history of fracture or osteoporosis in a first-degree relative.
  - White, Asian, or Hispanic ethnicity.
  - Low body weight (<127 pounds).
  - Smoking, heavy caffeine intake.
  - Late menarche, early menopause.
  - Low-calcium or high-phosphate intake.
  - Sedentary life-style.
  - Dementia and/or depression.
  - Medications (steroids, phenytoin, heparin, warfarin).

PATHOPHYSIOLOGY

Genetics

- 40% to 80% of the risk for osteoporosis is due to heredity—considered a complex polygenic process.
- Genes that have been implicated include vitamin D receptor (VDR), estrogen receptor, interleukin (IL)-6 androgen receptor, collagen type 1 and a1 gene polymorphisms.

Tissue Effects

- Maximum bone mass is achieved at ages 25 to 35 and is determined by genetics, amount of mechanical loading (exercise), nutrition (e.g., calcium intake), and hormone use.
- Normal bone architecture requires a remodeling process that maintains bone density and bone quality.
- Bone remodeling occurs constantly in the healthy adult at maturity with no net change in bone mass. Osteoclasts excavate erosion cavities on bone surfaces and osteoblasts fill in the cavities with new bone, giving it greater strength and repairing microfractures.
- Hormonal and cytokine factors that influence bone remodeling include estrogen, testosterone, calcitonin, parathyroid hormone (PTH), 1,25-dihydroxyvitamin D, IL-1 and IL-6, and tumor necrosis factor (TNF).
- In women, endogenous estrogen accelerates osteoclast apoptosis and prolongs the life of the osteoblasts. This preserves the balance between erosion and repair until menopause. In addition, estrogen increases intestinal and renal absorption of calcium and increases vitamin D–receptor activity.
- Bone mass declines steadily after age 35 until menopause, when the loss of bone accelerates. About one third of the lifetime loss of bone at the hip occurs before age 50. In the spine, bone loss is not significant until menopause. The most rapid loss of bone occurs in the first year after menopause. Overall, women lose 30% to 50% of their trabecular bone with aging. Not only is bone quantity lost, but the bone microarchitecture (quality) also is compromised.
- Estrogen deficiency after menopause accelerates bone turnover with increasing osteoclast activity. Interestingly, one of the mechanisms implicated in the activation of osteoclasts is the release of inflammatory mediators such as interleukins (IL-1, IL-6, IL-11) and TNF from osteoblasts. This stimulates hydrogen ion and protease release from osteoclasts. In addition, estrogen deficiency contributes to osteoblast apoptosis reducing their bone-building activities. These processes result in progressively greater surface of the bone being occupied by erosion cavities created by osteoclasts, and less effective filling and repair of these cavities by osteoblasts, leading to osteopenia and osteoporosis.
- Turnover is more rapid in trabecular (cancellous) bone (vertebral column, distal radius, proximal femur) than in cortical bone, with a loss of bone mineral density and disconnectivity of the trabecular elements leading to increased likelihood of fracture.
- Osteoporosis of trabecular bone increases the risk of vertebral compression fracture, fractures of the distal forearm, and hip fracture.

PATIENT PRESENTATION

History

Postmenopausal or surgical oophorectomy; older age; housebound; late menarche; family history; thin; white or Asian; poor diet (low in calcium, high in phosphates); smoking; caffeine; history of fractures; family history of fractures; dementia or depression; medications.

Symptoms

Loss of height; back pain; pain at fracture sites. More than 65% of individuals with compression fracture are asymptomatic.

Examination

Reduced height for weight; thin; "dowager hump"; evidence of fracture.

DIFFERENTIAL DIAGNOSIS

- Senile osteoporosis.
- Iatrogenic osteoporosis (drugs).
- Renal failure—associated bone disease.
- Multiple myeloma.
- Hyperthyroidism.

- Hyperparathyroidism.
- Cushing disease.
- Type 1 diabetes.
- Osteomalacia (low calcium, vitamin D deficiency).
- Rheumatic disease.

KEYS TO ASSESSMENT

- Identify at-risk patients—the National Osteoporosis Foundation recommends bone mineral density screening (see below) for all women older than age 65 or younger if the individual has one or more risk factors for osteoporosis (especially a history of fracture).
- Yearly height measurement.
- Consider measuring follicle-stimulating hormone (FSH) levels if perimenopausal.
- Laboratory evaluation to rule out other causes of osteopenia:
  - Glucose (diabetes).
  - Blood urea nitrogen (BUN) and creatinine (Cr).
  - Calcium, phosphorus (hyperparathyroidism).
  - T3, T4 (hyperthyroidism), parathyroid hormone (PTH).
  - Alkaline phosphatase (high in malignancy, multiple myeloma, Paget disease).
  - Consider serum protein electrophoresis (multiple myeloma).
  - Others as indicated by physical examination.
- Potential laboratory tests to confirm osteoporosis (still experimental, not reproducible enough for clinical use at this time):
  - Urinary type I collagen.
  - Cross-linked N-telopeptide (NTX).
- Diagnostic studies.
  - Dual-energy x-ray absorptiometry (DEXA) of the spine and hip is both the screening and the diagnostic modality of choice. It also can be used to monitor the effectiveness of therapy in women with known osteoporosis.
    1. DEXA provides two values, the Z score and the T score. The Z score compares the patient's bone mineral density (BMD) with age-matched subjects. The T score is used to diagnose osteoporosis by the WHO criteria through comparison of the patient's BMD to mean peak bone mass in a healthy young reference population.
    2. Recommendations for screening with DEXA according to the U.S. Preventive Services Task Force are that all women ages 65 and older be screened routinely for osteoporosis and that routine screening begin at age 60 for women at increased risk for osteoporotic fractures.
    3. Other indications can include adults with fragility fracture, adults taking a medication or adults with a disease or condition associated with low bone mass or bone loss, any individual being treated for low bone mass to monitor treatment effect, and any individual in whom evidence of bone loss would affect treatment decisions.
  - Radiographs are useful in evaluating for compression fractures, but osteopenia is evident only after 30% of the bone is lost. Phalangeal bone density can be done to predict hip fracture risk.
  - Other diagnostic studies.
    1. Magnetic resonance imaging (MRI).
    2. Quantitative ultrasound.
    3. Quantitative computed tomography (CT) scanning.

KEYS TO MANAGEMENT

- Prevention.
  - According to the National Osteoporosis Foundation, therapy for prevention of bone loss should be initiated for women without risk factors if the T score on DEXA is less than –2.0. If risk factors are present, therapy should be begun at a T score less than –1.5.

- Maintain adequate calcium intake:
    1. Important to begin in the prepubertal period and continue throughout life.
    2. Calcium citrate is the most easily absorbed; however, dairy products are more effective due to improved absorption with milk-based protein (MBP).
    3. Recommend 1 to 1.5 g/day of calcium intake.
    4. When combined with exercise can reduce hip fracture risk, but will not prevent spinal bone loss.
- Reduce phosphorus intake (soft drinks, prepared foods).
- Supplement vitamin D (400 to 800 international units daily).
- Exercise both pre- and postmenopausally.
    1. Exercise should be begun in youth to maximize bone density.
    2. Weight-bearing and resistance exercise increases total body calcium as well as vertebral bone density in postmenopausal women.
    3. Smoking cessation; avoid excessive caffeine intake.
    4. Avoid osteopenic medications (steroids, thyroxine) if possible.
    5. Fall protection measures should be implemented as needed.
- Pharmacologic prevention and treatment.
    - Bisphosphonates (alendronate, risedronate, ibandronate, etidronate, pamidronate, zoledronate).
        1. They suppress bone turnover by blocking osteoclast action on the bone; their function is sometimes described as a bone "shield."
        2. Alendronate and risedronate can be taken once per week for prevention of fracture and are well tolerated with few side effects except for esophageal and gastrointestinal irritation. They have been shown to reduce hip and spinal fractures by about 40% to 60% and increase bone mineral density significantly within 2 to 3 years.
        3. Ibandronate can be given orally once a month or as a cycle of 24 days of alternate-day drug followed by 2 months off, and reduces fracture rate by as much as 60%.
        4. Injectable etidronate, pamidronate, and zoledronate can also be used to prevent or treat osteoporosis and may be given every 3 months or yearly.
    - Selective estrogen receptor modulators (SERMs).
        1. Raloxifene is approved for use in osteoporosis and has been shown to significantly increase bone mineral density and provides a small reduction in the risk of vertebral fractures without increased risk for endometrial or breast cancer (see Chapters 9 and 25). It has not been shown to reduce the risk for hip fracture.
        2. Tibolone is a steroid receptor modulator that has been shown to be effective in some early studies at reducing fracture risk with few side effects, but its safety has not yet been fully determined and it has not yet been approved for use in the United States. One study in Europe did link tibolone with a 30% increase in risk for breast cancer.
        3. Baredoxifene is a SERM in worldwide phase III trials that may be effective for osteoporosis and safer than tibolone.
        4. Lasofoxifene is a new SERM that is in early trials but appears to be more potent for osteoporosis than raloxifene.
    - Parathyroid hormone (teriparatide).
        1. Daily injection provides noncontinuous parathyroid effects on bone that stimulate bone formation by increasing the number of osteoblasts.
        2. Indicated for prevention in individuals at high risk for fracture, that is, those with previous fracture, multiple risk factors, or intolerant of other preventive modalities for osteoporosis.
        3. Highly effective for treatment of osteoporosis with significant increases in both bone mineral density and improvements in bone microarchitecture.
        4. Increases bone mineral density in women with severe osteoporosis and reduces vertebral fracture risk by 65% and nonvertebral fracture risk by 53%.
        5. Requires daily subcutaneous injections, but nasal spray is now being evaluated and appears to be equally effective.

- Calcitonin.
    1. It is usually administered as a nasal spray.
    2. At a dose of 200 international units daily, it increases bone mass and decreases fracture rate by 33%.
    3. It can be used for its analgesic effect on painful osteoporotic bone fractures.
- Hormone replacement therapy (HRT).
    1. Estrogen is no longer considered front-line for therapy of osteoporosis, but can be considered for prevention.
    2. Significantly reduces risk for osteoporotic fracture.
    3. Inhibits osteoclasts and improves osteoblast function.
    4. Treatment should begin soon after menopause to maximize bone density.
    5. Risks for the use of conjugated equine estrogen plus medroxyprogesterone acetate are thought to outweigh the benefits for most women (although this is still controversial; see Chapter 25) thus other modalities are recommended unless fracture risk is high and other modalities are not tolerated.
    6. Some studies suggest that HRT can be combined with bisphophonates in women at high risk for fracture.

PATHOPHYSIOLOGY $\longrightarrow$	CLINICAL LINK
What is going on in the disease process that influences how the patient presents and how she should be managed?	*What should you do now that you understand the underlying pathophysiology?*
The risk of osteoporosis in postmenopausal women is related to the peak bone density achieved at age 35.	Adequate calcium intake, weight-bearing exercise, and oral contraceptives for secondary amenorrhea in young women can reduce the risk of osteoporosis later in life.
Osteoporosis affects trabecular bone more than cortical bone; the vertebrae, femoral necks, ribs, and distal radius are most often involved.	Patients may present first with fractures of the hip, wrist, or rib, or may complain of acute back pain with a history of no or little trauma.
Estrogen limits the activity of osteoclasts such that the balance is shifted to the osteoblastic filling in of bone.	Gonadal insufficiency due to menopause results in increased osteoclast activity and weaker bones; estrogen replacement results in increased bone density and reduced risk of fracture.
Many other conditions can cause osteopenia including hyperthyroidism, hyperparathyroidism, malignancies, and many others.	The differential diagnosis of osteopenia requires testing for other potentially treatable conditions. A careful history, physical examination, and laboratory testing are necessary to establish the cause.
Measurement of low bone mineral density is correlated with the risk of fracture. Osteopenia is not evident on plain radiograph until nearly a third of the bone density is lost.	Dual-energy x-ray absorptiometry (DEXA) is the best way to diagnose and monitor osteoporosis.
Calcium dietary deficiency results in bone resorption and decreased osteopenia.	Adequate dietary calcium is important for the prevention of osteoporosis.
The bisphosphonates inhibit the effect of osteoclasts on bone and significantly reduce fracture risk even within the first year of use.	Alendronate is an effective and well-tolerated alternative to hormonal treatment in selected patients.
Parathyroid hormone treatment increases the number of osteoblasts and significantly improves bone mineral density.	Parathyroid hormone treatment can be highly effective, especially in those individuals with osteoporotic fractures.

SUGGESTED READINGS

American College of Obstetricians and Gynecologists Women's Health Care Physicians. (2004). Osteoporosis. *Obstetrics & Gynecology, 104,* 66S-76S.

Asikainen, T. M., Kukkonen-Harjula, K., & Miilunpalo, S. (2004). Exercise for health for early postmenopausal women: a systematic review of randomised controlled trials. *Sports Medicine, 34,* 753-778.

Avci, D. & Bachmann, G. A. (2004). Osteoarthritis and osteoporosis in postmenopausal women: clinical similarities and differences. *Menopause, 11,* 615-621.

Bath, P. M. & Gray, L. J. (2005). Association between hormone replacement therapy and subsequent stroke: a meta-analysis. *British Medical Journal, 330,* 342.

Beitz, R. & Doren, M. (2004). Physical activity and postmenopausal health. *Journal of the British Menopause Society, 10,* 70-74.

Bouxsein, M. L., Kaufman, J., Tosi, L., Cummings, S., Lane, J., & Johnell, O. (2004). Recommendations for optimal care of the fragility fracture patient to reduce the risk of future fracture. *Journal of the American Academy of Orthopaedic Surgeons, 12,* 385-395.

Bukowski, J. F., Dascher, C. C., & Das, H. (2005). Alternative bisphosphonate targets and mechanisms of action. *Biochemical & Biophysical Research Communications, 328,* 746-750.

Calcitonin intranasal—unigene: salcatonin intranasal—unigene. (2004). *Drugs in R&D, 5,* 90-93.

Cappuzzo, K. A. & Delafuente, J. C. (2004). Teriparatide for severe osteoporosis. *Annals of Pharmacotherapy, 38,* 294-302.

Carrington, J. L. (2005). Aging bone and cartilage: cross-cutting issues. *Biochemical & Biophysical Research Communications, 328,* 700-708.

Cefalu, C. A. (2004). Is bone mineral density predictive of fracture risk reduction. *Current Medical Research & Opinion, 20,* 341-349.

DeHart, R. M. & Gonzalez, E. H. (2004). Osteoporosis: point-of-care testing. *Annals of Pharmacotherapy, 38,* 473-481.

Del Puente, A., Migliaccio, S., Esposito, A., Lello, S., & Ott, S. M. (2004). A reappraisal of therapeutic approaches to osteoporosis. *Aging-Clinical & Experimental Research, 16*(suppl), 42-46.

Devogelaer, J. P. (2004). A review of the effects of tibolone on the skeleton. *Expert Opinion on Pharmacotherapy, 5,* 941-949.

Dobnig, H. (2004). A review of teriparatide and its clinical efficacy in the treatment of osteoporosis. *Expert Opinion on Pharmacotherapy, 5,* 1153-1162.

Doggrell, S. A. (2004). Does the combination of alendronate and parathyroid hormone give a greater benefit than either agent alone in osteoporosis? *Expert Opinion on Pharmacotherapy, 5,* 955-958.

Ebeling, P. R. & Russell, R. G. (2003). Teriparatide (rhPTH 1-34) for the treatment of osteoporosis. *International Journal of Clinical Practice, 57,* 710-718.

Epstein, S. (2005). The roles of bone mineral density, bone turnover, and other properties in reducing fracture risk during antiresorptive therapy. *Mayo Clinic Proceedings, 80,* 379-388.

Eriksen, E. F. & Robins, D. A. (2004). Teriparatide: a bone formation treatment for osteoporosis. *Drugs of Today, 40,* 935-948.

Ettinger, B., San Martin, J., Crans, G., & Pavo, I. (2004). Differential effects of teriparatide on BMD after treatment with raloxifene or alendronate. *Journal of Bone & Mineral Research, 19,* 745-751.

Fadanelli, M. E. & Bone, H. G. (2004). Combining bisphosphonates with hormone therapy for postmenopausal osteoporosis. *Treatments in Endocrinology, 3,* 361-369.

Felsenberg, D. & Boonen, S. (2005). The bone quality framework: determinants of bone strength and their interrelationships, and implications for osteoporosis management. *Clinical Therapeutics, 27,* 1-11.

Flynn, C. A. (2004). Calcium supplementation in postmenopausal women. *American Family Physician, 69,* 2822-2823.

Francis, R. M. (2004). Non-response to osteoporosis treatment. *Journal of the British Menopause Society, 10,* 76-80.

Gambacciani, M. & Vacca, F. (2004). Postmenopausal osteoporosis and hormone replacement therapy. *Minerva Medica, 95,* 507-520.

Gandolini, G., Migliaccio, S., Bevilacqua, M., Lello, S., & Malavolta, N. (2004). Prevent, treat and maintain: a new goal for osteoporosis management in clinical practice. *Aging-Clinical & Experimental Research, 16*(suppl), 37-41.

Garnero, P. & Delmas, P. D. (2004). Contribution of bone mineral density and bone turnover markers to the estimation of risk of osteoporotic fracture in postmenopausal women. *Journal of Musculoskeletal Neuronal Interactions, 4,* 50-63.

Gennari, L., Merlotti, D., De, P. V., Calabro, A., Becherini, L., Martini, G., & Nuti, R. (2005). Estrogen receptor gene polymorphisms and the genetics of osteoporosis: a HuGE review. *American Journal of Epidemiology, 161,* 307-320.

Gruber, C. & Gruber, D. (2004). Bazedoxifene (Wyeth). *Current Opinion in Investigational Drugs, 5,* 1086-1093.

Harvey, N. & Cooper, C. (1929). The developmental origins of osteoporotic fracture. *Journal of the British Menopause Society, 10,* 14-15.

Iwamoto, J., Takeda, T., & Sato, Y. (2004). Effects of vitamin K_2 on osteoporosis. *Current Pharmaceutical Design, 10,* 2557-2576.

Jiang, Y., Zhao, J. J., Mitlak, B. H., Wang, O., Genant, H. K., & Eriksen, E. F. (2003). Recombinant human parathyroid hormone (1-34) [teriparatide] improves both cortical and cancellous bone structure. *Journal of Bone & Mineral Research, 18,* 1932-1941.

Kanis, J. A., Borgstrom, F., Johnell, O., & Jonsson, B. (2004). Cost-effectiveness of risedronate for the treatment of osteoporosis and prevention of fractures in postmenopausal women. *Osteoporosis International, 15,* 862-871.

Keller, M. I. (2004). Treating osteoporosis in post-menopausal women: a case approach. *Cleveland Clinic Journal of Medicine, 71,* 829-837.

Kessel, B. (2004). Hip fracture prevention in postmenopausal women. *Obstetrical & Gynecological Survey, 59,* 446-455.

Kleerekoper, M. (2004). Treatment of osteoporosis. *Clinical Obstetrics & Gynecology, 47,* 413-423.

Lanyon, L., Armstrong, V., Ong, D., Zaman, G., & Price, J. (2004). Is estrogen receptor alpha key to controlling bones' resistance to fracture? *Journal of Endocrinology, 182,* 183-191.

Laustsen, G. & Wimmett, L. (2005). 2004 drug approval highlights: FDA update. *Nurse Practitioner, 30,* 14-29.

Leib, E. S., Lewiecki, E. M., Binkley, N., Hamdy, R. C., & International Society for Clinical Densitometry. (2004). Official positions of the International Society for Clinical Densitometry. *Journal of Clinical Densitometry, 7,* 1-6.

Lewiecki, E. M. (2004). Low bone mineral density in premenopausal women. *Southern Medical Journal, 97,* 544-550.

Lindsay, R. (2004). Hormones and bone health in postmenopausal women. *Endocrine, 24,* 223-230.

Lobo, R. A. (2004). The rationale for low-dose hormonal therapy. *Endocrine, 24,* 217-221.

Lufkin, E. G., Sarkar, S., Kulkarni, P. M., Ciaccia, A. V., Siddhanti, S., Stock, J., & Plouffe, L., Jr. (2004). Antiresorptive treatment of postmenopausal osteoporosis: review of randomized clinical studies and rationale for the Evista alendronate comparison (EVA) trial. *Current Medical Research & Opinion, 20,* 351-357.

Madore, G. R., Sherman, P. J., & Lane, J. M. (2004). Parathyroid hormone. *Journal of the American Academy of Orthopaedic Surgeons*, 12, 67-71.

Mattsson, L. A., Skouby, S. O., Heikkinen, J., Vaheri, R., Maenpaa, J., & Timonen, U. (2004). A low-dose start in hormone replacement therapy provides a beneficial bleeding profile and few side-effects: randomized comparison with a conventional-dose regimen. *Climacteric*, 7, 59-69.

Mikkola, T. S., Clarkson, T. B., & Notelovitz, M. (2004). Postmenopausal hormone therapy before and after the women's health initiative study: what consequences? *Annals of Medicine*, 36, 402-413.

Munoz-Torres, M., Alonso, G., & Raya, M. P. (2004). Calcitonin therapy in osteoporosis. *Treatments in Endocrinology*, 3, 117-132.

Oglesby, A. K., Minshall, M. E., Shen, W., Xie, S., & Silverman, S. L. (2003). The impact of incident vertebral and non-vertebral fragility fractures on health-related quality of life in established postmenopausal osteoporosis: results from the teriparatide randomized, placebo-controlled trial in postmenopausal women. *Journal of Rheumatology*, 30, 1579-1583.

Parsons, L. C. (2005). Osteoporosis: incidence, prevention, and treatment of the silent killer. *Nursing Clinics of North America*, 40, 119-133.

Perez-Lopez, F. R. (2004). Postmenopausal osteoporosis and alendronate. *Maturitas*, 48, 179-192.

Phillips, E. M., Bodenheimer, C. F., Roig, R. L., & Cifu, D. X. (2004). Geriatric rehabilitation. 4. Physical medicine and rehabilitation interventions for common age-related disorders and geriatric syndromes. *Archives of Physical Medicine & Rehabilitation*, 85, S18-S22.

Reginster, J. Y. (2004). Prevention of postmenopausal osteoporosis with pharmacological therapy: practice and possibilities. *Journal of Internal Medicine*, 255, 615-628.

Roux, C., Garnero, P., Thomas, T., Sabatier, J. P., Orcel, P., Audran, M., & Comite Scientifique du, G. R. I. O. (2005). Recommendations for monitoring antiresorptive therapies in postmenopausal osteoporosis. *Joint, Bone, Spine: Revue du Rhumatisme*, 72, 26-31.

Schrager, S. (2004). Osteoporosis in women with disabilities. *Journal of Women's Health*, 13, 431-437.

Shea, B., Wells, G., Cranney, A., Zytaruk, N., Robinson, V., Griffith, L., Hamel, C., Ortiz, Z., Peterson, J., Adachi, J., Tugwell, P., Guyatt, G., Osteoporosis, M. G., & Osteoporosis Research, A. G. (2004). Calcium supplementation on bone loss in postmenopausal women. *Cochrane Database of Systematic Reviews*, CD004526.

Shepherd, A. J. (1992). An overview of osteoporosis. *Alternative Therapies in Health & Medicine*, 10, 26-33.

Shulman, L. P. (2004). The menopausal transition: how does route of delivery affect the risk/benefit ratio of hormone therapy? *Journal of Family Practice* (suppl), S13-S17.

Swegle, J. M. & Kelly, M. W. (2004). Tibolone: a unique version of hormone replacement therapy. *Annals of Pharmacotherapy*, 38, 874-881.

Tansavatdi, K., McClain, B., & Herrington, D. M. (2004). The effects of smoking on estradiol metabolism. *Minerva Ginecologica*, 56, 105-114.

Writing Group for the ISCD Position Development Conference. (2004). Indications and reporting for dual-energy x-ray absorptiometry. *Journal of Clinical Densitometry*, 7, 37-44.

Xenodemetropoulos, T., Davison, S., Ioannidis, G., & Adachi, J. D. (2004). The impact of fragility fracture on health-related quality of life: the importance of antifracture therapy. *Drugs & Aging*, 21, 711-730.

Yildirir, A. & Muderrisoglu, H. (2004). Non-lipid effects of statins: emerging new indications. *Current Vascular Pharmacology*, 2, 309-318.

Zanchetta, J. R., Bogado, C. E., Ferretti, J. L., Wang, O., Wilson, M. G., Sato, M., Gaich, G. A., Dalsky, G. P., & Myers, S. L. (2003). Effects of teriparatide [recombinant human parathyroid hormone (1-34)] on cortical bone in postmenopausal women with osteoporosis. *Journal of Bone & Mineral Research*, 18, 539-543.

Zizic, T. M. (2004). Pharmacologic prevention of osteoporotic fractures. *American Family Physician*, 70, 1293-1300.

Osteoporosis

INITIAL HISTORY

- 66-year-old female.
- Back pain for 6 to 8 weeks.
- Pain is constant and aggravated by activity.
- Ibuprofen provides temporary relief.

Question 1.   *What is the differential diagnosis at this time?*

Question 2.   *What additional questions would you like to ask her about her symptoms?*

ADDITIONAL HISTORY

- Patient denies any acute or previous injury to her back.
- States she has had a slight reduction in height.
- Denies change in weight.
- Denies any unusual bleeding.
- Denies fever or chills.
- Denies heat or cold intolerance or changes in her hair, skin, or nails.
- Denies any gastrointestinal symptoms.

□ **Leslie Buchanan, RN, MSN, ENP contributed this case study.**

- Denies genitourinary incontinence.
- Denies any extremity weakness.
- States there is no improvement of pain with position changes.

Question 3.   *What would you like to ask her about her medical history and family history?*

MEDICAL AND FAMILY HISTORY

- History of mild hypertension for which she takes an ACE inhibitor.
- No other long-term medications.
- Postmenopausal since age 48 but does not take hormones at the advice of her nurse practitioner.
- Denies endocrine or renal disease.
- Denies a personal history of breast cancer but has a family history in both her mother and sister.
- Mammogram last year was normal.
- Mother had a fractured hip from a fall 10 years ago.
- No previous fractures as an adult.

Question 4.   *What would you like to ask her about her life-style?*

LIFE-STYLE HISTORY

- Gets very little exercise, mostly light housework.
- Rarely gets outdoors.
- 20 pack/year smoking history.
- Drinks an occasional glass of wine.
- Drinks four or five caffeinated beverages per day.
- Does not take calcium or vitamin D supplements.

PHYSICAL EXAMINATION

- 66-year-old white female of slight stature, walking with normal gait and in no acute distress.
- Height = 5 feet, 3½ inches; weight = 54 kg.
- T = 37° C orally; P = 84 and regular; RR = 20 and unlabored; BP = 154/88 (sitting).

Skin, HEENT

- Dry skin; nails cracking.
- No areas of tenderness, slight thinning of hair.
- Tympanic membranes pearly without bulging or retraction.
- Conjunctivae clear, PERRLA, funduscopic without lesions.
- Clear without drainage or erythema.

Neck

- Moderate cervical lordosis.
- No bony tenderness.
- Full range of motion without pain elicited.
- Thyroid nontender without thyromegaly, no masses palpable.
- No adenopathy.

Chest

- Normal chest excursion, rhonchi throughout chest, all clear with cough.
- Cardiac examination with regular rate and rhythm without murmurs or gallops.

Abdomen, Neurologic

- Bowel sounds present throughout.
- No tenderness; no organomegaly; no masses.
- Alert and oriented ×3; recent and remote memory intact.
- Cranial nerves intact.
- No focal motor deficits; no gross sensory deficits.
- DTRs 1+ and symmetric throughout.
- Negative Kernig and Brudzinski signs.

Musculoskeletal

- Tenderness with palpation of the bony prominences of L1 and L2.
- Limited flexion and extension of the back.
- Lateral bending unlimited and nonpainful.
- No dorsal kyphosis (dowager hump).
- No deformity or swelling of joints.

Question 5.   *What are the pertinent positive and negative findings on physical examination?*

Question 6.   *What initial diagnostic testing is indicated?*

RADIOGRAPH RESULTS

- Osteopenia.
- Compression fracture of L2.
- Plain film of chest is negative.

Question 7. *Based on these results, what further diagnostic testing is indicated?*

LABORATORY RESULTS

- Serum chemistry levels, including phosphate and calcium, normal.
- CBC normal.
- Thyroid function test results normal.
- Rheumatoid factor negative.
- Serum and 24-hour urine alkaline phosphate level normal.
- Erythrocyte sedimentation rate and serum protein electrophoresis normal.
- DEXA T score 1.2.

Question 8. *Now what is your diagnosis?*

Question 9. *What is your treatment plan?*

Question 10. *What further care would you recommend?*

Chapter 25

Alterations During Menopause

DEFINITION

- Menopause is defined by the World Health Organization (WHO) as the permanent cessation of menstruation resulting from the loss of ovarian follicular activity. After 12 consecutive months of amenorrhea, the final menstrual period (FMP) is retrospectively designated as the time of menopause.
- The WHO further defines the perimenopause (climacteric) as the physiologic antecedents associated with the transition from premenopausal to postmenopausal follicular function and comprises the period (2 to 8 years) preceding the menopause and 1 year following the final menses. (Thus the last year of the perimenopause coincides with the first year of the postmenopause.)
- The Stages of Reproductive Aging Workshop (STRAW) of the National American Menopause Society has recommended redefining some of these terms:
  - Stages –2 (early) and –1 (late) menopausal transition begin with variations in menstrual cycle length and a monotropic rise in follicle-stimulating hormone (FSH) level. These stages end with the FMP.
  - Stages +1 (early) and +2 (late) postmenopause begin with the FMP. Stage +1 is further divided into segment a, the first 12 months after the FMP and segment b, the next 4 years. Stage +2 begins 5 years after the FMP and continues until death.
  - The perimenopause begins with stage –2 and ends after segment 1a of the postmenopause.

EPIDEMIOLOGY

- Women in the United States can now expect to spend one third of their lives postmenopausal.
- The average age of menopause is between 48 and 52 years (age 51 is most often quoted), but anytime between age 40 and 60 is normal.
- The factors associated with early menopause include smoking (average 1 to 2 years younger), menstrual cycles shorter than 26 days, higher body mass, noncontraceptive hormone use, presence of osteoporosis, and Asian descent.
- Although this is a natural process of aging, 90% of women are symptomatic and there are clear health implications.
  - The type and number of climacteric symptoms are related to race, ethnicity, education, perceived life stressors, and amount of exercise and leisure interests.
  - The onset of symptoms often occurs during the perimenopause before cessation of menses.

PATHOPHYSIOLOGY

Genetics

- There is to date relatively little understanding of the genetics associated with the menopause transition. Some genes have been associated with changes in level and sensitivity to endogenous estrogens (estrogen receptor polymorphism, PvuII, CYP17 polymorphism).
- Other relevant genes relate to the diseases that become more prevalent after the menopause transition such as genes that affect thrombosis, atherosclerosis, Alzheimer disease, and cancer risk.

Tissue Effects

- The transition to menopause occurs because of an interaction of central nervous system, endocrine, and ovarian events leading to an increase in the rate of loss of ovarian follicles and irregular reproductive cycles. Although the loss of ovarian estrogen release is key to the symptoms of the climacteric, several discoveries suggest that there is a more complex interaction of events.
    - Inhibin A and inhibin B are ovarian and pituitary compounds that form a secondary negative feedback loop on the hypothalamic-pituitary axis that is independent of hormone levels. Neuroendocrine changes (e.g., increased FSH) are seen prior to ovarian failure when inhibin B levels decline (beginning up to 10 years before the menopause) and while estradiol and progesterone levels remain normal and menstrual cycles are regular.
    - Desynchronization of neural signals with changes in the daily and monthly rhythmicity of hormone levels has been documented before measurable primary ovarian dysfunction occurs. This can result in hot flashes and sleep disturbances (felt to be more directly related to hypothalamic dysfunction than to pure estrogen deficiency) that may begin as early as age 40 even when estradiol and cycles remain normal.
- Menopausal transition.
    - Early menopausal transition is characterized by regular menstrual cycles, but they are of shorter length (change by 7 days or more).
        1. FSH levels begin to rise and inhibin B levels start to fall (elevation in FSH is the first measurable sign of reproductive aging).
        2. Early symptoms include hot flashes and breast tenderness.
    - Late menopausal transition is characterized by more than two skipped periods (an interval of amenorrhea >60 days).
        1. Unpredictable variations in cycle length are due to erratic maturation of the remaining ovarian follicles, with some ovulatory cycles (estrogen rise followed by luteinizing hormone [LH] and progesterone secretion) mixed with anovulatory cycles (no LH and progesterone surge).
        2. FSH levels rise significantly.
- Postmenopause.
    - There is no ovulation and estradiol levels fall.
    - The ovarian stroma produces androgens (androstenedione, testosterone) that are converted to estrone and estradiol in peripheral fat cells so that there is some protective estrogen effect until late in life.
- Effects of estrogen deficiency.
    - Genitourinary atrophy and dysfunction: Atrophic vaginitis, urethritis, incontinence, uterovaginal prolapse. Proposed mechanisms include vaginal wall atrophy, increases in vaginal pH, thinning of the urethral mucosa, decreased sensitivity of the α-adrenergic receptors at the bladder neck, and atrophy of the bladder trigone.
    - Cognitive defects, dementia, and mood alterations: The proposed mechanisms for changes in cognition after menopause include dysregulation of numerous neurotransmitters (norepinephrine, dopamine, serotonin); altered monamine oxidase (MAO) activity; decreased neuronal growth factors; decreased cerebral blood flow; increased silent cerebral ischemic events; and altered sleep patterns (sleep-related

disordered breathing, insomnia). Recently, estrogen deficiency has been linked to changes in amyloid precursor proteins that are associated with Alzheimer disease.

- Vasomotor instability (hot flash): Affects 80% to 85% of U.S. women and begins in the perimenopause.
  1. It is a specific thermoregulatory disorder triggered by a neuroendocrine imbalance from the hypothalamus that is associated with estrogen withdrawal.
  2. There is dysfunction of the thermoregulatory center in the medial preoptic area of the hypothalamus that is responsible for determining core body temperature and the thermoregulatory "zone." Women with hot flashes have a thermoregulatory zone that is shifted downward (heat intolerant) and is narrowed (small changes in core body temperature trigger heat retention or heat loss mechanisms).
     a. Norepinephrine, which is tonically inhibited by endorphins and catecholestrogen, becomes elevated in perimenopausal women and causes a lowering of the thermoregulatory zone and an increase in core body temperature.
     b. Core body temperature rises slightly approximately 15 minutes before the onset of hot flash symptoms in about 60% of events. A rise in temperature of even as little as 0.01° C above the upper limit of the thermoregulatory zone will trigger the heat loss mechanisms that are experienced as symptomatic hot flashes.
     c. Exercise, which lowers norepinephrine levels, can reduce vasomotor symptoms in the majority of symptomatic women.
  3. Although there is no correlation with baseline LH, FSH, or gonadotropin-releasing hormone (GnRH) levels, periodic surges in LH are seen during the perimenopause that are correlated with many (but not all) hot flashes.
  4. Estrogen withdrawal is associated with decreased serotonin levels and with up-regulation of some serotonin receptors in the hypothalamus. An imbalance in the amount and type of serotonin receptor activation can trigger hot flashes. It has been demonstrated that selective serotonin reuptake inhibitors (SSRIs) are effective in reducing hot flashes in many women treated with these medications.
  5. Clinically, episodes of temperature elevation are correlated with flushing of the skin, perspiration, palpitations, nausea, and dizziness. Peripheral vasodilation is followed by vasoconstriction and shivering. These symptoms can disturb sleep and are associated with an increased risk for osteoporosis and other metabolic abnormalities such as hyperglycemia.
- Atherosclerotic cardiovascular disease: There is an increased risk of coronary and cerebrovascular disease after menopause. Proposed mechanisms include decreased ability to heal vascular injury; decreased endogenous vasodilators (e.g., nitric oxide); decreased insulin sensitivity; decreased high-density lipoprotein (HDL) and increased low-density lipoprotein (LDL) (especially small dense LDL); down-regulation of hepatic LDL receptors; increased Lp(a); increased adhesion molecule activity; increased oxidant activity; increased thrombogenic factors (fibrinogen, factor VII, plasminogen-activator inhibitor-1); increased homocysteine, and increased smooth muscle cell proliferation. Estrogen deficiency is also associated with decreased atherosclerotic plaque stability, a key component of the risk for acute coronary syndromes.
- Osteoporosis: Increased osteoclast activity (see Chapter 24).
- Other: Increases in intra-abdominal fat; decreases in skeletal muscle contractility; alterations in integument structure.

PATIENT PRESENTATION

History

Woman in her late 40s or early 50s; menstrual cycle changes with shortened cycles followed by erratic cycles; smoking; chemotherapy; surgery; hormone use.

Symptoms

- Perimenopausal symptomatology involves the following three interacting factors:
  - Abnormalities in hypothalamic, endocrine, and neurotransmitter function.
  - Sociologic changes in aging.
  - Psychologic changes in aging.
- Perimenopausal and menopausal symptomatology:
  - Hot flashes, perspiration, night sweats.
  - Vaginal dryness, vaginal discharge, dyspareunia.
  - Uterovaginal prolapse, urethritis, stress incontinence.
  - Decreased cognitive ability, memory loss.
  - Fatigue, insomnia, anxiety, mood lability.
  - Decreased muscle strength.
  - Osteoporosis, fractures.
  - Alopecia, hirsutism, skin dryness, pruritus, wrinkles.

Examination

Dry skin; alopecia; hirsutism; loss of height; vaginal dryness and discharge; uterine prolapse; evidence of atherosclerotic disease; evidence of vertebral compression.

KEYS TO ASSESSMENT

- If the patient is younger than 40 years of age, evaluate for possible causes of premature menopause such as gynecologic surgery (especially with oophorectomy), chemotherapy, or congenital abnormalities (e.g., Turner syndrome).
- Obtain a careful menstrual history including menarche, perimenopause, and any postmenopausal bleeding.
- Assess the patient's risk for cardiovascular disease and osteoporosis.
- Carefully review for perimenopausal symptoms and be sure and ask about sleep disturbance, fatigue, and mood changes. Also ask about exercise, smoking, and diet.
- Assess for medical contraindications for hormone replacement (breast or endometrial cancer, active thrombotic disease, undiagnosed uterine bleeding, hepatic failure).
- Perform a careful physical examination, with special attention to cardiovascular and gynecologic examinations; vaginal maturation index may indicate postmenopausal state.
- Perform laboratory evaluation for osteoporosis (see Chapter 24).
- Measure serum FSH level (may be elevated).
- Measure inhibin B level if uncertainty exists (level may be decreased).

KEYS TO MANAGEMENT

- Nonpharmacologic therapies.
  - Exercise has been shown to result in improvement in hot flashes, mood, muscle strength, bone mineral density, and overall quality of life, while decreasing postmenopausal cardiac risk.
  - Further recommendations for general health promotion should include smoking cessation, weight control, and healthy diet to reduce cardiovascular disease and cancer risks.
  - Help the patient identify and avoid stimuli that trigger vasomotor flashes including alcohol, caffeine, and hot spicy foods; layered clothing may help with temperature control.
  - Herbs and vitamins such as black cohosh, St. John's wort, ginseng, chasteberry, dong quai, evening primrose oil, wild yam root, fennel, licorice, tea of sage or motherwort, bee pollen, vitamin E, vitamin B complex, and vitamin C have not been consistently shown to be effective, but may be used by individuals with varying effectiveness.
  - Phytoestrogens are estrogen-like compounds created by the intestinal bacterial conversion of isoflavonoids (found in soybean products) and lignins (found in cereals,

seeds, and nuts). They have been found to have either no or slight effect on hot flashes and may improve lipid profile, but there are conflicting results as to whether their estrogenic properties reduce or increase the risk for breast cancer.

- Educate the patient about using vaginal lubricants.
- Create a safe and caring environment with open discussion about symptoms, aging, and relationship concerns.
- Hormone replacement therapy (HRT).
    - HRT is a term used to describe numerous types of estrogen and/or progesterone treatments for the management of menopausal symptoms. These medications are generally very effective in managing hot flashes and genitourinary symptoms, and reducing the risk for osteoporosis and colon cancer.
    - The mechanisms by which HRT affects body systems are highly complex and depend on many factors, for example, the type of estrogen and progesterone used, the age of the individual being treated, genetic influences on numerous associated physiologic processes (clot formation, cell division), and the timing of hormone administration (how soon after menopause, how long treatment is continued). Other factors that confound an individual's response to HRT include reproductive and family history, smoking history, and the presence of diseases (e.g., collagen vascular disease, diabetes, hepatic disease, cancer).
    - It is difficult to interpret the results of the many clinical trials that have been conducted to assess the risks and benefits of HRT because of differences in methodology and the type of HRT used. The Women's Health Initiative is the largest prospective trial of HRT to date. This trial compared placebo with oral conjugated equine estrogen (CEE) plus medroxyprogesterone acetate (MPA) in one arm of the trial and to CEE alone in the other arm. It is interesting to note that two thirds of the participants were older than age 60 when they were begun on HRT, tended to be obese, and almost half were past or current smokers. Although there remains great controversy over whether this study truly reflects the majority of women who seek treatment with HRT and whether an accurate interpretation of the results has been reported, the following listing of risks and benefits is based on the results of that trial.
        1. Risks.
            a. Breast cancer (see Chapter 9): Increase in risk in the combined CEE and MPA arm. There was no increase in risk in the CEE-alone arm.
            b. Atherosclerotic cardiovascular disease: Transient increase in risk for in the first few years of combined CEE and MPA. There was no effect on cardiovascular risk in the CEE-alone arm.
            c. Venous thromboembolism: Risk increased significantly.
            d. Stroke risk: A small but significant increase.
            e. Gallbladder disease (especially gallstones): Risk increased significantly.
            f. Dementia: A slightly greater risk of developing dementia was observed (Women's Health Initiative Memory Study [WHIMS]).
        2. Benefits.
            a. Decreased hot flashes.
            b. Improved urogenital symptoms.
            c. Reduced risk for osteoporotic fracture (see Chapter 24).
            d. Reduced risk of colon cancer.
    - Additional considerations from other studies.
        1. Unopposed estrogen (without progesterone) increases the risk for endometrial cancer.
        2. HRT may worsen hepatic failure in those with underlying hepatic disease.
        3. HRT may worsen migraines.
        4. HRT is associated with improved carbohydrate metabolism (improves insulin sensitivity and diabetic control) and reduces the risk of diabetes.
        5. Oral HRT can improve lipid profile: decreases LDL and Lp(a) and increases HDL. But it also increases C-reactive protein (CRP) by as much as fourfold, which

          is an important indicator of cardiovascular risk. Transdermal HRT does not increase CRP.

6. Transdermal HRT does not increase the risk of venous thromboembolism.
7. HRT may increase muscle strength and may improve mood and libido.

- Currently, decisions about HRT or alternatives should be collaborative with the patient and should be made after careful assessment of the risks versus the benefits for each individual. In general, HRT should be used only for the treatment of menopausal symptoms (hot flashes, genitourinary changes) for the shortest time possible and only in women without a history of heart disease, cancer, stroke, or venous thromboembolism. For the management of heart disease, osteoporosis, or other complications of the postmenopausal state, other appropriate forms of therapy (e.g., statins, bisphosphonates) should be used.
- Low-dose formulations of HRT, transdermal patches, estrogen lotions, and intravaginal rings can be considered for relief of hot flashes and urogenital complaints.
- Progestins alone can help reduce hot flashes, but are associated with dysfunctional uterine bleeding, mood changes, and worsening of vaginal atrophy.
- Androgens are used with estrogen in some women to increase libido, decrease breast tenderness, and decrease migraines. There is no indication for androgens alone. Primary side effects are hirsutism and acne.
- Research continues into other forms of hormonal treatment for the complications of menopause, including new types of estrogens and progesterones, as well as innovative modes of hormone administration. The growing understanding of genetic influences on health, disease, and response to medications (e.g., presence of ER-α IVS1-401 C/C genotype) may make it possible to use the optimal form of hormone treatment for a specific individual.

- Alternatives to HRT.
  - The selective estrogen receptor modulators (SERMs) are an expanding group of drugs that have estrogenic effects on some tissues and antiestrogenic effects on others. One example of a SERM is raloxifene, which treats osteoporosis, reduces the risk of breast cancer, reduces the risk of heart disease, and does not increase risk for endometrial cancer, but unfortunately increases hot flashes and the risk for venous thromboembolism. Better drugs are in development.
  - Venlafaxine is a new antidepressant that improves catecholamine and serotonin balance and reduces vasomotor symptoms by 60% to 75%.
  - Selective serotonin reuptake inhibitors (SSRIs), especially fluoxetine and paroxetine, have been shown to decrease vasomotor symptoms by as much as 65%; some controversy over their effectiveness remains here.
  - Other drugs include gabapentin, clonidine, cetrizine, and drospirenone—all have been shown to be effective in small trials.

PATHOPHYSIOLOGY →	CLINICAL LINK
What is going on in the disease process that influences how the patient presents and how she should be managed?	*What should you do now that you understand the underlying pathophysiology?*
Perimenopause is characterized by fewer oocytes with decreased follicular estradiol production.	Premenopausal causes of increased oocyte loss (e.g., chemotherapy) can result in early onset menopause.
Decreasing inhibin levels and desynchronization of the neuroendocrine pathways precede changes in FSH and estradiol.	Symptoms of menopause can precede the cessation of menses and documented changes in serum FSH and estradiol. Thus the climacteric may be significantly symptomatic for patients before the onset of menopause itself can be clinically documented.
Estrogen is important for maintaining normal functioning of the skin, neurons, blood vessels, bones, muscles, and the urogenital epithelium.	Perimenopausal estrogen deficiency is characterized by thin, dry skin; decreased cognitive ability; increased cardiovascular risk; osteoporosis; decreased muscle strength; and atrophic vaginitis.
The climacteric is characterized by neuroendocrine changes involving a shift in the thermoregulatory zone associated with norepinephrine, serotonin, and LH levels.	Vasomotor instability (hot flashes) occurs frequently in perimenopausal women and may be relieved with exercise (reduces norepinephrine), SSRIs, and/or hormone replacement.
Endogenous estrogen and progesterone affect different receptors in tissues at different times and in complex ways.	HRT is not really hormone "replacement." In its current form, HRT is the use of non-physiologic types and doses of hormones such that for most women its benefits (e.g., decreased hot flashes, osteoporotic fractures) are not outweighed by its risks (e.g., increased risk of heart attack, strokes, breast cancer, thromboembolism).
Selective estrogen receptor modulators have antiestrogen effects in the breast, and have variable effects on estrogen receptors in bone, heart, liver, and endometrium.	Alternatives to HRT are available that may reduce the risk of breast cancer and improve osteoporotic and cardiovascular risk; however, better drugs are needed.

SUGGESTED READINGS

Amin, S. H., Kuhle, C. L., & Fitzpatrick, L. A. (2003). Comprehensive evaluation of the older woman. *Mayo Clinic Proceedings, 78,* 1157-1185.

Andreen, L., Sundstrom-Poromaa, I., Bixo, M., Andersson, A., Nyberg, S., & Backstrom, T. (2005). Relationship between allopregnanolone and negative mood in postmenopausal women taking sequential hormone replacement therapy with vaginal progesterone. *Psychoneuroendocrinology, 30,* 212-224.

Ay, A. & Yurtkuran, M. (2005). Influence of aquatic and weight-bearing exercises on quantitative ultrasound variables in postmenopausal women. *American Journal of Physical Medicine & Rehabilitation, 84,* 52-61.

Bath, P. M. & Gray, L. J. (2005). Association between hormone replacement therapy and subsequent stroke: a meta-analysis. *British Medical Journal, 330,* 342.

Bhavnani, B. R. (2003). Estrogens and menopause: pharmacology of conjugated equine estrogens and their potential role in the prevention of neurodegenerative diseases such as Alzheimer's. *Journal of Steroid Biochemistry & Molecular Biology, 85,* 473-482.

Bibbins-Domingo, K., Lin, F., Vittinghoff, E., Barrett-Connor, E., Hulley, S. B., Grady, D., & Shlipak, M. G. (2005). Effect of hormone therapy on mortality rates among women with heart failure and coronary artery disease. *American Journal of Cardiology, 95,* 289-291.

Brewer, D. & Nashelsky, J. (329). What nonhormonal therapies are effective for postmenopausal vasomotor symptoms? *Journal of Family Practice, 52,* 324-325.

Bukowski, J. F., Dascher, C. C., & Das, H. (2005). Alternative bisphosphonate targets and mechanisms of action. *Biochemical & Biophysical Research Communications, 328,* 746-750.

Carrington, J. L. (2005). Aging bone and cartilage: cross-cutting issues. *Biochemical & Biophysical Research Communications, 328,* 700-708.

Casadesus, G., Atwood, C. S., Zhu, X., Hartzler, A. W., Webber, K. M., Perry, G., Bowen, R. L., & Smith, M. A. (2005). Evidence for the role of gonadotropin hormones in the development of Alzheimer disease. *Cellular & Molecular Life Sciences, 62,* 293-298.

Chiechi, L. M. (2004). Estrasorb. *Drugs, 7,* 860-864.

Cirillo, D. J., Wallace, R. B., Rodabough, R. J., Greenland, P., LaCroix, A. Z., Limacher, M. C., & Larson, J. C. (2005). Effect of estrogen therapy on gallbladder disease. *Journal of the American Medical Association, 293,* 330-339.

Colacurci, N., Manzella, D., Fornaro, F., Carbonella, M., & Paolisso, G. (2003). Endothelial function and menopause: effects of raloxifene administration. *Journal of Clinical Endocrinology & Metabolism, 88,* 2135-2140.

Colacurci, N., Zarcone, R., Borrelli, A., De Franciscis, P., Fortunato, N., Cirillo, M., & Fornaro, F. (2004). Effects of soy isoflavones on menopausal neurovegetative symptoms. *Minerva Ginecologica, 56,* 407-412.

Craig, M. C., Maki, P. M., & Murphy, D. G. (2005). The Women's Health Initiative Memory Study: findings and implications for treatment. *Lancet Neurology, 4,* 190-194.

De Castro, F., Moron, F. J., Montoro, L., Galan, J. J., Real, L. M., & Ruiz, A. (2005). Re: polymorphisms associated with circulating sex hormone levels in postmenopausal women. *Journal of the National Cancer Institute, 97,* 152-153.

Dick, I. M., Devine, A., Beilby, J., & Prince, R. L. (2005). Effects of endogenous estrogen on renal calcium and phosphate handling in elderly women. *American Journal of Physiology—Endocrinology & Metabolism, 288,* E430-E435.

Doty, T. J. (2005). Postmenopausal hormone replacement therapy after the Women's Health Initiative. *JAAPA, 18,* 30-37.

Dunkin, J., Rasgon, N., Wagner-Steh, K., David, S., Altshuler, L., & Rapkin, A. (2005). Reproductive events modify the effects of estrogen replacement therapy on cognition in healthy postmenopausal women. *Psychoneuroendocrinology, 30,* 284-296.

Ebeling, P. R. & Russell, R. G. (2003). Teriparatide (rhPTH 1-34) for the treatment of osteoporosis. *International Journal of Clinical Practice, 57,* 710-718.

Evans, M. L., Pritts, E., Vittinghoff, E., McClish, K., Morgan, K. S., & Jaffe, R. B. (2005). Management of postmenopausal hot flushes with venlafaxine hydrochloride: a randomized, controlled trial. *Obstetrics & Gynecology, 105,* 161-166.

Freeman, R. & Lewis, R. M. (2004). The therapeutic role of estrogens in postmenopausal women. *Endocrinology & Metabolism Clinics of North America, 33,* 771-789.

Fugate, S. E. & Church, C. O. (2004). Nonestrogen treatment modalities for vasomotor symptoms associated with menopause. *Annals of Pharmacotherapy, 38,* 1482-1499.

Gass, M. S., Rebar, R. W., Cuffie-Jackson, C., Cedars, M. I., Lobo, R. A., Shoupe, D., Judd, H. L., Buyalos, R. P., & Clisham, P. R. (2004). A short study in the treatment of hot flashes with buccal administration of 17-beta estradiol. *Maturitas, 49,* 140-147.

Gorodeski, G. I., Hopfer, U., Liu, C. C., & Margles, E. (2005). Estrogen acidifies vaginal pH by up-regulation of proton secretion via the apical membrane of vaginal-ectocervical epithelial cells. *Endocrinology, 146,* 816-824.

Henderson, V. W., Benke, K. S., Green, R. C., Cupples, L. A., Farrer, L. A., & MIRAGE, S. G. (2005). Postmenopausal hormone therapy and Alzheimer's disease risk: interaction with age. *Journal of Neurology, Neurosurgery & Psychiatry, 76,* 103-105.

Herrington, D. M. & Klein, K. P. (2003). Randomized clinical trials of hormone replacement therapy for treatment or prevention of cardiovascular disease: a review of the findings. *Atherosclerosis, 166,* 203-212.

Iwamoto, I., Fujino, T., Douchi, T., & Nagata, Y. (2003). Association of estrogen receptor alpha and beta3-adrenergic receptor polymorphisms with endometrial cancer. *Obstetrics & Gynecology, 102,* 506-511.

Kligler, B. (2003). Black cohosh. *American Family Physician, 68,* 114-116.

Krebs, E. E., Ensrud, K. E., MacDonald, R., & Wilt, T. J. (2004). Phytoestrogens for treatment of menopausal symptoms: a systematic review. *Obstetrics & Gynecology, 104,* 824-836.

Kreijkamp-Kaspers, S., Kok, L., Bots, M. L., Grobbee, D. E., Lampe, J. W., & van der Schouw, Y. T. (2005). Randomized controlled trial of the effects of soy protein containing isoflavones on vascular function in postmenopausal women. *American Journal of Clinical Nutrition, 81,* 189-195.

Kuller, L. H. & Women's Health Initiative. (2003). Hormone replacement therapy and risk of cardiovascular disease: implications of the results of the Women's Health Initiative. *Arteriosclerosis, Thrombosis & Vascular Biology, 23,* 11-16.

Maclennan, A. H., Broadbent, J. L., Lester, S., & Moore, V. (2004). Oral oestrogen and combined oestrogen/progestogen therapy versus placebo for hot flushes. [Update of *Cochrane Database Systematic Reviews* 2001;(1):CD002978; PMID: 11279791]. *Cochrane Database of Systematic Reviews,* CD002978.

Mattsson, L. A., Skouby, S. O., Heikkinen, J., Vaheri, R., Maenpaa, J., & Timonen, U. (2004). A low-dose start in hormone replacement therapy provides a beneficial bleeding profile and few side-effects: randomized comparison with a conventional-dose regimen. *Climacteric, 7,* 59-69.

Mazer, N. A. & Shifren, J. L. (2003). Transdermal testosterone for women: a new physiological approach for androgen therapy. *Obstetrical & Gynecological Survey*, 58, 489-500.

McLay, R. N., Maki, P. M., & Lyketsos, C. G. (2003). Nulliparity and late menopause are associated with decreased cognitive decline. *Journal of Neuropsychiatry & Clinical Neurosciences*, 15, 161-167.

Moe, K. E. (2004). Hot flashes and sleep in women. *Sleep Medicine Reviews*, 8, 487-497.

Olsson, H., Bladstrom, A., & Ingvar, C. (2003). Are smoking associated cancers prevented or postponed in women using hormone replacement therapy? *Obstetrics & Gynecology*, 102(3), 565-570.

Paoletti, R. & Wenger, N. K. (2003). Review of the International Position Paper on Women's Health and Menopause: a comprehensive approach. *Circulation*, 107, 1336-1339.

Parsons, L. C. (2005). Osteoporosis: incidence, prevention, and treatment of the silent killer. *Nursing Clinics of North America*, 40, 119-133.

Perez, D. G., Loprinzi, C. L., Barton, D. L., Pockaj, B. A., Sloan, J., Novotny, P. J., & Christensen, B. J. (2004). Pilot evaluation of mirtazapine for the treatment of hot flashes. *The Journal of Supportive Oncology*, 2, 50-56.

Pockaj, B. A., Loprinzi, C. L., Sloan, J. A., Novotny, P. J., Barton, D. L., Hagenmaier, A., Zhang, H., Lambert, G. H., Reeser, K. A., & Wisbey, J. A. (2004). Pilot evaluation of black cohosh for the treatment of hot flashes in women. *Cancer Investigation*, 22, 515-521.

Prestwood, K. M. (2003). Editorial: The search for alternative therapies for menopausal women: estrogenic effects of herbs. *Journal of Clinical Endocrinology & Metabolism*, 88, 4075-4076.

Raine-Fenning, N. J., Brincat, M. P., & Muscat-Baron, Y. (2003). Skin aging and menopause: implications for treatment. *American Journal of Clinical Dermatology*, 4, 371-378.

Robinson, D. & Cardozo, L. D. (2003). The role of estrogens in female lower urinary tract dysfunction. *Urology*, 62, 45-51.

Roughead, Z. K., Hunt, J. R., Johnson, L. K., Badger, T. M., & Lykken, G. I. (2005). Controlled substitution of soy protein for meat protein: effects on calcium retention, bone, and cardiovascular health indices in postmenopausal women. *Journal of Clinical Endocrinology & Metabolism*, 90, 181-189.

Schult, T. M., Ensrud, K. E., Blackwell, T., Ettinger, B., Wallace, R., & Tice, J. A. (2004). Effect of isoflavones on lipids and bone turnover markers in menopausal women. *Maturitas*, 48, 209-218.

Schurmann, R., Holler, T., & Benda, N. (2004). Estradiol and drospirenone for climacteric symptoms in postmenopausal women: a double-blind, randomized, placebo-controlled study of the safety and efficacy of three dose regimens. *Climacteric*, 7, 189-196.

Seibel, M. M. (2003). Treating hot flushes without hormone replacement therapy. *Journal of Family Practice*, 52, 291-296.

Sherwin, B. B. (2003). Estrogen and cognitive functioning in women. *Endocrine Reviews*, 24, 133-151.

Shulman, L. P. (2004). The menopausal transition: how does route of delivery affect the risk/benefit ratio of hormone therapy? *Journal of Family Practice* (Suppl), S13-S17.

Sikon, A. & Thacker, H. L. (2004). Treatment options for menopausal hot flashes. *Cleveland Clinic Journal of Medicine*, 71, 578-582.

Simpkins, J. W., Yang, S. H., Wen, Y., & Singh, M. (2005). Estrogens, progestins, menopause and neurodegeneration: basic and clinical studies. *Cellular & Molecular Life Sciences*, 62, 271-280.

Soares, C. N., Poitras, J. R., & Prouty, J. (2003). Effect of reproductive hormones and selective estrogen receptor modulators on mood during menopause. *Drugs & Aging*, 20, 85-100.

Speroff, L. (2003). Efficacy and tolerability of a novel estradiol vaginal ring for relief of menopausal symptoms. *Obstetrics & Gynecology*, 102, 823-834.

Stahlberg, C., Pedersen, A. T., Lynge, E., & Ottesen, B. (2003). Hormone replacement therapy and risk of breast cancer: the role of progestins. *Acta Obstetricia et Gynecologica Scandinavica*, 82, 335-344.

Taylor, M. (2003). Alternatives to HRT: an evidence-based review. *International Journal of Fertility & Womens Medicine*, 48, 64-68.

Tice, J. A., Ettinger, B., Ensrud, K., Wallace, R., Blackwell, T., & Cummings, S. R. (2003). Phytoestrogen supplements for the treatment of hot flashes: the Isoflavone Clover Extract (ICE) Study: a randomized controlled trial. *Journal of the American Medical Association*, 290, 207-214.

Vogel, R. A. (2003). The changing view of hormone replacement therapy. *Reviews in Cardiovascular Medicine*, 4, 68-71.

von Schoultz, E., Rutqvist, L. E., & Stockholm Breast Cancer Study Group. (2005). Menopausal hormone therapy after breast cancer: the Stockholm randomized trial. *Journal of the National Cancer Institute*, 97, 533-535.

Wattanakumtornkul, S., Pinto, A. B., & Williams, D. B. (2003). Intranasal hormone replacement therapy. *Menopause*, 10, 88-98.

Welnicka-Jaskiewicz, M. & Jassem, J. (2003). The risks and benefits of hormonal replacement therapy in healthy women and in breast cancer survivors. *Cancer Treatment Reviews*, 29, 355-361.

Wesstrom, J., Ulfberg, J. & Nilsson, S. (2005). Sleep apnea and hormone replacement therapy: a pilot study and a literature review. *Acta Obstetricia et Gynecologica Scandinavica*, 84, 54-57.

Wiegratz, I. & Kuhl, H. (2004). Progestogen therapies: differences in clinical effects? *Trends in Endocrinology & Metabolism*, 15, 277-285.

Wihlback, A. C., Nyberg, S., Backstrom, T., Bixo, M., & Sundstrom-Poromaa, I. (2005). Estradiol and the addition of progesterone increase the sensitivity to a neurosteroid in postmenopausal women. *Psychoneuroendocrinology*, 30, 38-50.

Wise, P. M. (2003). Impact of menopause on the brain. *Alzheimer Disease & Associated Disorders*, 17(suppl 2), S48-S50.

Wyon, Y., Wijma, K., Nedstrand, E., & Hammar, M. (2004). A comparison of acupuncture and oral estradiol treatment of vasomotor symptoms in postmenopausal women. *Climacteric*, 7, 153-164.

Zegura, B., Keber, I., Sebestjen, M., & Borko, E. (2003). Orally and transdermally replaced estradiol improves endothelial function equally in middle-aged women after surgical menopause. *American Journal of Obstetrics & Gynecology*, 188, 1291-1296.

Alterations During Menopause

INITIAL HISTORY

- 54-year-old white female.
- Complaining of fatigue, hot flashes, perivaginal itching, dyspareunia, and vaginal discharge.
- Periods stopped 15 months ago after several months of erratic cycles.
- Has had no vaginal bleeding in the past year.

Question 1. *What would you like to ask this patient about her symptoms?*

ADDITIONAL HISTORY

- Fatigue has increased gradually over the past 2 years.
- Has hot flashes many times during the day and is frequently awakened at night.
- Vaginal symptoms have occurred gradually and are not accompanied by abdominal pain or dysuria.
- Denies any history of vaginal infections.
- Has had one sexual partner for 20 years.

Question 2. *What would you like to ask about her medical history?*

MEDICAL HISTORY

- No history of migraines, gallbladder disease, deep venous thrombosis, or hepatic disease.
- Long history of hypercholesterolemia, but has never had chest pain or been diagnosed with heart or cerebrovascular disease.
- No personal or family history of breast cancer.
- Mammogram last year was normal.
- Takes no medications and has no known allergies.

Question 3. *What would you like to ask her about her life-style?*

LIFE-STYLE HISTORY

- Patient eats a low-fat diet and tries to watch her weight and cholesterol, but she admits her diet is low in calcium and high in phosphate.
- Used to walk regularly but got "out of the habit."
- Does not smoke cigarettes or drink alcohol.

PHYSICAL EXAMINATION

- Alert, thin female with no acute distress; mild kyphosis especially at the upper thoracic spine.
- T = 37° C orally; P = 80 and regular; RR = 15 and unlabored; BP = 142/75 right arm.

HEENT, Skin
- Skin is thin and dry without rashes.
- PERRL, fundi without hemorrhages or exudates.
- Pharynx clear.

Lungs, Cardiac
- Good chest excursion; lungs clear to auscultation and percussion.
- Cardiac with RRR without murmurs or gallops.

Abdomen, Extremities
- Abdomen soft, nontender, without organomegaly or masses.
- Extremities with full pulses without edema.

Breasts, Pelvic
- Breasts symmetric without masses, tenderness, or nipple discharge; axillae without adenopathy.
- Pelvic with dry perivaginal and vaginal tissues; decreased estrogen effect; Pap pending; no uterine or adnexal masses.

Neurologic
- Oriented ×4.
- Strength and sensation normal and symmetric.
- DTR 2+ and symmetric.
- Gait normal.

Question 4. *What are the pertinent positives and negatives on examination?*

Question 5. *What laboratory tests would you order?*

LABORATORY RESULTS

- FSH level increased.
- Chemistries, including calcium and phosphate levels, normal.
- CBC, including HCT, normal.
- Liver function normal.
- Lipid profile shows increased LDL and decreased HDL.
- Mammogram consistent with postmenopause and without masses or abnormal calcifications.
- Dual-energy x-ray absorptiometry (DEXA) consistent with decreased bone mineral density.

Question 6. *What recommendations for management should be made for this patient?*

Chapter 26

Allergic Rhinitis

DEFINITION

- Allergic rhinitis is a clinical condition of increased humoral immunity that is immunoglobulin E (IgE)—mediated (type I hypersensitivity) and occurs in response to environmental antigens, resulting in inflammation of the upper respiratory tract.
- Previous classification schemes described seasonal, perennial, or occupational categories; newer classification schemes use the terms "intermittent" versus "persistent" and describe symptom severity as "mild" or "moderate/severe." These newer classification schemes provide the basis for a stepwise approach to therapy.

EPIDEMIOLOGY

- Allergic (sometimes called atopic) rhinitis is the most common allergic condition. Its prevalence is estimated at 20% of the U.S. population. Up to 40% of those with allergic rhinitis also have asthma.
- It is becoming more common, especially in industrialized countries.
- Peak symptoms occur in the second, third, and fourth decades, but children (average age 10) are also affected.
- There is a clear genetic predisposition for allergic disease; a 13% prevalence if neither parent is atopic, 30% if one is atopic, and 50% if both parents are atopic.
- Intrauterine and childhood exposure to allergens increases the risk of allergic rhinitis and other allergic disorders such as asthma.
- Common allergens include:
  - Seasonal aeroallergens (5 to 70 μm in size): pollen from flowering plants, trees, grasses, ragweed; fungus spores.
  - Perennial aeroallergens: dust mites, animal dander, roaches, latex, mice feces and urine.
  - Food allergens: eggs, milk, corn, nuts, shellfish.
- The bedroom is the location of allergen exposure that correlates with the greatest risk for allergic disease.
- Childhood infections with some intracellular pathogens (e.g., hepatitis A, *Toxoplasma gondii*, *Helicobacter pylori*) are associated with less risk for developing allergies, whereas a history of vaccination to hepatitis B, pertussis, and polio increases the risk of allergy. Theoretically, the infections prime the immune system to respond to environmental antigens with cellular immunity, whereas vaccinations prime for increased humoral immunity such as that seen in allergic disease.
- Exposure to environmental pollutants such as nitrogen dioxide and sulfur dioxide can increase the severity of the response to allergens.

PATHOPHYSIOLOGY

Genetics

- More than 20 genes have been implicated in allergic disease including interleukin (IL)-4, IL-4 receptor, cytokine, interferon gamma (INF-γ), β-adrenergic receptor, 5 lipoxygenase, and leukotriene C4 synthetase genes.

Tissue Effects

- Allergens inhaled into the upper respiratory tract are ingested by macrophages, dendritic cells, and B lymphocytes (antigen presenting cells [APCs]). They are then processed and presented on the surface of these cells for interaction with T helper lymphocytes (CD4 cells) (Figure 26-1).
- Irritants can directly stimulate airway cells to promote allergic reactions as well.
- T helper (CD4) cells release two major groups of cytokines, TH_1 (interferon and interleukin [IL]-2), which promote cellular immunity, and TH_2 (IL-4, IL-5, IL-8, IL-13), which promote humoral immunity (antibodies).
- In allergic patients, the number of dendritic cells and B lymphocytes in the respiratory mucosa is increased. B lymphocyte and dendritic cell antigen presentation favors TH_2 cytokine release by the T helper (CD4) cell, thus allergic individuals are predisposed to antibody production in response to environmental allergens.
    - IL-4 stimulates B lymphocte proliferation and an "isotype switch" such that the B lymphocyte changes from producing IgM to producing huge amounts of IgE.
    - IL-5 recruits and activates eosinophils, promotes mucus hypersecretion, activates fibroblasts, and promotes release of toxic neuropeptides (e.g., major basic protein).
    - IL-8 activates polymorphonucleocytes (PMNs) and promotes adhesion molecule expression on endothelial and epithelial cells, leading to more migration of inflammatory cells.
    - IL-13 impairs mucociliary clearance, induces release of TGF-β from epithelial cells leading to scarring, induces production of anaphylatoxins, impairs $β_2$-adrenergic receptor–mediated relaxation of airway smooth muscle, and contributes to inflammation.
- IgE binds to the mast cell via high-affinity Fc receptors, with resultant mast cell degranulation and release of vasoactive (e.g., histamine), chemotactic, and inflammatory mediators (e.g., prostaglandins, leukotrienes).

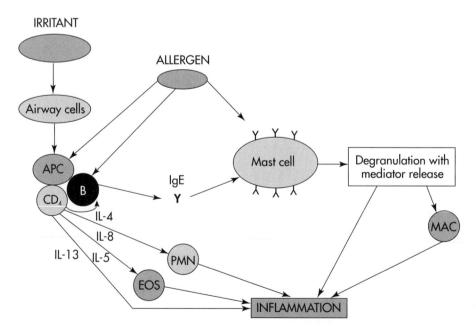

FIGURE **26-1** **Cellular Interactions in Allergy.**

- The allergic response then is one of vascular and cellular responses that cause inflammation. This process occurs episodically in response to allergen exposures, but can lead to chronic changes in the upper respiratory mucosa, with persistent symptoms.
- The clinical presentation depends on the allergen, the individual, and the tissue most targeted for allergic response. In allergic rhinitis:
    - The nasal mucosa becomes edematous with increased mucus production.
    - Inspiratory effort with negative nasal airway pressure results in nasal collapse and airway obstruction. Eustachian tube blockage can result in serous otitis and can lead to otitis media.
    - Upper respiratory inflammation is associated with lower airway inflammatory responses and can be associated with asthma.
    - There is often a late-phase response mediated by memory T cells and eosinophils in which symptoms recur 4 to 12 hours after the initial exposure.

Summary of Allergic Rhinitis Pathophysiology

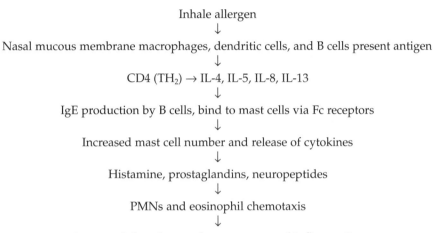

Inhale allergen
↓
Nasal mucous membrane macrophages, dendritic cells, and B cells present antigen
↓
CD4 (TH$_2$) → IL-4, IL-5, IL-8, IL-13
↓
IgE production by B cells, bind to mast cells via Fc receptors
↓
Increased mast cell number and release of cytokines
↓
Histamine, prostaglandins, neuropeptides
↓
PMNs and eosinophil chemotaxis
↓
Acute and chronic vascular responses and inflammation
↓
Nasal mucosal edema and mucus production, interaction with lower airway inflammation
↓
Inspiratory effort → negative nasal airway pressure → nasal collapse → airway obstruction

PATIENT PRESENTATION

History

Family history of allergy; allergen exposure; perennial or seasonal symptoms; underlying respiratory disease; childhood infections and vaccinations.

Symptoms

Nasal congestion; rhinorrhea; postnasal drainage; sore throat; cough (especially when lying down); hoarseness; sneezing; itchy nose; watery eyes; headache; earache; loss of smell and taste; fatigue; daytime somnolence.

Examination

Shiners; Dennie-Morgan infraorbital creases; allergic salute; swollen, pale nasal mucous membranes; nasal and pharyngeal erythema; nasal polyps; serous otitis; children may develop high-arched palate and dental overbite (facial remodeling due to persistent mouth breathing).

DIFFERENTIAL DIAGNOSIS

- Infectious rhinitis (rhinovirus, adenovirus).
- Rhinitis medicamentosa.

- Gustatory, vasomotor, atrophic, or drug-induced rhinitis.
- Sinusitis.
- Cerebrospinal fluid rhinorrhea.
- Adenoidal hyperplasia.
- Nasal polyps.
- Septal deviation; adenocarcinoma of the nasal mucosa.
- Foreign bodies.
- Otitis media.
- Ciliary dyskinesia syndrome.

KEYS TO ASSESSMENT

- Perform anterior rhinoscopy using a speculum and mirror.
- Nasal endoscopy may be indicated to look for nasal and sinus pathologic changes.
- Obtain a nasal smear; the presence of numerous eosinophils confirms allergy.
- Spirometry is indicated to rule out associated airway obstruction due to asthma.
- Perform allergy testing.
    - Skin testing: Prick and puncture tests (anaphylaxis is a small risk).
        1. The size of the response correlates with degree of symptoms.
        2. False-positive (sensitization to an allergen without actual symptoms from it) and false-negative results can occur.
    - Measurement of total serum IgE is not useful in rhinitis and should no longer be used as a diagnostic tool; however, the measurement of allergen-specific IgE in serum is indicated.
    - Nasal challenge with allergens is indicated when there are discrepancies between the history and allergy testing. Symptom scores are combined with objective measures to determine response: counting sneezes, measuring volume of nasal excretion, nasal airflow, and airflow resistance.
- Plain sinus radiographs can be used to evaluate for associated sinusitis but are not indicated for the diagnosis of allergic rhinitis. Computed tomography is indicated to eliminate other conditions, exclude chronic sinusitis, and to evaluate patients who do not respond to treatment or have unilateral rhinitis.

KEYS TO MANAGEMENT

- Allergen avoidance.
    - Encase mattress, pillow, and quilt in impermeable covers; decontaminate surfaces.
    - Wash all bedding weekly in a hot cycle (55° to 60° C).
    - Replace carpets with linoleum or wooden flooring.
    - Use a vacuum cleaner with integral high-efficiency particulate air (HEPA) filter and double-thickness bags.
    - Hot wash or freeze soft toys.
    - Provide pet-free areas (especially the bedrooms).
    - Use dehumidifiers; wear a mask when vacuuming.
- Nasal douching with a traditional alkaline nasal douche or a sterile saltwater spray has been shown to improve symptoms of rhinitis.
- Antihistamine therapies.
    - In general, use antihistamines alone for seasonal rhinitis, and in combination with decongestants (pseudoephedrine, naphazoline, oxymetazoline) for perennial rhinitis.
    - "First-generation" antihistamines (e.g., diphenhydramine) can cause irritability, insomnia, hypertension, arrhythmias, and seizures.
    - "Second-generation" antihistamines (azelastine, cetirizine, fexofenadine, loratadine) are more effective with fewer side effects and may decrease associated asthma symptoms. New antihistamines have been approved in recent months with even fewer side effects and more efficacy.

- Anti-inflammatory therapies.
  - Nasal steroids provide symptomatic relief in up to 90% of patients and are superior to antihistamines in relieving nasal symptoms.
  - Leukotriene antagonists (e.g., montelukast) can also be effective in relieving symptoms.
  - Oral steroids should be used only for intolerable symptoms such as total nasal obstruction and impaired sleep; "steroid bursts" (e.g., 30 mg × 3 days) or long-acting injections are an option during highly symptomatic periods.
- Anticholinergic therapy.
  - Intranasal ipratropium effectively relieves rhinorrhea but overall effectiveness is debated.
- Immunotherapy (allergy shots).
  - Decreases histamine and IgE, induces T cell anergy, produces IgG antibodies that block IgE activity, and causes a shift away from antibody production.
  - Dosing schedules require several injections per week for several weeks, then weekly or biweekly injections for the duration of the season (or continuously for perennial rhinitis); continue for at least 2 years.
  - Provides excellent long-term allergy control and may prevent future asthma.
  - Generally safe; 3% of individuals will get some reaction during their course of therapy (50% of which are due to dosing errors); monitor patients for 20 minutes after injection.
  - New nasal or sublingual immunotherapy can be done at home safely and effectively.
- Omalizumab nasal spray (humanized monoclonal antibody to IgE) is being developed. Subcutaneous injection is currently approved for asthma and is highly effective for treating allergic rhinitis symptoms.
- Future therapies.
  - Humanized monoclonal antibody to IL-4 and IL-5.
  - Allergen-specific DNA vaccines.
  - Cytokine blockers (e.g., CCR3).

PATHOPHYSIOLOGY →	CLINICAL LINK
What is going on in the disease process that influences how the patient presents and how he or she should be managed?	*What should you do now that you understand the underlying pathophysiology?*
Strong genetic component to the risk for allergic disease. In addition, an increased risk for allergic disease can begin with intrauterine allergen exposure.	A family history is important, and pregnant mothers with a family history of allergies should consider reducing their allergen exposure.
The amount of allergen exposure during childhood is correlated with the risk for allergic disease. The exposure of greatest risk occurs in the bedroom.	Children with a family history of allergies should have their allergen exposure limited as much as possible, especially in the bedroom.
Allergy is type I (IgE-mediated) hypersensitivity and is the result of a powerful humoral immune response.	Childhood infections with intracellular pathogens stimulate cellular immunity and may reduce the risk of allergies. Certain vaccinations, which work through stimulating humoral immune responses, may increase the risk for allergic disease. Future decisions about the risk/benefit ratio of new immunizations should take into account potential effects on the overall immune response.
Antigen presentation to the immune system results in activation of the T helper (CD4) cells that produce large amounts of IL-4, which in turn stimulates the production of IgE by B lymphocytes.	New therapies for allergy include monoclonal antibodies that block the activity of IL-4 and IgE.
IgE binding to the surface of mast cells causes the release of histamine and other cytokines. This, along with activation of PMNs and eosinophils, results in vascular and cellular responses that cause inflammation.	Antihistamines and anti-inflammatories are the mainstays of pharmacologic management for allergic rhinitis. Intranasal steroids are the most effective form of treatment, along with second-generation antihistamines such as loratadine. The leukotriene antagonists offer another anti-inflammatory alternative.
Inflammation of the nasal mucosa results in the symptoms of allergic rhinitis, including nasal congestion and serous otitis.	Decongestants such as pseudoephedrine can be used in combination with antihistamines and anti-inflammatory drugs to relieve nasal congestion and open the eustachian tubes.

SUGGESTED READINGS

Agrawal, D. K. (2004). Anti-inflammatory properties of desloratadine. *Clinical & Experimental Allergy*, 34, 1342-1348.

Alfaro, V. (2004). Role of histamine and platelet-activating factor in allergic rhinitis. *Journal of Physiology & Biochemistry*, 60, 101-111.

Asero, R. (2004). Food additives intolerance: does it present as perennial rhinitis? *Current Opinion in Allergy & Clinical Immunology*, 4, 25-29.

Bachert, C. (2004). Persistent rhinitis—allergic or nonallergic? *Allergy*, 59(suppl 76), 11-15.

Bachert, C., Vignola, A. M., Gevaert, P., Leynaert, B., van Cauwenberge, P., & Bousquet, J. (2004). Allergic rhinitis, rhinosinusitis, and asthma: one airway disease. *Immunology & Allergy Clinics of North America*, 24, 19-43.

Benson, M. (2005). Pathophysiological effects of glucocorticoids on nasal polyps: an update. *Current Opinion in Allergy & Clinical Immunology*, 5, 31-35.

Blaiss, M. (2004). Current concepts and therapeutic strategies for allergic rhinitis in school-age children. *Clinical Therapeutics*, 26, 1876-1889.

Borchers, A. T., Keen, C. L., & Gershwin, M. E. (2004). Fatalities following allergen immunotherapy. *Clinical Reviews in Allergy & Immunology*, 27, 147-158.

Bousquet, J., Bindslev-Jensen, C., Canonica, G. W., Fokkens, W., Kim, H., Kowalski, M., Magnan, A., Mullol, J., & van Cauwenberge, P. (2004). The ARIA/EAACI criteria for antihistamines: an assessment of the efficacy, safety and pharmacology of desloratadine. *Allergy*, 59(suppl 77), 4-16.

Bousquet, J., Jacot, W., Vignola, A. M., Bachert, C., & van Cauwenberge, P. (2004). Allergic rhinitis: a disease remodeling the upper airways? *Journal of Allergy & Clinical Immunology*, 113, 43-49.

Brownell, J. & Casale, T. B. (2000). Anti-IgE therapy. *Immunology & Allergy Clinics of North America*, 24, 551-568.

Bush, R. K. (2004). Etiopathogenesis and management of perennial allergic rhinitis: a state-of-the-art review. *Treatments in Respiratory Medicine*, 3, 45-57.

Busse, W. & Kraft, M. (2005). Cysteinyl leukotrienes in allergic inflammation: strategic target for therapy. *Chest*, 127, 1312-1326.

Casale, T. B. & Prous, S. (2004). Omalizumab: an effective anti-IgE treatment for allergic asthma and rhinitis. *Drugs of Today*, 40, 367-376.

Ciprandi, G. (2004). Treatment of nonallergic perennial rhinitis. *Allergy*, 59(suppl 76), 16-22.

Cowart, M., Altenbach, R., Black, L., Faghih, R., Zhao, C., & Hancock, A. A. (2004). Medicinal chemistry and biological properties of non-imidazole histamine H3 antagonists. *Mini-Reviews in Medicinal Chemistry*, 4, 979-992.

Craig, T. J., McCann, J. L., Gurevich, F., & Davies, M. J. (2004). The correlation between allergic rhinitis and sleep disturbance. *Journal of Allergy & Clinical Immunology*, 114, S139-S145.

Creticos, P. S., Chen, Y. H., & Schroeder, J. T. (2000). New approaches in immunotherapy: allergen vaccination with immunostimulatory DNA. *Immunology & Allergy Clinics of North America*, 24, 569-581.

Currie, G. P., Srivastava, P., Dempsey, O. J., & Lee, D. K. (2005). Therapeutic modulation of allergic airways disease with leukotriene receptor antagonists. *QJM*, 98, 171-182.

D'Amato, G., Liccardi, G., Noschese, P., Salzillo, A., D'Amato, M., & Cazzola, M. (2004). Anti-IgE monoclonal antibody (omalizumab) in the treatment of atopic asthma and allergic respiratory diseases. *Current Drug Targets—Inflammation & Allergy*, 3, 227-229.

Ellegard, E. K. (2004). Clinical and pathogenetic characteristics of pregnancy rhinitis. *Clinical Reviews in Allergy & Immunology*, 26, 149-159.

Fabbri, L., Peters, S. P., Pavord, I., Wenzel, S. E., Lazarus, S. C., Macnee, W., Lemaire, F., & Abraham, E. (2005). Allergic rhinitis, asthma, airway biology, and chronic obstructive pulmonary disease in AJRCCM in 2004. *American Journal of Respiratory & Critical Care Medicine*, 171, 686-698.

Finegold, I. (2004). Immunotherapy in the age of anti-IgE. *Clinical Reviews in Allergy & Immunology*, 27, 75-82.

Fisher, L., Ghaffari, G., Davies, M., & Craig, T. (2005). Effects of poor sleep in allergic rhinitis. *Current Opinion in Allergy & Clinical Immunology*, 5, 11 16.

Fraunfelder, F. W. (2004). Epinastine hydrochloride for atopic disease. *Drugs of Today*, 40, 677-683.

Gelfand, E. W. (2004). Inflammatory mediators in allergic rhinitis. *Journal of Allergy & Clinical Immunology*, 114, S135-S138.

Gendo, K. & Larson, E. B. (2004). Evidence-based diagnostic strategies for evaluating suspected allergic rhinitis. *Annals of Internal Medicine*, 140, 278-289.

Golightly, L. K. & Greos, L. S. (2005). Second-generation antihistamines: actions and efficacy in the management of allergic disorders. *Drugs*, 65, 341-384.

Greenberger, P. A. (2004). Interactions between rhinitis and asthma. *Allergy & Asthma Proceedings*, 25, 89-93.

Greisner, W. A., III. (2004). Onset of action for the relief of allergic rhinitis symptoms with second-generation antihistamines. *Allergy & Asthma Proceedings*, 25, 81-83.

Hansen, I., Klimek, L., Mosges, R., & Hormann, K. (2004). Mediators of inflammation in the early and the late phase of allergic rhinitis. *Current Opinion in Allergy & Clinical Immunology*, 4, 159-163.

Helm, R. M. (2004). Diet and the development of atopic disease. *Current Opinion in Allergy & Clinical Immunology*, 4, 125-129.

Holgate, S., Casale, T., Wenzel, S., Bousquet, J., Deniz, Y., & Reisner, C. (2005). The anti-inflammatory effects of omalizumab confirm the central role of IgE in allergic inflammation. *Journal of Allergy & Clinical Immunology*, 115, 459-465.

Huggins, J. L. & Looney, R. J. (2004). Allergen immunotherapy. *American Family Physician*, 70, 689-696.

Hussain, I. & Kline, J. N. (2004). DNA, the immune system, and atopic disease. *Journal of Investigative Dermatology, Symposium Proceedings*, 9, 23-28.

Jones, N. (2004). Allergic rhinitis: aetiology, predisposing and risk factors. *Rhinology*, 42, 49-56.

Kaliner, M. A. (2004). Omalizumab and the treatment of allergic rhinitis. *Current Allergy & Asthma Reports*, 4, 237-244.

Keles, N. (2004). Treatment of allergic rhinitis during pregnancy. *American Journal of Rhinology*, 18, 23-28.

Kirtsreesakul, V. & Naclerio, R. M. (2004). Role of allergy in rhinosinusitis. *Current Opinion in Allergy & Clinical Immunology*, 4, 17-23.

Malling, H. J. (2004). Immunotherapy for allergic rhino-conjunctivitis. *Clinical Allergy & Immunology*, 18, 495-509.

Meltzer, E. O., Szwarcberg, J., & Pill, M. W. (2004). Allergic rhinitis, asthma, and rhinosinusitis: diseases of the integrated airway. *Journal of Managed Care Pharmacy*, 10, 310-317.

Miranowski, A. C. & Ditto, A. M. (2004). Allergic rhinitis. *Allergy & Asthma Proceedings*, 25, S11-S12.

Nayak, A. (2004). A review of montelukast in the treatment of asthma and allergic rhinitis. *Expert Opinion on Pharmacotherapy*, 5, 679-686.

Nelson, H. S. (2004). Advances in upper airway diseases and allergen immunotherapy. *Journal of Allergy & Clinical Immunology*, 113, 635-642.

Norman, P. S. (2004). Immunotherapy: 1999-2004. *Journal of Allergy & Clinical Immunology*, 113, 1013-1023.

Passalacqua, G., Lombardi, C., & Canonica, G. W. (2004). Sublingual immunotherapy: an update. *Current Opinion in Allergy & Clinical Immunology*, 4, 31-36.

Pawankar, R. (2004). Allergic rhinitis and asthma: the link, the new ARIA classification and global approaches to treatment. *Current Opinion in Allergy & Clinical Immunology, 4,* 1-4.

Portnoy, J. M., Van Osdol, T., & Williams, P. B. (2004). Evidence-based strategies for treatment of allergic rhinitis. *Current Allergy & Asthma Reports, 4,* 439-446.

Sheikh, A., Panesar, S. S., & Dhami, S. (2004). Seasonal allergic rhinitis. *Clinical Evidence,* 694-709.

Simons, F. E. (2004). Advances in H1-antihistamines. *New England Journal of Medicine, 351,* 2203-2217.

Spergel, J. M. (2005). Atopic march: link to upper airways. *Current Opinion in Allergy & Clinical Immunology, 5,* 17-21.

Stanaland, B. E. (2004). Once-daily budesonide aqueous nasal spray for allergic rhinitis: a review. *Clinical Therapeutics, 26,* 473-492.

Stanaland, B. E. (2004). Therapeutic measures for prevention of allergic rhinitis/asthma development. *Allergy & Asthma Proceedings, 25,* 11-15.

Storms, W. W. (2004). Pharmacologic approaches to daytime and nighttime symptoms of allergic rhinitis. *Journal of Allergy & Clinical Immunology, 114,* S146-S153.

Taramarcaz, P. & Gibson, P. G. (2004). The effectiveness of intranasal corticosteroids in combined allergic rhinitis and asthma syndrome. *Clinical & Experimental Allergy, 34,* 1883-1889.

Till, S. J., Francis, J. N., Nouri-Aria, K., & Durham, S. R. (2004). Mechanisms of immunotherapy. *Journal of Allergy & Clinical Immunology, 113,* 1025-1034.

Venge, P. (2004). Monitoring the allergic inflammation. *Allergy, 59,* 26-32.

Wang, D. Y., Raza, M. T., & Gordon, B. R. (2004). Control of nasal obstruction in perennial allergic rhinitis. *Current Opinion in Allergy & Clinical Immunology, 4,* 165-170.

Wheeler, A. W. & Woroniecki, S. R. (2004). Allergy vaccines—new approaches to an old concept. *Expert Opinion on Biological Therapy, 4,* 1473-1481.

Wilson, A. M., O'Byrne, P. M., & Parameswaran, K. (2004). Leukotriene receptor antagonists for allergic rhinitis: a systematic review and meta-analysis. *American Journal of Medicine, 116,* 338-344.

Wilson, D. R., Lima, M. T., & Durham, S. R. (2005). Sublingual immunotherapy for allergic rhinitis: systematic review and meta-analysis. *Allergy, 60,* 4-12.

Allergic Rhinitis

INITIAL HISTORY

- A 27-year-old female graduate nursing student presents in December with a 5-week history of itchy eyes and nasal congestion with watery nasal discharge.
- She also complains of a "tickling" cough, especially at night.

Question 1. *What is your differential diagnosis based on the information you now have?*

Question 2. *What other questions would you like to ask this patient about her symptoms?*

ADDITIONAL HISTORY

- Patient complains of repetitive sneezing and has recently developed earache, especially on the right.
- Seems to get "colds" that last for weeks every winter; her symptoms seem to improve in the spring.
- Has a cat, but is not aware of any allergies.
- Cough is somewhat productive of clear phlegm, but she can tell that the phlegm comes down from the back of her throat.
- Nasal congestion is worse at night.

- Denies any trauma to her face.
- No significant medical history and is on no medications.

Question 3.   *What questions would you like to ask her about her family and her childhood?*

FAMILY AND CHILDHOOD HISTORY

- Mother had asthma as a child, and her sister has multiple allergies.
- Patient was always sick during the winter months as a child.
- Mother had cats in the house during her pregnancy and throughout the patient's childhood; they routinely slept at the foot of her bed.
- Grew up in Chicago.
- Never had any serious childhood infections and received the usual vaccinations.

Question 4.   *How would you interpret her history at this point?*

PHYSICAL EXAMINATION

- Well-appearing 27-year-old white female in no acute distress; sniffling frequently.
- Afebrile, T = 37° C orally; RR = 18 and unlabored (breathing through her mouth at rest); BP = 125/70 (sitting).

Skin
- Without rashes.

HEENT
- PERRL; fundi benign.
- Sclera red and slightly swollen with frequent tearing.
- Outer nares with red irritated skin.
- Internal nares with red, boggy, moist mucosa, no purulent discharge seen; no evidence of polyps on anterior rhinoscopy.
- Pharynx erythematous without exudate; purulent postnasal drainage visible.
- Both tympanic membranes with mild serous otitis.

Neck
- No palpable cervical, supraclavicular, infraclavicular, or axillary adenopathy.
- Thyroid nonpalpable.

Chest
- Lungs clear to auscultation and percussion.
- No wheezing even on forced expiration.

Cardiac, Abdomen, Extremities, Neurologic
- Examination unremarkable.

Question 5.   *What do you think of her examination findings?*

Question 6.   *What diagnostic tests would you obtain?*

LABORATORY RESULTS

- Nasal smear positive for eosinophils.
- Nasal endoscopy confirms findings of anterior rhinoscopy; no specific sinus pathologic changes noted.
- Allergy skin testing positive for house dust mite and cat dander.
- Spirometry normal.

Question 7.   *How would you interpret these laboratory results?*

Question 8. *How would you manage this patient now?*

Chapter 27

Human Immunodeficiency Virus (HIV) Disease

DEFINITION

- HIV disease is a clinical condition caused by infection with the human immunodeficiency virus (HIV). With few exceptions, HIV infection leads to the acquired immunodeficiency syndrome (AIDS).
- AIDS is defined by the Centers for Disease Control and Prevention as HIV infection with an associated indicator disease including (1) certain opportunistic infections; (2) certain cancers such as Kaposi sarcoma, lymphomas, and invasive cervical or anal carcinomas; (3) wasting syndrome; (4) associated neurologic diseases; and (5) recurrent pneumonias; or HIV infection and a CD4 cell count less than 200 (or CD4% less than 14).

EPIDEMIOLOGY

- The two major types of lentiviruses that infect humans are HIV-1 and HIV-2. It is believed that zoonotic transfer of these simian immunodeficiency viruses may have occurred several times, giving rise to genetically distinct HIV strains.
- Both HIV-1 and HIV-2 are spread principally by intimate sexual contact, perinatal transmission, or via infected blood or body fluids (intravenous drug use [IVDU], transfusion). Patterns of sexual transmission vary in different societies and cultures. In most of the world, heterosexual intercourse and perinatal transmission are the most common forms of transmission.
- The global epidemic (or pandemic) of HIV-1 infection continues and is growing most rapidly in the nations of Central and South America, Southeast Asia, the former Soviet Republics in eastern Europe, and in the subcontinent of India, although the largest number of HIV-infected people is still found in sub-Saharan Africa.
- In the United States, the percentage of AIDS cases acquired through sexual intercourse between men who have sex with men and the percentage acquired through IVDU have declined.
- The overall incidence of AIDS in the United States peaked in 1993 and has since declined.
- The proportion of those infected with HIV who are black or Hispanic continues to grow; now more than 50% of the people with AIDS in the United States are non-Hispanic blacks and Hispanics.
- Mortality from AIDS in the United States has decreased dramatically since more effective antiretroviral drugs became available; however, most people with HIV disease do not have access to optimal drug therapy and medical care.
- More than 40% of newborns who are infected with HIV have strains of HIV that are partially or completely resistant to existing antiretroviral drugs.

- There are several HIV-1 groups (M, N, O) of which M is the most common, and there are subtypes (clades) of HIV-1 M (A to J) distributed in differing proportions around the world. These subtypes are different from one another in important ways. For example, HIV-1E (more common in Thailand) may be more readily transmitted through heterosexual intercourse compared with HIV-1B (most common in Europe and the United States).
- There is no HIV-2 pandemic; it is still mostly restricted to West Africa (e.g., Cameroon, Ivory Coast, Senegal). Compared with HIV-1, people can be infected with HIV-2 for much longer periods without developing disease. There is evidence that HIV-2–infected people may be at a decreased risk for acquiring HIV-1 infection.

PATHOPHYSIOLOGY

Genetics

- Genetic association analyses implicate a minimum of 14 AIDS restriction genes whose polymorphic variants affect HIV-1 cell entry, acquired and innate immunity, and cytokine defenses to HIV-1. A sampling of implicated genes includes RANTES chemokine variants, class I and II HLA alleles (e.g., the A2/6802 supertype is associated with a greatly decreased risk for HIV infection), CCR5 (see below), CCR2, CCL5, CXCR6, CEM15, vitamin D receptor (VDR), IL-10, FAS, and interferon-γ. Other genes affect responsiveness to medications (e.g., *CYP2B6, M41L, L210W, K65R* allelic variants).

Binding of HIV to Host Cells

- HIV is a retrovirus with single-stranded ribonucleic acid (RNA) contained within a capsid and an envelope, as well as three important enzymes (reverse transcriptase, integrase, and protease) (Figure 27-1).
- The viral envelope has on its surface a **glycop**rotein (**gp**120) in combination with gp41—this molecule binds to the CD4 receptor on T helper lymphocytes and on macrophages and dendritic cells. HIV-1 viruses specialize in infecting either T helper (CD4) lymphocytes (T-cell trophic) or macrophages and dendritic cells (monocyte trophic).

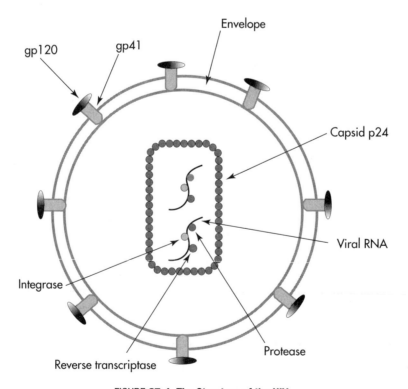

FIGURE **27-1 The Structure of the HIV.**

- HIV cannot bind and penetrate unless there are appropriate coreceptors present on the surface of the host cell. Macrophages, dendritic cells, and T helper cells all have CD4 molecules on their surfaces. Macrophages and dendritic cells also have CCR5 coreceptors and T helper cells have CXCR4 coreceptors.
- Macrophages and dendritic cells are the primary sites of initial infection via mucosal exposure. Dendritic cells infected with HIV travel to lymph nodes and display cell surface molecules that concentrate the virus and enable transmission to resident T helper cells.
- Fusion of the virus to the host cell requires three steps:
  - Binding of gp120/gp41 to the CD4 molecule on macrophages, dendritic cells, and T helper cells.
  - After binding of the gp120 molecule on the virus with the CD4 molecule, conformational changes of the bound molecules occur that expose the viral molecules to coreceptors on the T helper cell surface. A new class of antiretroviral drugs has been released that prevent this conformational change and therefore inhibit viral fusion with the host cells (fusion inhibitors).
  - This conformational change is followed by interaction of the virus with the chemokine coreceptors on the host cells—CCR5 on macrophages (monocyte trophic) and CXCR4 (fusin) on CD4 cells.
    1. CCR5 is a molecule found on normal macrophages and dendritic cells that participates in the release of cytokines and T cell and eosinophil activation; 10% of whites are heterozygous for a CCR5 mutation and have a slower rate of infection and disease progression; 1% of whites are homozygous for this mutation and resistant to infection.
    2. CXCR4 is a molecule found on normal T cells that participates in T cell activation; a small number of individuals have been identified with a SDF-13A mutation that is associated with a slower rate of HIV disease progression.
    3. A new class of antiretroviral drugs known as chemokine antagonists is being investigated. These drugs block these coreceptors, thereby either preventing infection or slowing the progression of disease.

Viral Replication

- HIV contains **reverse transcriptase** such that when it enters the cell it can make DNA from its RNA, which then integrates (using **integrase**) into the host DNA. The integrated HIV genome reproduces more viral RNA and makes a large polypeptide that is then cleaved into its active parts (by **protease**). The cell then assembles new copies of the virus and sheds them into body fluids and tissues.
- The virus also produces regulatory proteins (called tat, rev, and nef) that modulate the production of viral RNA by the integrated viral DNA. Other genes code for infectivity and drug resistance.
- There is enormous genetic diversity of HIV-1 due to the incredible rate of HIV replication and a high mutation rate (one out of every three replication cycles results in the production of a mutant form of the virus). This allows the virus to adapt rapidly to any selective pressures that it may encounter, including antiretroviral drugs and host immune responses. Drug resistance mutations have been identified for all of the currently available antiretroviral drugs. In any one individual, approximately 3300 viruses with one of these mutations are produced each day.
- This viral diversity limits the likelihood of finding an effective vaccine and means that multiple drug combinations and the sequenced use of a variety of agents at different times are necessary to prevent the acquisition of partial or complete resistance to antiretroviral drugs.

NATURAL HISTORY AND IMMUNOLOGY OF HIV INFECTION

- Primary infection occurs most commonly through mucous membranes. Significant viremia occurs within 2 to 3 days with extensive seeding of the lymphoid system.

- Symptomatic primary infection (acute retroviral syndrome) occurs in 80% to 90% of HIV-infected patients. The time from infection to the onset of symptoms is usually 2 to 4 weeks. Symptoms include fever, adenopathy, pharyngitis, rash, myalgias, and headache.
- Once infection has occurred, viral replication begins at an astonishing pace with billions of viruses produced daily.
- The half-life of HIV in plasma is 1 to 2 days; 30% of HIV in plasma is replaced daily by viral replication such that the entire HIV population turns over in 14 days.
- HIV replication is maintained from newly infected CD4 cells such that 99% of the virus in the bloodstream at any moment is from newly infected cells. Billions of CD4 cells are produced, infected, and destroyed daily.
- The virus establishes long-term, latent, nonproductive infection in inactive CD4 cells (memory cells), precursor lymphocyte cells in the bone marrow, dendritic cells of the lymph nodes, and the glial cells of the central nervous system (CNS). These cells are not accessible to the immune system and provide "sanctuary" for the virus. Infection of these sanctuary sites has been found to occur very early during the course of the primary infection and makes eradication of the virus very difficult.
- Reactivation of the virus from these sanctuary sites may occur when there are coinfecting pathogens that activate HIV gene expression. Inflammatory cytokines and T cell activation lead to accelerated HIV replication and spread to other tissues. T cells produce RANTES, MIP-1α, MIP-1β, and SDF-1 that normally control macrophage and T cell activation, but as HIV infection progresses, the balance is lost.
- Cellular immunity is the primary mode of viral (and CD4 cell) killing.
    - T cytotoxic lymphocytes (CD8 cells) recognize infected T helper (CD4) cells and macrophages and directly destroy these cells and the viruses they contain.
    - Cellular immunity is facilitated by the secretion of cytokines from uninfected CD4 cells called the TH$_1$ cytokines. During the course of HIV infection, the virus induces many of the CD4 cells to shift from the TH$_1$ mode of cytokine production (favors cellular immunity) to the TH$_2$ cytokine profile (favors humoral immunity). Humoral immunity is less effective for HIV killing. This makes it more difficult to develop effective HIV vaccines.
- It is postulated that the virus can also contribute to decreasing CD4 cell numbers and function by other mechanisms including the following:
    - HIV appears to be directly cytopathic to some T cells, and may result in a greater proportional decrease in lymphocytes in the gastrointestinal mucosa than in circulating levels, thus rendering the gastrointestinal tract as a prime target for opportunistic infection.
    - HIV can contribute to decreasing production of T helper cells through infection of the bone marrow.
- After several weeks, a steady state and clinical latency is achieved in which the immune system is able to decrease the amount of virus in the blood by killing infected CD4 cells, and the bone marrow is able to maintain production of adequate numbers of newly produced and functional CD4 cells.
- Viral replication continues at a very high rate in the blood, and at a slower rate in lymph nodes and other sanctuary sites. The level at which the viral load or viral titer (the measured number of copies of the virus per unit volume of blood) stabilizes—sometimes called the "set point"—is determined by the capacity of the immune system to kill infected lymphocytes. The set point predicts the rate of clinical deterioration; the higher the set point, the more rapid the progression to AIDS.
- Over time, the ability of the marrow to produce CD4 cells falls below that necessary to replenish the killed CD4 cells, and immunosuppression results. Without treatment, the clinically latent phase gives way to a 2- to 4-year phase of chronic symptoms and rising viral titers, but not yet life-threatening illness.
- Late in the clinical latent period, the structure of lymph nodes begins to break down, releasing more active virus into the circulation. Viral titers rise dramatically, and CD4 levels fall below the level necessary to prevent life-threatening opportunistic infections (<200, AIDS).

TABLE **27-1**   Clinical Staging of HIV Infection

Category A	Category B	Category C
One or more of the following conditions in an adolescent or adult (>13 yr) with documented HIV infection: Asymptomatic HIV infection Persistent generalized lymphadenopathy Acute (primary) HIV infection with accompanying illness or history of acute HIV	Symptomatic disease including: Thrush Vulvovaginal candidiasis Seborrheic dermatitis Eosinophilic folliculitis Cervical dysplasia Fever Diarrhea Oral hairy leukoplakia Varicella zoster Pelvic inflammatory disease Listeriosis Peripheral neuropathy	Presence of an AIDS indicator condition: Candida of esophagus or lung Invasive cervical cancer Extrapulmonary histoplasmosis Coccidioidomycosis or cryptococcosis Cryptosporidiosis CMV Extracutaneous, herpes simplex HIV-associated dementia HIV-associated wasting Kaposi sarcoma CNS lymphoma Non-Hodgkin lymphoma *Mycobacterium avium* complex (MAC) *Mycobacterium tuberculosis* Nocardiosis *Pneumocystis jiroveci* pneumonia (PCP) Progressive multifocal leukoencephalopathy Salmonella septicemia Strongyloidiasis Toxoplasmosis
Conditions listed in categories B and C must not have occurred	Conditions in category C must not have occurred	

From The Centers for Disease Control and Prevention (CDC) and the World Health Organization (WHO) classification of HIV and AIDS.

AIDS

- Loss of normal CD4 cell activity disrupts virtually every aspect of immune function, especially cellular immunity.
- The complex immune deficits in AIDS leave the body vulnerable to many common opportunistic infectious agents, including fungi, parasites, mycobacteria, viruses, and bacteria, as well as AIDS-associated malignancies (Table 27-1).
- HIV-Associated Wasting Syndrome.
  - Defined as the involuntary loss of 10% of body weight with chronic fever, weakness, or diarrhea in the absence of other related illnesses contributing to the weight loss. The newer expanded definition includes malnutrition as well as metabolic causes.
  - Correlates with poor prognosis and may occur early in disease progression.
  - Causes include anorexia (depression, financial difficulties, oropharyngeal disease, side effect of medications), malabsorption (gastrointestinal diseases), and metabolic abnormalities (low testosterone or growth hormone, cytokine abnormalities [especially tumor necrosis factor, TNF]).
- AIDS Dementia Complex (ADC).
  - HIV infection is frequently complicated by CNS effects including decreased cognitive function.
  - HIV infects the microglial cells that surround neurons and release neurotoxic substances.
  - Many opportunistic infections can occur in the CNS, and these must be differentiated from ADC.

PATIENT PRESENTATION

History

History of exposures (number of incidents of unprotected sex, sexual networks, specific sexual activities, use of condoms, IVDA, transfusions); other sexually transmitted diseases (STDs); pregnancy; menstrual history; addiction history; recurrent infections; coinfections such as hepatitis B or C; opportunistic infections; neoplasms; depression; changes in sleep patterns; family, living, and work environment; vaccination history.

Symptoms

Fever; night sweats; weakness; adenopathy; pharyngitis; rash; myalgias; headache; weight loss; seborrhea; skin rashes and pain; mouth pain; anal pain; dysphagia; dyspnea; cough; chest pain; abdominal pain; diarrhea; vaginal bleeding, blurred vision; diarrhea; memory loss; confusion.

Examination

Fever, muscle wasting; rashes; skin lesions; oral lesions; perianal lesions; adenopathy; pulmonary consolidation (crackles); pleural rub; cardiac dysfunction (cardiomegaly, S_3, pericardial rub); abdominal tenderness; abdominal or pelvic masses; evidence of sexually transmitted diseases or cervical disease on pelvic examination; focal neurologic deficits; cognitive deficits.

DIFFERENTIAL DIAGNOSIS

- Other viral infections: Mononucleosis, influenza, hepatitis.
- Other immunocompromised states (congenital or drug induced).
- Opportunistic infections (listed earlier).
- Malignancies.
- Depression.

KEYS TO ASSESSMENT

Screening

- The CDC recommends that all patients in hospitals that have a high rate of newly diagnosed AIDS patients (1/1000 discharges) should be tested, as well as all pregnant women.
- Other indications for testing include:
    - People with STDs.
    - Individuals at high risk (IVDU, men who have sex with men with a history of high-risk behavior).
    - Heterosexuals with more than one partner in the past 12 months.
    - People with active TB.
    - Occupationally exposed people.
    - Blood or tissue donors.
- The average time from exposure to seroconversion is 70 days; more than 95% of infected individuals will seroconvert by 6 months. Because individuals may not become seropositive for the antibodies for several weeks or months after primary infection, there may be a "window period" during which they may be infectious to others but still be HIV-antibody negative.
- Although a salivary swab testing and home-use rapid test for HIV are available, it is still important to provide appropriate counseling before and after testing for HIV.

Diagnosis of HIV Infection

- Measuring anti-HIV antibodies remains the most commonly used screening and diagnostic test for HIV.
- The enzyme-linked immunosorbent assay (ELISA) test has high sensitivity but lower specificity, thus may result in "false positives," which means that the test falsely detects antibodies in the blood even when infection is not present. The number of false positives is decreased by doing an additional test called a Western blot, which is more specific than the ELISA for HIV infection and therefore helps to confirm the actual presence of infection.
- Viral titers (polymerase chain reaction [HIV RNA PCR] or branched chain DNA [bDNA]), also called viral load, can be measured within hours to days of infection.
    - This test is expensive and complicated, and is not yet appropriate for general screening of the population.

- Used to monitor the progression of infection and the response to treatment in those already known to be infected with HIV.
- AIDS is defined as documented HIV infection with an associated indicator disease including (1) certain opportunistic infections; (2) certain cancers such as Kaposi sarcoma, lymphomas, and invasive cervical or anal carcinomas; (3) wasting syndrome; (4) associated neurologic diseases; and (5) recurrent pneumonias; or HIV infection and a CD4 (T helper) cell count of <200 cells/mL.

Laboratory Testing Once HIV Infection Is Confirmed

- Viral load assay (HIV RNA PCR or bDNA).
- CD4 cell count.
- Complete blood count (CBC) with differential and platelet count.
- Chemistry panel including fasting lipid profile (some antiretroviral drugs affect lipid metabolism).
- Urinalysis.
- Chest radiograph.
- Pap smear in women.
- Serologies to detect potential opportunistic infections (e.g., syphilis; toxoplasmosis; hepatitis A, B, and C; cytomegalovirus [CMV], varicella-zoster).
- PPD.

Clinical Staging of HIV Infection (see Table 27-1)

- These categories can be further subdivided 1 through 3, depending on the associated CD4 cell count.

PREVENTION

- There is accurate information with which to educate all individuals about how to prevent infection with HIV. However, prevention requires not just information but also skills and community support. Social and cultural norms and values may facilitate or inhibit successful HIV prevention education and practices.
- In pregnant women infected with HIV, perinatal transmission can be reduced through the proper use of antiviral medications. Cesarean section reduces risk further, and infected mothers should not breast-feed.
- Vaccine development continues, but has been limited by (a) the rapid rate of viral mutation, (b) geographic specificity of viral strains, and (c) inability to generate enough humoral and cellular immunity to neutralize virus.
- Live attenuated viral vaccines have been tested in animals and do provide some cellular immunity, but have been complicated by an unacceptable incidence of actually causing HIV infection.

MANAGEMENT

- When to begin antivirals in adults and adolescents is still controversial. It is recognized that eradication of HIV infection cannot be achieved with current antiretroviral therapy, that active antiretroviral therapy is associated with substantial toxicity, and that the difficulty of long-term adherence to current treatment regimens leads to the development of drug resistance.
- Decisions about initiating treatment for HIV disease should be made after careful consideration of the patient's wishes and preferences in the context of the patient's HIV RNA levels, CD4 cell counts, and clinical symptoms.
- The CDC recommends:
    - Antiretroviral therapy is recommended for all patients with history of an AIDS-defining illness or severe symptoms of HIV infection regardless of CD4+ T cell count.
    - Antiretroviral therapy is also recommended for asymptomatic patients with <200 CD4+ T cells/mm^3.

- Asymptomatic patients with CD4+ T cell counts of 201 to 350 cells/mm^3 should be offered treatment.
- For asymptomatic patients with CD4+ T cell counts of >350 cells/mm^3 and plasma HIV RNA >100,000 copies/mL, most experienced clinicians defer therapy but some clinicians may consider initiating treatment.
- Therapy should be deferred for patients with CD4+ T cell counts of >350 cells/mm^3 and plasma HIV RNA <100,000 copies/mL.
- The goals of treatment are to reduce the amount of HIV in the plasma to undetectable (<50 copies/mL) and to achieve the recovery of immunity (increased CD4 count).
- Treatment requires careful monitoring for drug levels, CD4 and HIV levels, drug toxicities, and other complications of the infection.
- Antiretroviral treatment requires the simultaneous initiation of combinations of at least three drugs to prevent resistance (highly active antiretroviral therapy [HAART]). Current antiretroviral drugs include:
  - Those that inhibit reverse transcriptase activity.
    1. Nucleoside reverse transcriptase inhibitors (NRTIs) such as AZT (zidovudine), 3TC (lamivudine), didanosine (ddI), zalcitabine (ddC), stavudine (d4T), abacavir (ABC), and emtricitabine (FTC).
    2. Non-nucleoside reverse transcriptase inhibitors (NNRTIs) such as nevirapine, delavirdine, efavirenz, and capravirine.
  - Those that inhibit protease activity (protease inhibitors, [PI]) such as indinavir, ritonavir, saquinavir, nelfinavir, amprenavir, and tripranavir.
  - A new class of antiretroviral drugs has recently been approved for the treatment of HIV. These drugs are called fusion inhibitors.
    1. Prevent conformational change at gp120/gp41 and CD4 binding, thus preventing coreceptor interaction.
    2. Enfuvirtide (Fuzeon) is the first drug approved in this class and is indicated for use in combination with other antiretrovirals in treatment-experienced individuals with HIV-1 infection.
- The CDC recommends several preferred regimens, but acknowledges that patient or provider preferences or the presence of other disease may make alternative regimens preferable in specific cases. The panel recommends that an initial regimen contain two NRTIs and either a NNRTI or a ritonavir-boosted or unboosted PI.
- Combination antiretrovirals are available that include more than one drug from more than one class. Tenofovir + lamivudine (or emtricitabine) are now recommended as a 2-NRTI backbone for both NNRTI- and PI-based regimens.
- All antiretroviral drugs produce toxicity. Toxicities vary with specific drugs, and may include diarrhea, pancytopenia, dyslipidemias, lipodystrophy, lactic acidemia, hypertriglyceridemia, nephrolithiasis, and insulin resistance.
- Adherence is a crucial issue because even short viral bursts can result in increased seeding of lymphoid reservoirs and increased likelihood of drug resistance. However, even excellent adherence to these complicated drug regimens cannot prevent the eventual development of drug resistance.
- Management of patients who develop resistance includes sequencing of antivirals, newer agents, and multiple combinations of drugs.
- Many experimental drugs that attack other steps in viral replication (e.g., attachment inhibitors, chemokine antagonists, integrase inhibitors, fusion inhibitors) or that bolster immune function (e.g., interleukin 2 (IL-2), interferons) are being evaluated.
- Prophylaxis to prevent opportunistic infections (TB, MAC, PCP, and CMV) is begun when the CD4 count falls to specified levels. Immune restoration (increase in CD4 counts to >200/mm^3) allows for cessation of these prophylactic drugs so long as the CD4 counts remain adequate.
- Vaccinations should include hepatitis A and B, *Haemophilus influenzae*, Pneumovax, influenza, and tetanus-diphtheria—most of these are most effective if given when CD4 counts are greater than 200/mm^3.

- Women should receive optimal therapy regardless of pregnancy status.
  - Perinatal transmission prevention is optimized by the use of combination therapy using two or three drugs (with possible delay of PI until after first trimester) and can reduce transmission rates from 25% to 2%. In countries where HAART is not available, concentrated treatment with AZT during the intrapartum period reduces transmission significantly.
  - Cesarean birth reduces risk further and infected mothers should not breast-feed.
- People with HIV infection, even when they have no symptoms and their viral loads are undetectable, are infectious and should take consistent and appropriate precautions to prevent the transmission of HIV to others.
- CDC recommendations for postexposure prophylaxis (PEP):
  - Antiretroviral medications should be initiated as soon as possible after exposure.
  - For people seeking care 72 hours or less after nonoccupational exposure to blood, genital secretions, or other potentially infectious body fluids of a person known to be HIV infected and when that exposure represents a substantial risk for transmission, a 28-day course of highly active antiretroviral therapy (HAART) is recommended.
  - For occupational exposure, a basic 4-week regimen of two drugs for most HIV exposures and an expanded regimen that includes the addition of a third drug for HIV exposures that pose an increased risk for transmission. When the source person's virus is known or suspected to be resistant to one or more of the drugs considered for the PEP regimen, the selection of drugs to which the source person's virus is unlikely to be resistant is recommended.

PATHOPHYSIOLOGY ⟶	CLINICAL LINK
What is going on in the disease process that influences how the patient presents and how he or she should be managed?	*What should you do now that you understand the underlying pathophysiology?*
HIV is not one virus—it is many viruses, including HIV-1, HIV-2, and several subgroups and clades with differing geographic distributions and virulence factors. ⟶	Worldwide transmission patterns of HIV differ and are constantly changing. New types of HIV infection are being described and it is unlikely that a true "global" vaccine will be developed.
HIV infection involves binding of the viral envelope to the target cells (macrophages, CD4 lymphocytes) via a complex series of steps that require the interaction of numerous viral and host cell receptors and chemokines. ⟶	Fusion inhibitors prevent HIV entry into cells. Genetic alterations in viral and host cell surface characteristics may explain some of the differences observed in infectivity. Furthermore, purposeful alterations in these factors may provide future therapies to prevent HIV infection.
Three important enzymes are coded by the viral RNA: reverse transcriptase, integrase, and protease. Activity of each of these enzymes is necessary for viral reproduction inside the host cell. ⟶	Current therapies for HIV include two classes of drugs that inhibit reverse transcriptase and drugs that inhibit protease. Integrase inhibitors are in development.
HIV replication occurs at an incredible rate and is associated with numerous mutations. These mutations can lead to increased virulence and to drug resistance. ⟶	In any individual, the virus present in his or her body is constantly changing. Careful drug adherence is necessary to prevent the development of resistance. Unprotected sex is ill II advised even between two HIV-positive adults. Furthermore, an individual's initial infection may be with a virus that is already drug resistant.
HIV killing by the immune system relies on CD8 cell–mediated cellular immunity that destroys infected CD4 cells. HIV tends to shift the immune system from the TH_1 cytokine pattern, which promotes cellular immunity, to the TH_2 pattern of humoral immunity. Humoral immunity is less effective for HIV killing. ⟶	Experimental therapies for HIV include immune-modulating drugs (e.g., IL-2, interferons) that shift the TH_2 cytokine pattern back to the TH_1 pattern, thus improving cellular immunity and viral killing.
Immunodeficiency occurs when killing of infected CD4 cells exceeds bone marrow replenishment with healthy cells, and when lymph nodes break down and release virus. When CD4 cell levels fall below 200/mL and the viral load rises, opportunistic infections develop that have a very high morbidity and mortality. ⟶	Monitoring the CD4 cell count and viral load are crucial to initiating antiviral therapy, evaluating responses to therapy, and predicting the occurrence of the many infections of AIDS. Aggressive antiretroviral therapy and prophylaxis for opportunistic infections have improved quality of life and outcomes for many patients, but drug toxicities are often severe.

SUGGESTED READINGS

Ambrus, J. L., Sr. & Ambrus, J. L., Jr. (2004). Nutrition and infectious diseases in developing countries and problems of acquired immunodeficiency syndrome. *Experimental Biology & Medicine,* 229, 464-472.

Andersen, J. L. & Planelles, V. (2005). The role of Vpr in HIV-1 pathogenesis. *Current HIV Research,* 3, 43-51.

Anthony, N. J. (2004). HIV-1 integrase: a target for new AIDS chemotherapeutics. *Current Topics in Medicinal Chemistry,* 4, 979-990.

Asboe, D. (2004). Enfuvirtide: antiretroviral class 4, drug 1. *HIV Clinical Trials,* 5, 1-6.

Bafica, A., Scanga, C. A., Schito, M., Chaussabel, D., & Sher, A. (2004). Influence of coinfecting pathogens on HIV expression: evidence for a role of Toll-like receptors. *Journal of Immunology,* 172, 7229-7234.

Baraz, L. & Kotler, M. (2004). The Vif protein of human immunodeficiency virus type 1 (HIV-1): enigmas and solutions. *Current Medicinal Chemistry,* 11, 221-231.

Barbaro, G., Scozzafava, A., Mastrolorenzo, A., & Supuran, C. T. (2005). Highly active antiretroviral therapy: current state of the art, new agents and their pharmacological interactions useful for improving therapeutic outcome. *Current Pharmaceutical Design,* 11, 1805-1843.

Becker, Y. (2004). The changes in the T helper 1 (Th1) and T helper 2 (Th2) cytokine balance during HIV-1 infection are indicative of an allergic response to viral proteins that may be reversed by Th2 cytokine inhibitors and immune response modifiers—a review and hypothesis. *Virus Genes,* 28, 5-18.

Becker, Y. (2005). CpG ODNs treatments of HIV-1 infected patients may cause the decline of transmission in high risk populations—a review, hypothesis and implications. *Virus Genes,* 30, 251-266.

Belyakov, I. M. & Berzofsky, J. A. (2004). Immunobiology of mucosal HIV infection and the basis for development of a new generation of mucosal AIDS vaccines. *Immunity,* 20, 247-253.

Benito, J. M., Lopez, M., & Soriano, V. (2004). The role of CD8+ T-cell response in HIV infection. *AIDS Reviews,* 6, 79-88.

Blankson, J. N. (2005). Primary HIV-1 infection: to treat or not to treat. *AIDS Reader,* 15, 245-246.

Borkow, G. & Lapidot, A. (2005). Multi-targeting the entrance door to block HIV-1. *Current Drug Targets—Infectious Disorders,* 5, 3-15.

Boska, M. D., Mosley, R. L., Nawab, M., Nelson, J. A., Zelivyanskaya, M., Poluektova, L., Uberti, M., Dou, H., Lewis, T. B., & Gendelman, H. E. (2004). Advances in neuroimaging for HIV-1 associated neurological dysfunction: clues to the diagnosis, pathogenesis and therapeutic monitoring. *Current HIV Research,* 2, 61-78.

Bukrinskaya, A. G. (2004). HIV-1 assembly and maturation. *Archives of Virology,* 149, 1067-1082.

Cahn, P. (2004). Emtricitabine: a new nucleoside analogue for once-daily antiretroviral therapy. *Expert Opinion on Investigational Drugs,* 13, 55-68.

Cheung, P. K., Wynhoven, B., & Harrigan, P. R. (2004). 2004: which HIV-1 drug resistance mutations are common in clinical practice? *AIDS Reviews,* 6, 107-116.

Coakley, E., Petropoulos, C. J., & Whitcomb, J. M. (2005). Assessing chemokine co-receptor usage in HIV. *Current Opinion in Infectious Diseases,* 18, 9-15.

Cooper, D. A. & Lange, J. M. (2004). Peptide inhibitors of virus-cell fusion: enfuvirtide as a case study in clinical discovery and development. *The Lancet Infectious Diseases,* 4, 426-436.

De Milito, A. (2004). B lymphocyte dysfunctions in HIV infection. *Current HIV Research,* 2, 11-21.

Demonte, D., Quivy, V., Colette, Y., & Van Lint, C. (2004). Administration of HDAC inhibitors to reactivate HIV-1 expression in latent cellular reservoirs: implications for the development of therapeutic strategies. *Biochemical Pharmacology,* 68, 1231-1238.

den Uyl, D., van der Horst-Bruinsma, I, & van Agtmael, M. (2004). Progression of HIV to AIDS: a protective role for HLA-B27? *AIDS Reviews,* 6, 89-96.

DeVico, A. L. & Gallo, R. C. (2004). Control of HIV-1 infection by soluble factors of the immune response. *Nature Reviews, Microbiology,* 2, 401-413.

Dezube, B. J., Pantanowitz, L., & Aboulafia, D. M. (2003). Management of AIDS-related Kaposi sarcoma: advances in target discovery and treatment. *AIDS Reader,* 14, 236-238.

Dines, I., Rumjanek, V. M., & Persechini, P. M. (2004). What is going on with natural killer cells in HIV infection? *International Archives of Allergy & Immunology,* 133, 330-339.

Donaghy, H., Stebbing, J., & Patterson, S. (2004). Antigen presentation and the role of dendritic cells in HIV. *Current Opinion in Infectious Diseases,* 17, 1-6.

Feikin, D. R., Feldman, C., Schuchat, A., & Janoff, E. N. (2004). Global strategies to prevent bacterial pneumonia in adults with HIV disease. *The Lancet Infectious Diseases,* 4, 445-455.

Fittipaldi, A. & Giacca, M. (2005). Transcellular protein transduction using the Tat protein of HIV-1. *Advanced Drug Delivery Reviews,* 57, 597-608.

Fraaij, P. L., Rakhmanina, N., Burger, D. M., & de Groot, R. (2004). Therapeutic drug monitoring in children with HIV/AIDS. *Therapeutic Drug Monitoring,* 26, 122-126.

Frenkel, L. M. & Tobin, N. H. (2004). Understanding HIV-1 drug resistance. *Therapeutic Drug Monitoring,* 26, 116-121.

Gaillard, P., Fowler, M. G., Dabis, F., Coovadia, H., Van Der, H. C., Van Rompay, K., Ruff, A., Taha, T., Thomas, T., De Vincenzi, I., Newell, M. L., & Ghent IAS Working Group on HIV in Women and Children. (2004). Use of antiretroviral drugs to prevent HIV-1 transmission through breast-feeding: from animal studies to randomized clinical trials. *Journal of Acquired Immune Deficiency Syndromes: JAIDS,* 35, 178-187.

Galvin, S. R. & Cohen, M. S. (2004). The role of sexually transmitted diseases in HIV transmission. *Nature Reviews, Microbiology,* 2, 33-42.

Garber, D. A., Silvestri, G., & Feinberg, M. B. (2004). Prospects for an AIDS vaccine: three big questions, no easy answers. *The Lancet Infectious Diseases,* 4, 397-413.

Giri, M., Ugen, K. E., & Weiner, D. B. (2004). DNA vaccines against human immunodeficiency virus type 1 in the past decade. *Clinical Microbiology Reviews,* 17, 370-389.

Gonzalez-Scarano, F. & Martin-Garcia, J. (2005). The neuropathogenesis of AIDS. *Nature Reviews, Immunology,* 5, 69-81.

Gorry, P. R., Churchill, M., Crowe, S. M., Cunningham, A. L., & Gabuzda, D. (2005). Pathogenesis of macrophage tropic HIV-1. *Current HIV Research,* 3, 53-60.

Goulder, P. J. & Watkins, D. I. (2004). HIV and SIV CTL escape: implications for vaccine design. *Nature Reviews, Immunology,* 4, 630-640.

Greene, W. C. (2004). The brightening future of HIV therapeutics. *Nature Immunology,* 5, 867-871.

Gulzar, N. & Copeland, K. F. (2004). CD8+ T-cells: function and response to HIV infection. *Current HIV Research,* 2, 23-37.

Hamer, D. H. (2004). Can HIV be cured? Mechanisms of HIV persistence and strategies to combat it. *Current HIV Research,* 2, 99-111.

Hamers, F. F. & Downs, A. M. (2004). The changing face of the HIV epidemic in western Europe: what are the implications for public health policies. *Lancet,* 364, 83-94.

Huigen, M. C., Kamp, W., & Nottet, H. S. (2004). Multiple effects of HIV-1 trans-activator protein on the pathogenesis of HIV-1 infection. *European Journal of Clinical Investigation,* 34, 57-66.

Johnson, A. A., Marchand, C., & Pommier, Y. (2004). HIV-1 integrase inhibitors: a decade of research and two drugs in clinical trial. *Current Topics in Medicinal Chemistry,* 4, 1059-1077.

John-Stewart, G., Mbori-Ngacha, D., Ekpini, R., Janoff, E. N., Nkengasong, J., Read, J. S., Van de, P. P., Newell, M. L., & Ghent IAS Working Group on HIV in Women and Children. (2004). Breast-feeding and transmission of HIV-1. *Journal of Acquired Immune Deficiency Syndromes: JAIDS,* 35, 196-202.

Joseph, J. & Behar, T. (2004). Viral and host genetic factors regulating HIV/CNS disease. *Journal of Neurovirology,* 10(suppl 1), 1-6.

Kao, A. W. & Price, R. W. (2004). Chemokine receptors, neural progenitor cells, and the AIDS dementia complex. *Journal of Infectious Diseases,* 190, 211-215.

Karakousis, P. C., Moore, R. D., & Chaisson, R. E. (2004). *Mycobacterium avium* complex in patients with HIV infection in the era of highly active antiretroviral therapy. *The Lancet Infectious Diseases,* 4, 557-565.

Kaslow, R. A., Dorak, T., & Tang, J. J. (2005). Influence of host genetic variation on susceptibility to HIV type 1 infection. *Journal of Infectious Diseases,* 191(suppl 1), S68-S77.

Kaul, M. & Lipton, S. A. (2004). Signaling pathways to neuronal damage and apoptosis in human immunodeficiency virus type 1-associated dementia: chemokine receptors, excitotoxicity, and beyond. *Journal of Neurovirology,* 10(suppl 1), 97-101.

Kennedy, P. G. (2004). Neurological infection. *Lancet Neurology,* 3, 13.

Kinlaw, W. B. & Marsh, B. (2004). Adiponectin and HIV-lipodystrophy: taking HAART. *Endocrinology,* 145, 484-486.

Kinloch-de Loes, S. (2004). Role of therapeutic vaccines in the control of HIV-1. *Journal of Antimicrobial Chemotherapy,* 53, 562-566.

Kino, T. & Chrousos, G. P. (2004). Human immunodeficiency virus type-1 accessory protein Vpr: a causative agent of the AIDS-related insulin resistance/lipodystrophy syndrome? *Annals of the New York Academy of Sciences,* 1024, 153-167.

Klasse, P. J. & Moore, J. P. (2004). Is there enough gp120 in the body fluids of HIV-1-infected individuals to have biologically significant effects. *Virology,* 323, 1-8.

Kopnisky, K. L., Stoff, D. M., & Rausch, D. M. (2004). Workshop report: The effects of psychological variables on the progression of HIV-1 disease. *Brain, Behavior, & Immunity,* 18, 246-261.

Kuritzkes, D. R. (2004). Preventing and managing antiretroviral drug resistance. *AIDS Patient Care & STDs,* 18, 259-273.

Lawn, S. D. (2004). AIDS in Africa: the impact of coinfections on the pathogenesis of HIV-1 infection. *Journal of Infection,* 48, 1-12.

Levesque, K., Finzi, A., Binette, J., & Cohen, E. A. (2004). Role of CD4 receptor down-regulation during HIV-1 infection. *Current HIV Research,* 2, 51-59.

Li, F. & Wild, C. (2005). HIV-1 assembly and budding as targets for drug discovery. *Current Opinion in Investigational Drugs,* 6, 148-154.

Lichterfeld, M., Yu, X. G., Le Gall, S., & Altfeld, M. (2005). Immunodominance of HIV-1-specific CD8(+) T-cell responses in acute HIV-1 infection: at the crossroads of viral and host genetics. *Trends in Immunology,* 26, 166-171.

Lopalco, L. (2004). Humoral immunity in HIV-1 exposure: cause or effect of HIV resistance? *Current HIV Research,* 2, 127-139.

Lyons, F., Prendiville, W., & Mulcahy, F. (2004). Cervical disease in HIV-1-positive women: a review. *International Journal of STD & AIDS,* 15, 89-92.

Manji, H. & Miller, R. (2004). The neurology of HIV infection. *Journal of Neurology, Neurosurgery & Psychiatry,* 75(suppl 1), i29-i35.

Mastroianni, C. M., d'Ettorre, G., Forcina, G., & Vullo, V. (2004). Teaching tired T cells to fight HIV: time to test IL-15 for immunotherapy? *Trends in Immunology,* 25, 121-125.

Matthews, T., Salgo, M., Greenberg, M., Chung, J., DeMasi, R., & Bolognesi, D. (2004). Enfuvirtide: the first therapy to inhibit the entry of HIV-1 into host CD4 lymphocytes. *Nature Reviews, Drug Discovery,* 3, 215-225.

Medina, C. & Johnson, W. (2004). HIV/AIDS prevention in Latino and African-American communities. *Journal of the National Medical Association,* 96, 9S-11S.

Mehta, N. & Reilly, M. (2005). Atherosclerotic cardiovascular disease risk in the HAART-treated HIV-1 population. *HIV Clinical Trials,* 6, 5-24.

Menendez-Arias, L. & Este, J. A. (2004). HIV-resistance to viral entry inhibitors. *Current Pharmaceutical Design,* 10, 1845-1860.

Modrzejewski, K. A. & Herman, R. A. (2004). Emtricitabine: a once-daily nucleoside reverse transcriptase inhibitor. *Annals of Pharmacotherapy,* 38, 1006-1014.

Moore, J. P., Kitchen, S. G., Pugach, P., & Zack, J. A. (2004). The CCR5 and CXCR4 coreceptors—central to understanding the transmission and pathogenesis of human immunodeficiency virus type 1 infection. *AIDS Research & Human Retroviruses,* 20, 111-126.

Mueller, A. & Strange, P. G. (2004). The chemokine receptor, CCR5. *International Journal of Biochemistry & Cell Biology,* 36, 35-38.

Muthumani, K., Desai, B. M., Hwang, D. S., Choo, A. Y., Laddy, D. J., Thieu, K. P., Rao, R. G., & Weiner, D. B. (2004). HIV-1 Vpr and anti-inflammatory activity. *DNA & Cell Biology,* 23, 239-247.

Noe, A., Plum, J., & Verhofstede, C. (2005). The latent HIV-1 reservoir in patients undergoing HAART: an archive of pre-HAART drug resistance. *Journal of Antimicrobial Chemotherapy,* 55, 410-412.

Obaro, S. K., Pugatch, D., & Luzuriaga, K. (2004). Immunogenicity and efficacy of childhood vaccines in HIV-1-infected children. *The Lancet Infectious Diseases,* 4, 510-518.

O'Brien, S. J. & Nelson, G. W. (2004). Human genes that limit AIDS. *Nature Genetics,* 36, 565-574.

Ohtaka, H. & Freire, E. (2005). Adaptive inhibitors of the HIV-1 protease. *Progress in Biophysics & Molecular Biology,* 88, 193-208.

Oluwole, S. F., Ali, A. O., Shafaee, Z., & DePaz, H. A. (2005). Breast cancer in women with HIV/AIDS: report of five cases with a review of the literature. *Journal of Surgical Oncology,* 89, 23-27.

Pantaleo, G. & Koup, R. A. (2004). Correlates of immune protection in HIV-1 infection: what we know, what we don't know, what we should know. *Nature Medicine,* 10, 806-810.

Petrovas, C., Mueller, Y. M., & Katsikis, P. D. (2004). HIV-specific CD8+ T cells: serial killers condemned to die? *Current HIV Research,* 2, 153-162.

Pommier, Y., Johnson, A. A., & Marchand, C. (2005). Integrase inhibitors to treat HIV/AIDS. *Nature Reviews, Drug Discovery,* 4, 236-248.

Post, F. A. & Easterbrook, P. J. (2005). Antiretroviral therapy in advanced HIV-1 infection. *Journal of the International Association of Physicians in AIDS Care: JIAPAC,* 4, 8-10.

Rambaut, A., Posada, D., Crandall, K. A., & Holmes, E. C. (2004). The causes and consequences of HIV evolution. *Nature Reviews Genetics,* 5, 52-61.

Regulier, E. G., Reiss, K., Khalili, K., Amini, S., Rappaport, J., Zagury, J. F., & Katsikis, P. D. (2004). T-cell and neuronal apoptosis in HIV infection: implications for therapeutic intervention. *International Reviews of Immunology*, 23, 25-59.

Richman, D. D. (2004). Benefits and limitations of testing for resistance to HIV drugs. *Journal of Antimicrobial Chemotherapy*, 53, 555-557.

Ruhnke, M. (2004). Mucosal and systemic fungal infections in patients with AIDS: prophylaxis and treatment. *Drugs*, 64, 1163-1180.

Ruibal-Ares, B. H., Belmonte, L., Bare, P. C., Parodi, C. M., Massud, I., & de Bracco, M. M. (2004). HIV-1 infection and chemokine receptor modulation. *Current HIV Research*, 2, 39-50.

Ruxrungtham, K., Brown, T., & Phanuphak, P. (2004). HIV/AIDS in Asia. *Lancet*, 364, 69-82.

Safrit, J. T., Ruprecht, R., Ferrantelli, F., Xu, W., Kitabwalla, M., Van Rompay, K., Marthas, M., Haigwood, N., Mascola, J. R., Luzuriaga, K., Jones, S. A., Mathieson, B. J., Newell, M. L., & Ghent IAS Working Group on HIV in Women and Children. (2004). Immunoprophylaxis to prevent mother-to-child transmission of HIV-1. *Journal of Acquired Immune Deficiency Syndromes: JAIDS*, 35, 169-177.

Scarlatti, G. (2004). Mother-to-child transmission of HIV-1: advances and controversies of the twentieth centuries. *AIDS Reviews*, 6, 67-78.

Schiavoni, I., Muratori, C., Piacentini, V., Giammarioli, A. M., & Federico, M. (2004). The HIV-1 Nef protein: how an AIDS pathogenetic factor turns to a tool for combating AIDS. *Current Drug Targets—Immune Endocrine & Metabolic Disorders*, 4, 19-27.

Schols, D. (2004). HIV co-receptors as targets for antiviral therapy. *Current Topics in Medicinal Chemistry*, 4, 883-893.

Schrofelbauer, B., Yu, Q., & Landau, N. R. (2004). New insights into the role of Vif in HIV-1 replication. *AIDS Reviews*, 6, 34-39.

Schwartz, R. A. (2004). Kaposi's sarcoma: an update. *Journal of Surgical Oncology*, 87, 146-151.

Shaheen, F. & Collman, R. G. (2004). Co-receptor antagonists as HIV-1 entry inhibitors. *Current Opinion in Infectious Diseases*, 17, 7-16.

Shiver, J. W. & Emini, E. A. (2004). Recent advances in the development of HIV-1 vaccines using replication-incompetent adenovirus vectors. *Annual Review of Medicine*, 55, 355-372.

Siliciano, J. D. & Siliciano, R. F. (2004). A long-term latent reservoir for HIV-1: discovery and clinical implications. *Journal of Antimicrobial Chemotherapy*, 54, 6-9.

Smith, R. A., Loeb, L. A., & Preston, B. D. (2005). Lethal mutagenesis of HIV. *Virus Research*, 107, 215-228.

Sommerfelt, M. A., Nyhus, J., & Sorensen, B. (2004). Novel peptide-based HIV-1 immunotherapy. *Expert Opinion on Biological Therapy*, 4, 349-361.

Stebbing, J., Gazzard, B., & Douek, D. C. (2004). Where does HIV live? *New England Journal of Medicine*, 350, 1872-1880.

Stephens, H. A. (2005). HIV-1 diversity versus HLA class I polymorphism. *Trends in Immunology*, 26, 41-47.

Stoff, D. M. (2004). Mental health research in HIV/AIDS and aging: problems and prospects. *AIDS*, 18(suppl 1), S3-S10.

Stone, V. E. & Smith, K. Y. (2004). Improving adherence to HAART. *Journal of the National Medical Association*, 96, 27S-29S.

Stratov, I., DeRose, R., Purcell, D. F., & Kent, S. J. (2004). Vaccines and vaccine strategies against HIV. *Current Drug Targets*, 5, 71-88.

Tang, J. W. & Pillay, D. (2004). Transmission of HIV-1 drug resistance. *Journal of Clinical Virology*, 30, 1-10.

Temesgen, Z., Cainelli, F., Warnke, D., Koirala, J., & Collaborative Research Network, C. (2004). Initial anti-retroviral therapy in chronically-infected HIV-positive adults. *Expert Opinion on Pharmacotherapy*, 5, 595-612.

Tershakovec, A. M., Frank, I., & Rader, D. (2004). HIV-related lipodystrophy and related factors. *Atherosclerosis*, 174, 1-10.

Tolstrup, M., Ostergaard, L., Laursen, A. L., Pedersen, S. F., & Duch, M. (2004). HIV/SIV escape from immune surveillance: focus on Nef. *Current HIV Research*, 2, 141-151.

Tremblay, C. (2004). Effects of HIV-1 entry inhibitors in combination. *Current Pharmaceutical Design*, 10, 1861-1865.

Valcour, V. G., Shikuma, C. M., Watters, M. R., & Sacktor, N. C. (2004). Cognitive impairment in older HIV-1-seropositive individuals: prevalence and potential mechanisms. *AIDS*, 18(suppl 1), S79-S86.

Verani, A., Gras, G., & Pancino, G. (2005). Macrophages and HIV-1: dangerous liaisons. *Molecular Immunology*, 42, 195-212.

Verucchi, G., Calza, L., Manfredi, R., & Chiodo, F. (2004). Human immunodeficiency virus and hepatitis C virus coinfection: epidemiology, natural history, therapeutic options and clinical management. *Infection*, 32, 33-46.

Whitney, J. B. & Ruprecht, R. M. (2004). Live attenuated HIV vaccines: pitfalls and prospects. *Current Opinion in Infectious Diseases*, 17, 17-26.

Wilflingseder, D., Banki, Z., Dierich, M. P., & Stoiber, H. (2005). Mechanisms promoting dendritic cell-mediated transmission of HIV. *Molecular Immunology*, 42, 229-237.

Winnock, M., Salmon-Ceron, D., Dabis, F., & Chene, G. (2004). Interaction between HIV-1 and HCV infections: towards a new entity? *Journal of Antimicrobial Chemotherapy*, 53, 936-946.

Wolkowicz, R. & Nolan, G. P. (2005). Gene therapy progress and prospects: novel gene therapy approaches for AIDS. *Gene Therapy*, 12, 467-476.

Yang, O. O. (2004). CTL ontogeny and viral escape: implications for HIV-1 vaccine design. *Trends in Immunology*, 25, 138-142.

Yazdanpanah, Y., Sissoko, D., Egger, M., Mouton, Y., Zwahlen, M., & Chene, G. (2004). Clinical efficacy of anti-retroviral combination therapy based on protease inhibitors or non-nucleoside analogue reverse transcriptase inhibitors: indirect comparison of controlled trials. *British Medical Journal*, 328, 249.

Yu, X. G., Lichterfeld, M., Addo, M. M., & Altfeld, M. (2005). Regulatory and accessory HIV-1 proteins: potential targets for HIV-1 vaccines? *Current Medicinal Chemistry*, 12, 741-747.

HIV Disease

INITIAL HISTORY

- A 32-year-old white female is admitted to the hospital with a 5-day history of fever, dyspnea, productive cough, and right-sided pleuritic chest pain
- States she has had pneumonia several times in the past 3 years.
- She is currently on oral contraceptives but is taking no other medications and has no known allergies.

Question 1.   *What else would you like to ask this patient about her history of present illness and past medical history?*

ADDITIONAL HISTORY

- Denies any chills, vomiting, headache, or rashes.
- She was told that her previous pneumonias were "just the usual kind" and were effectively treated with antibiotics.
- She has not smoked since she left college 10 years ago.
- Denies any history of lung disease, heart disease, or other hospitalizations.
- Long history of vaginal yeast infections and was recently told that her Pap smear was abnormal but "not cancer."
- States her overall health has not been good lately, with fatigue and a 7-pound unintentional weight loss over the past 6 months.

Question 2.   *What about her history concerns you, and what else would you like to ask her now?*

ADDITIONAL HISTORY

- Has had occasional night sweats and has had mild anorexia for the past few months.
- Denies any recent travel and does not know anyone with tuberculosis or other unusual infections; her PPD was last checked while she was in college and was negative.
- Has had four sexual partners in the past year and has had occasional unprotected sex with each.
- Has no children and works as an accountant in a large local firm.
- Denies any history of toxin exposure.

PHYSICAL EXAMINATION

- Thin, ill-appearing female with occasional productive cough.
- T = 39° C orally, RR = 25, BP = 110/70 (sitting).

Skin
- Seborrhea around the nose, cheeks, and scalp.

HEENT
- PERRL; fundi without lesions.
- Nares and tympanic membranes without lesions.
- Pharynx reveals a thick cheesy exudate on the soft palate and tongue.

Neck
- Palpable cervical adenopathy.
- Thyroid nonpalpable.

Chest
- Lungs with dullness to percussion, increased tactile fremitus, inspiratory crackles, and egophony over the right lower lobe.
- Cardiac rhythm regular without murmurs or gallops.

Abdomen, Extremities, Neurologic
- No abdominal masses or tenderness.
- No pedal edema; pulses full; palpable inguinal adenopathy.
- Alert and oriented; neurologic examination nonfocal.

Pelvic
- Erythema and mild excoriation of the perineum.
- Thick, white vaginal discharge.
- No adnexal masses.
- Pap smear obtained.

Question 3.   *What do you think of her additional history and her examination findings?*

Question 4.   *What diagnostic tests would you obtain?*

LABORATORY RESULTS

- HIV ELISA positive.
- White blood count (WBC) = 9000/mm^3 with 90% PMNs; Hct = 37%; PLTs = 190,000/mm^3.
- Serum chemistries normal.
- Chest radiograph reveals right lower lobe infiltrate consistent with lobar pneumonia.
- Sputum gram-positive for numerous PMNs and gram-positive diplococci.
- Sputum culture positive for *S. pneumoniae.*
- Blood cultures negative.
- Oxygen saturation = 96%.
- PPD negative.
- Hepatitis serology negative.
- Oral and vaginal smear KOH positive for yeast.
- Pap smear reveals inflammation and mild dysplasia without carcinoma.

Question 5.   *How would you interpret these laboratory results and what would you do next?*

HOSPITAL COURSE

- The patient responds to antibiotics, and hydration.
- Western blot test result is positive.

Question 6.   *What additional laboratory tests would you order now?*

ADDITONAL LABORATORY RESULTS

- HIV RNA PCR = 25,000 copies/mL.
- CD4 count = 400/mm^3.
- Lipid profile normal.
- Serologies all negative.

Question 7.   *How should this patient be managed?*